A CLINICAL GUIDE TO

Nutrition Care
in End-Stage
Renal Disease

SECOND EDITION

THE AMERICAN DIETETIC ASSOCIATION

Library of Congress Cataloging-in-Publication Data
A Clinical guide to nutrition care in end-stage renal disease /
editor-in-chief, Jean Stover.— 2nd ed.
      p. cm.
      "A cooperative project of the Council on Renal
Nutrition of the National Kidney Foundation, Inc. and the
Renal Practice Group of The American Dietetic
Association."
      Includes bibliographical references and index.
      ISBN 0–88091–124–7
      1. Chronic renal failure—Nutritional aspects. 2.
Chronic renal failure—Diet therapy. I. Stover, Jean. II.
National Kidney Foundation. Council on Renal Nutrition.
III. American Dietetic Association. Renal Practice
Group.
      [DNLM: 1. Kidney Failure, Chronic—diet therapy.
WJ 342 C641 1993]
RC918.R4C63 1993
616.6'140654—dc20
DNLM/DLC
for Library of Congress
                             93–31214
                                CIP

Printed in the United States of America.

The views expressed in this publication are those of the
authors and are not necessarily those of The American
Dietetic Association. Mention of product names in this publication does not constitute endorsement by the authors or by
The American Dietetic Association.

First edition published in 1987.

CONTRIBUTORS

Eleanor Brown, RD[†]
Formerly of Dialysis Clinics Inc
Atlanta, Georgia

Simone P. Camel, MS, RD
Hermann Hospital
Texas Medical Center
Houston, Texas

Pat Collins-Thayer, MS, RD
Renal Dialysis of St. Louis Inc
St. Louis, Missouri

Marcia Davis, RD
Regional Kidney Disease Program
Minneapolis, Minnesota

Jean Gardner, RD
Mount Carmel Mercy Hospital
Detroit, Michigan

Diane Gillit, MS, RD
Formerly of South Plains Dialysis Center
Lubbock, Texas

Peggy Wright Harris, RD
Shreveport Regional Dialysis
Shreveport, Louisiana

Peggy Harum, RD
Miami, Florida

Susan Hood, MS, RD
Burlington County Dialysis Center
Mt. Holly, New Jersey

Sally LePage-Barclay, RD
Formerly of University of Wisconsin Hospital
and Clinics
Madison, Wisconsin

Susan Levine Lewis, MS, RD
Marriott Corporation
Medway, Massachusetts

Carol Liftman, MS, RD
Pennsylvania Hospital
Franklin Dialysis Center Inc
Philadelphia, Pennsylvania

Linda McCann, RD
Formerly of Satellite Dialysis Centers Inc
Menlo Park, California

Irene Muth, RD
Formerly of Temple University Hospital
Philadelphia, Pennsylvania

Polly Nelson, RD
UCLA Medical Center
Los Angeles, California

Kathy Norwood, MS, RD
Chromalloy American Kidney Center
St. Louis, Missouri

Joni J. Pagenkemper MS, RD
Department of Nutrition and Dietetics
School of Allied Health Professions
Loma Linda University
Loma Linda, California

[†]Deceased.

iii

Heidi Combs Peacey, MS, RD
Puget Sound Kidney Center
Everett, Washington

Charlotte Roberts, MS, RD
VA Wadsworth Medical Center
Los Angeles, California

Sharon Schatz, MS, RD
Playa del Rey, California

Jean Stover, RD
University of Pennsylvania Medical Center
Philadelphia, Pennsylvania

Barbara E. Wendland, RPDt
Mt. Sinai Hospital
Toronto, Ontario, Canada

Contents

FOREWORD

I am pleased to have had the opportunity to review and endorse the second edition of *A Clinical Guide to Nutrition Care in End-Stage Renal Disease.* The importance of nutrition assessment and management of the patient with renal disease has been well recognized over the past several years. The challenges of improving and maintaining adequate nutritional status for this population are great!

Although recommendations for nutritional requirements of patients with renal disease vary in the literature, it is hoped that dietitians will be able to use this manual as a guide to develop and promote practical goals for the patients. The intent of this manual is to provide information that can be used by students and dietitians new to the field of renal nutrition, as well as by those who have been renal dietitians for a number of years.

Members of both the Renal Dietitians dietetic practice group of The American Dietetic Association and the National Kidney Foundation Council on Renal Nutrition who wrote and reviewed the contents of this manual are to be commended for their worthwhile contributions.

Marsha Wolfson, MD
Chief, Nephrology Section
Portland VA Medical Center
Associate Professor, Department of Medicine
Oregon Health Sciences University
Portland, Oregon

INTRODUCTION

In 1983, the Council on Renal Nutrition of the National Kidney Foundation and the Renal Dietitians dietetic practice group of The American Dietetic Association began an ambitious project. This project was the development of a clinical guide to assist professionals in the fields of nutrition and allied health in caring for people with end-stage renal disease (ESRD).

More than 300 renal dietitians were surveyed to determine the content of the guide. Respondents identified three objectives, which were as follows:

1. It must be practical and contain information that would be useful in practice, but contain a minimum of theoretical background information.
2. The guide must represent a consensus formed by clinical practitioners, on the bases of current scientific literature and experience.
3. It must recognize the uniqueness of the patient with ESRD, a "terminally ill" person who might live for many years on a complex medical and dietary regimen.

The first edition of this clinical guide was developed with these objectives in mind. Now it has been updated and expanded in an effort to keep pace with issues in the field of nephrology that specifically affect renal nutrition practice. After reading this text, a practitioner should have a broad overview of the nomenclature and concepts involved in the care of patients with ESRD, as well as those with other medical conditions such as urolithiasis.

This guide should provide a sound foundation on which to build a knowledge inventory for further continuing education. It must be noted, however, that nutrient recommendations throughout this text are only *guidelines* for renal dietitians. They may differ somewhat among various researchers and practitioners at any given time. References are provided when such recommendations are made, unless the recommendations have been formed on the basis of the chapter authors' clinical experience.

It is also beyond the scope of this manual to provide an in-depth study of kidney function or the causes of ESRD. Additional continuing education opportunities for dietitians practicing in the field of renal nutrition include the following:

1. Physician-staff conferences in the dialysis unit. These conferences may be a formal in-service program, or, more frequently, are an informal part of the general rounds or staff meetings when patient care plans are developed. Practitioners should be present to gain an understanding of the patient care philosophy of the physician and nursing staff and new developments within nephrology practice.
2. Current literature and texts on renal disease. The nephrologists with whom the practitioner works are the best sources of information concerning the journals and texts available. Many of the more common nephrology journals are cited in this text, including the *Journal of Renal Nutrition*.
3. Membership in the Council on Renal Nutrition of the National Kidney Foundation and the Renal Dietitians dietetic practice group of The American Dietetic Association. A summary of each organization's structure and their membership benefits can be found in appendix J.

4. Membership in local Council on Renal Nutrition groups and attendance at local educational meetings sponsored by National Kidney Foundation affiliates and ESRD networks. The dialysis administrator, head nurse, and/or social worker may be good resources for the last. Other renal dietitians in a practitioner's area are often helpful in providing information on local Council on Renal Nutrition membership.

Acknowledgments

This manual of nutrition care for people with renal failure has had many reviewers in addition to those who contributed by writing specific sections. The following professionals deserve recognition for their time, effort, and assistance with this project.

Carolyn Cochran, MS, RD

Charlene Compher, MS, RD

Anne Diefendorf, RD

Nancy Ginsberg, MS, RD

Lauren Hudson, RD

Susan Kohl, RD

Joel Kopple, MD

Nancy Mathews, RD

Sherry Medford, MS, RD

Kathy Schiro, MS, RD

Nancy Spinozzi, RD

Kathy Steppacher, MS, RD

Marsha Wolfson, MD

The following professionals deserve special thanks for their hours of intensive review of this manual.

Karla Giles, RD

Mary Kay Hensley, MS, RD

Linda McCann, RD

Lois Shroeder, PhD, RD

Susan Weil, RD

1. OVERVIEW: THE NORMAL AND DISEASED KIDNEY

Basic Kidney Function

The kidneys are located in the abdomen, in the small of the back. Each kidney is approximately the size of a fist and weighs about 6 oz. The primary functions of the kidneys include the following:

■ Removal of excess fluid and waste products. More than 200 waste products are normally excreted by the kidney, including urea, creatinine, sodium, and potassium

■ Maintenance of the acid-base balance of the body

■ Regulation of blood pressure through production of the hormone renin and maintenance of salt and water balance

■ Stimulation of red blood cell production by production of the hormone erythropoietin

■ Maintenance of normal bone health by regulation of calcium and phosphorus metabolism, which is accomplished by activation of vitamin D and excretion of excess phosphorus

■ Removal of some drugs and poisons

A person suffering from advanced impairment of kidney function usually experiences edema, uremia (accumulation of waste products in the blood), metabolic acidosis, hypertension, anemia, bone disease, and an increased sensitivity to many drugs.

Types of Kidney Failure

Renal failure may be either acute (ARF) or chronic (CRF), both of which require intervention with dietary management, dialysis, or both. Patients with ARF are expected to regain kidney function, while those with CRF eventually must rely on dietary management and dialysis or kidney transplantation for survival.

Acute Renal Failure

Patients with ARF generally present with a sudden onset of symptoms. When evaluated radiologically, the kidneys and urinary tract appear normal in size. The medical history includes a recent, isolated insult to the kidneys. The most common causes include:

■ Shock, that is, a sudden loss of blood supply to the kidneys as a result of trauma, surgical complications, or hypotension

■ Exposure to a nephrotoxic chemical or drug such as radiologic contrast medium, cleaning solvent, pesticide, or specific antibiotics

■ Recent streptococcal infection

Because the insult occurred to previously healthy kidneys (although it is sometimes found superimposed over the early stages of chronic kidney disease), the kidneys usually repair if the patient can be supported by way of dietary management and/or dialysis. Dialysis is usually a temporary therapeutic strategy for these patients.

Chronic Renal Failure

CRF results from the progressive deterioration of kidney tissue over several months or years. In its most simplistic form, CRF results from the substitution of scar tissue for viable kidney tissue. The kidneys may appear shrunken at radiologic evaluation, except in the case of polycystic kidney disease, in which cysts cause enlargement. With the loss of about 90% or more of kidney function, the patient reaches end-stage renal disease (ESRD). Some of the most common causes of ESRD include:

■ Diseases of the glomeruli, causing glomerulonephritis

■ Damage to the renal blood vessels caused by nephrosclerosis resulting from hypertension

■ Obstructive diseases, such as recurrent kidney stones, and congenital birth defects of the kidney and urinary tract

■ Systemic and/or metabolic diseases in which kidney disease is one part of the disease process, including conditions such as diabetes mellitus, systemic lupus erythematosus, and hyperuricemia

■ Abuse of analgesic or "street" drugs

When it has been determined that a patient has ESRD, various treatment modalities are available. They include conservative management, hemodialysis, peritoneal dialysis, and renal transplantation. Each of these modalities and its relevant nutrition-related aspects is discussed in chapters contained in this manual.

The Nephrotic Syndrome

The *nephrotic syndrome* is a term that refers to a group of findings in patients in whom an alteration of the glomerular basement membrane of the kidney leads to the persistent loss of large amounts of protein into the urine. Clinical characteristics include the following:

■ Albuminuria of greater than 3 g/d (proportional amounts for children)

■ Hypoalbuminemia

■ Hyperlipidemia

■ Edema

This disease state affecting the kidneys may be reversible through treatment with corticosteroid or immunosuppressive medications. On the other hand, disease in some patients is resistant to treatment and gradually may progress to CRF. The nephrotic syndrome also can be part of another disease process. Among the numerous causes are primary glomerular disease and conditions secondary to multisystemic diseases, infections, medications, neoplasia, allergens, and familial and metabolic diseases.

The nutrition concerns relative to protein recommendations for patients with the nephrotic syndrome may be found in chapter 3, Conservative Management—Dietary

Treatment in Early Stages of Chronic Renal Failure, and chapter 7, Nutrition Management of the Patient With Diabetes and Renal Disease. These recommendations are the same for all diseases in which the nephrotic syndrome is present.

It is beyond the scope of this manual to go into further detail about normal kidney function or the impact of specific kidney diseases. For further information, suggested readings on normal and abnormal kidney function, ARF, and nephrotic syndrome are included. Additional references on abnormal kidney function are included at the end of many of the chapters contained in this manual.

Suggested Readings

The Normal and Diseased Kidney

Abuela JB. *Renal Pathophysiology, the Essentials.* Baltimore, Md: Williams & Wilkins; 1989.

Klahr S. *The Kidney and Body Fluids in Health and Disease.* New York, NY: Plenum; 1984.

Kopple JD. Nutrition, diet, and the kidney. In: Shils M, Young V, eds. *Modern Nutrition in Health and Disease.* 7th ed. Philadelphia, Pa: Lea & Febiger; 1988.

Reed GM, Sheppard VF. *Regulation of Fluid and Electrolyte Balance: A Programmed Instruction in Clinical Physiology.* 2nd ed. Philadelphia, Pa: WB Saunders; 1971.

Smith K. *Fluids and Electrolytes: A Conceptual Approach.* New York, NY: Churchill Livingstone; 1980.

Williams SR. *Nutrition and Diet Therapy.* St. Louis, Mo: Mosby; 1989.

ARF

Corwin HL, Bonventre JV. Acute renal failure in the intensive care unit. *Intensive Care Med.* 1988;14:86–96.

Corwin HL, Bonventre JV. Acute renal failure. *Med Clin North Am.* 1986;70:1037–1054.

Feinstein EI. Parenteral nutrition in acute renal failure. *Am J Nephrol.* 1985;5:145–149.

Gaudio KN, Seigel NJ. Pathogenesis and treatment of acute renal failure. *Pediatr Clin North Am.* 1987;34:771–787.

Kopple JD. Nutritional therapy in kidney failure. *Nutr Rev.* 1981;39:193–206.

Meguid NM, Campos AC, Hammond WG, et al. Nutritional support in surgical practice. Part II. *Am J Surg.* 1990;159:427–443.

Popovtzer NM, Michael VF, Ogden DA, et al. Acute renal failure. *Int J Artific Org.* 1986;8:13–24.

Proietti R, Pelosi G, Santori R, et al. Nutrition in acute renal failure. *Resuscitation.* 1983;10:159–166.

Schneeweiss B, Graninger W, Stockenhuber F, et al. Energy metabolism in acute and chronic renal failure. *Am J Clin Nutr.* 1990;52:596–601.

Spreiter SC, Myers BD, Swenson RS, et al. Protein-energy requirements in subjects with acute renal failure receiving intermittent hemodialysis. *Am J Clin Nutr.* 1980;33:1433–1437.

Stefee WP. Nutritional support in renal failure. *Surg Clin North Am.* 1981;61:661–670.

Teschner M, Heidland A. Hypercatabolism in acute renal failure mechanisms and therapeutic approaches. *Blood Purif.* 1989;7:16–27.

Tolkoff-Rubin N. *Acute Renal Failure* (videocassette). Boston, Mass: Department of Continuing Education of Harvard Medical School and Massachusetts General Hospital Emergency Training Course.

The Nephrotic Syndrome

Alavi N. Reduction of proteinuria by indomethacin in patients with nephrotic syndrome. *Am J Kidney Dis.* 1986;8:397–403.

Bernard D. Extrarenal complications of the nephrotic syndrome. *Kidney Int.* 1988;3:1184–1202.

Coggins CH, Cornell BF. Nutritional management of nephrotic syndrome. In: Mitch WE, Klahr W, eds. *Nutrition and the Kidney.* Boston, Mass: Little, Brown and Co; 1988;239–249.

Grundy SM, Vega GL. Rationale and management of hyperlipidemia of the nephrotic syndrome. *Am J Med.* 1989;87:3N–11N.

Guarini GF. Nutritional state in patients on long-term protein diet or with nephrotic syndrome. *Kidney Int.* 1989;35(suppl):5195–5200.

Kaysen G. Albumin metabolism in the nephrotic syndrome. *Am J Kidney Dis.* 1988;12:461.

Kaysen G. Effect of dietary protein intake on albumin homeostasis in nephrotic patients. *Kidney Int.* 1986;29:572–577.

Kaysen G, Don B, Schambelan M. Proteinuria, albumin synthesis, and hyperlipidemia in the nephrotic syndrome. *Nephrol Dial Transplant* 1991;6:141–149.

Kaysen GA. Nutritional management of nephrotic syndrome. *J Renal Nutr.* 1992;2:50–58.

Kopple JD. Nutrition, diet and the kidney. In: Shils M, Young V, eds. *Modern Nutrition in Health and Disease.* 7th ed. Philadelphia, Pa: Lea & Febiger; 1988.

Monsey H. Effect of a high protein diet in patients with the nephrotic syndrome. *Clin Sci.* 1989;77:445–451.

Olmer M. Protein diet and nephrotic syndrome. *Kidney Int.* 1989; 36 (suppl):152–153.

2. Nutrition Assessment in Chronic Renal Failure

Assessment of the nutritional status of a renal patient involves the evaluation of multiple parameters, including anthropometric measurements, biochemical and hematologic values, medical and dietary history, metabolic status, and results of a physical examination.

The following material covers the use of these parameters as they apply to the renal patient. Sample assessment forms can be used as worksheets for the collection of patient information. (See appendix F, Forms and Documentation.)

Anthropometric Evaluation

Anthropometric measurements provide information about adequacy of a patient's weight status and the distribution of body fat and skeletal mass. They can be used to identify nutritional excesses or deficiencies in kilocalorie or somatic protein reserves. These measurements also can be used to compare one or more people with people in other population groups or to record changes in one person over time. In one study, anthropometric standards used for the general population were found to apply to a majority of stable patients undergoing hemodialysis, with the exception of nondiabetic female patients who were significantly thinner.[1] Other studies have shown that body weight, triceps skinfold (TSF), and midarm circumference (MAC) measurements were lower in patients undergoing dialysis.[2,3]

Because methods for obtaining anthropometric measures and charts for evaluation of healthy clients are available elsewhere,[4-6] the following discussion of anthropometric indices will focus primarily on information relative to patients with renal disease.

Actual Body Weight

The actual weight of the renal patient must be estimated. Dry weight or estimated dry weight is the actual body weight at normal hydration (minus extra fluid).[7] This estimation is adjusted as necessary, usually by the physician, but the dietitian should recommend changes if significant changes in dietary intake are reported. Serial measurements of MAC and bioelectric impedance analysis to assess total body water may also be helpful in recommending dry weight changes.[8] Fluid status always must be considered when body weight is evaluated.

Height

Initial measurement of height is essential. For patients who are unable to stand, recumbent bed height, arm span, or knee height measurements may provide an estimate of stature.[9]

Yearly measurement of height for those who are able to stand is important because decreasing stature may reflect bone disease.

Estimation of Frame Size

Frame size is used with height and weight tables and may be estimated by either wrist circumference or elbow breadth. Procedures for making these measurements can be found elsewhere.[6]

Desirable Body Weight

A desirable body weight must be established for a patient with renal failure, to assess the actual weight. Currently, a variety of methods and tables are used to determine this desirable "normalized" or "ideal" body weight.[10]

One simple method to use is the Hamwi formula. The ideal body weight of a person with a medium frame can be calculated by using 100 lb for women and 106 lb for men for the first 5 ft in height, and adding 5 lb for each additional inch in height for women and 6 lb for each additional inch for men. Ten percent of that weight is added for a large-framed individual, and 10% is subtracted for a small-framed individual.[11]

Ideal body weight or weight range may be also derived from sources such as the tables of the Metropolitan Life Insurance Company, the NHANES percentiles, or provisional weight standards for the elderly published by Masters et al.[9,10]

Once the desirable weight or weight range is established, a relative body weight (RBW) percentage can be determined to assess the actual weight.[9]

$$RBW\% = \frac{\text{measured weight (kg)}}{\text{desirable weight (kg) or midpoint of desirable weight range (kg)}} \times 100$$

Another method to assess actual or measured weight is the body mass index (BMI).[9]

$$BMI = \frac{\text{measured weight (kg)}}{[\text{height (m)}]^2}$$

Some practitioners prefer to use the patient's usual or premorbid weight (if the patient is not obese) when establishing weight goals. Also, adjustment for amputation(s) must be considered.[9]

Estimation of Body Fat and Protein Reserves

The TSF thickness is an indicator of body fat composition, and midarm muscle circumference (MAMC) and midarm muscle area may be used to estimate muscle or protein reserves.[10] Decreased TSF measurements have been documented in some hemodialysis patient groups.[2,3]

Excess fluid in body tissues may affect the measurement of TSF; thus, it is recommended that measurements be obtained after dialysis, when dry weight is achieved. Results may also be more accurate when an arm without a vascular access in place is used.

Other tools can help with evaluation of body composition, if they are available. Bioelectric impedance analysis is used to assess lean body mass, fat reserves, and total body water. Infrared interactance is used in determining percentage of body fat. Use of the latter method is unaffected by extraneous fluid.[8]

Anthropometric Measurements of Children

Monitoring growth is an essential part of ongoing management in children with renal disease. Measurements should be obtained frequently (at least monthly for dialysis patients) and by the same practitioner, if possible. Children with CRF frequently exhibit growth retardation. All of the causes are not known, but some factors include age of onset of renal disease, glomerluar filtration rate, adequacy of nutrient intake, presence of osteodystrophy, and a variety of metabolic and hormonal imbalances.

Height (or length) should be measured regularly according to standardized methods for infants and children and plotted on the appropriate growth chart for age and sex.[12] Because of seasonal variation in growth rates, a minimum of 6 months of serial measurements should be observed when evaluating overall linear growth.

Weight also should be measured regularly, by using consistent techniques and equipment. Estimated dry weight is used to document body weight, as in the adult population. However, because there is no precise way to determine the dry weight for a person with edema (as the term "estimated" implies), weight changes relative to growth are difficult to interpret. Regardless, weight for age, as well as height for age and weight for height, are plotted serially on standardized growth charts. Head circumference is measured for children 36 months of age or younger, and these measurements are plotted serially as well.

MAC, MAMC, TSF, and subscapular skinfold tests can be obtained to provide additional information regarding the nutritional status of the child. Again, these are most useful when they are performed consistently by the same practitioner by using standardized techniques and equipment.

No normal anthropometric values for children with renal disease are yet available for evaluation of growth and development of such patients. Therefore, standards for normal children are used and serial values are monitored for each patient.

Clinical Signs of Nutrient Deficiency

Most clinical signs of nutrient deficiency are mild and not specific to people with renal failure. Physical signs do not appear until malnutrition has been prolonged and severe, and these are best used in diagnosis as part of a group of symptoms common to a particular nutrient deficiency or problem. A listing of clinical signs and associated nutrient deficiencies is given in reference 13.

The Diet History

A diet history is used to collect information about the patient's nutritional, social, and medical status, to make a valid assessment of nutritional needs, and to formulate a workable plan for implementation of an appropriate diet prescription.

The interview segment is often the first step in building a relationship between patient and dietitian. It is as important for the renal dietitian to establish a positive rapport with the patient as it is to collect the data. An explanation of why the questions are being asked and how the answers will be used will help the patient feel more at ease. Finishing the session with a brief explanation and reasons for any immediate plans for change helps set the tone for future teaching. Clarification of the role of the renal dietitian as an empathic helper rather than a "diet cop" is important.

The interview should be conducted with the patient if possible, and can include a family member or other caretaker, depending on the circumstances.

Sample data collection forms included in appendix F of this manual may help a dietitian to develop a form that will suit the needs of his or her facility and specific patient population. The forms should include the following information:

- Current nutrient needs
- Previous diet restrictions
- Factors that may interfere with adequate intake, such as chewing, swallowing, nausea, vomiting, diarrhea, and/or allergies
- Identification of resources such as family and other support systems
- Current medications
- Meal planning information, such as food preferences, cultural influences, and seasonings commonly used
- Meal patterns, including food frequencies, meals away from home, snacks, and portion sizes commonly used

Evaluation of the Diet History

The dietitian can estimate the patient's usual nutrient intake by analyzing the typical meal pattern and other information. The data generated should be summarized for use in developing an initial plan of care. It will also be helpful when establishing the educational needs of each individual patient.

Evaluation of Biochemical Parameters

Because neither hemodialysis nor peritoneal dialysis can completely replace natural kidney function, laboratory values cannot be interpreted by the same standards that are in use for the general population.

Dialysis units determine their own ranges for acceptable laboratory values on the basis of type of analyzing equipment used, as well as adult and pediatric criteria screens established by the Health Care Financing Administration. These criteria screens address nutritional status, osteodystrophy, anemia, potassium, adequacy of dialysis, blood pressure, and interdialytic weight gain.[14] The dietitian must be aware of the facility's guidelines for biochemical parameters.

Serum Proteins

There is no "perfect" measure of protein status for any population group. Total protein, transferrin, albumin, and prealbumin levels are all used as nutritional indicators, but in patients with renal disease, almost all are influenced by other factors. Transferrin, albumin, and prealbumin levels are all affected by hydration status, and the transferrin level may change, depending on iron deficiency or overload. Prealbumin, because it has a shorter half-life than albumin, is a more sensitive nutritional measure but may be falsely elevated in the euvolemic patient with CRF.[15] Changes in serum levels of prealbumin are directly correlated to changes in nutritional status, however, and may be serially evaluated for change in one patient.[15,16]

Current research indicates that insulin-like growth factor-1, which is a serum protein with mitogenic properties and insulin-like activities, may be an improved biochemical indicator of nitrogen balance.[17]

Blood Urea Nitrogen

Blood urea nitrogen (BUN) is a nitrogenous waste product of protein metabolism and most commonly becomes elevated with increased protein intake, catabolism (from infection, surgery, poor nutrition, and/or glucocorticoid usage), gastrointestinal bleeding, and/or decreased efficiency of dialysis.[18] High BUN levels may lead to uremic symptoms such as nausea, vomiting, diarrhea, lethargy, and confusion.[19] A decreased BUN level may be an indication of decreased protein intake, loss of protein through emesis or diarrhea, frequent dialysis, protein anabolism, or overhydration.[14,20] Thus, the BUN level cannot be used as an isolated parameter to assess nutritional status or the adequacy of dialysis. Currently, Health Care Financing Administration screens recommend a specific percentage of reduction of BUN levels before and after hemodialysis.[14] If reduction is insufficient, ineffective dialysis treatments may be the cause.

Creatinine

Creatinine is a nitrogenous waste product of muscle metabolism. Unlike BUN, it is not directly affected by dietary protein intake. For this reason, creatinine levels are used to assess renal function. A twice-normal serum creatinine level suggests a 50% nephron loss.[18]

Serum creatinine can also be used as a guide in evaluation of the effectiveness of dialysis. A renal patient's creatinine level usually stabilizes in an approximate range once a dialysis regimen has been established. Any sudden increases noted, especially in conjunction with elevated BUN and potassium levels, may be attributed to changes in the dialysis regimen (missing or shortening scheduled treatments), lowered blood flow, recirculation in the vascular access, or loss of residual kidney function.

Creatinine is produced daily in proportion to the body's muscle mass.[21] This level can sometimes be used as a parameter in nutrition assessment, because lowered levels over time may reflect reduced muscle mass. This is only true, however, if no change has occurred in the residual renal function or dialysis treatment plan.

Potassium

Potassium is found primarily in the intracellular fluid, but it is also present in extracellular fluid. Extracellular potassium is important because of its influence on muscle activity, especially the cardiac muscle.[22] Hypokalemia *or* hyperkalemia may induce muscle weakness, and cardiac arrhythmias and hyperkalemia can cause cardiac arrest.

Hypokalemia may be caused by the use of potassium-depleting diuretics, overall decreased nutritional intakes, vomiting, diarrhea, excessive use of the potassium-binding resin, and/or dialysis against a low- or zero-potassium dialysate.[20]

Causes of hyperkalemia include the following: excessive overall nutritional intake, including nutritional supplements; constipation; infection; gastrointestinal bleeding; insulin deficiency; metabolic acidosis (low serum CO_2 level), drug content or interactions (ie, the effects of beta-blocking drugs or drugs inhibiting angiotensin-converting enzyme); inadequate dialysis; and catabolism of malnutrition and/or cell damage caused by injury or surgery.[15, 20, 22] It is also wise to check the validity of laboratory values, especially if the blood sample is hemolyzed.

Sodium

Sodium is the principal cation of extracellular fluid. Functions of sodium include preservation of normal muscle function, maintenance of acid-base balance, osmotic pressure of body fluids, and permeability of cells.[23]

Serum sodium level is not a reliable indicator of sodium intake. Fluid retention can dilute an elevated level, making it appear normal. Serum levels must be interpreted in conjunction with the patient's current fluid status.

Hyponatremia may be caused by the following: fluid overload or excessive use of intravenous fluid without electrolytes, sodium depletion due to severe sodium restriction, sodium-wasting nephropathies, and cirrhosis with ascites. Spurious hyponatremia may exist with hyperlipidemia or hyperglycemia. Serum sodium levels decrease by 3 mEq/L relative to every 100 mg/dL increase in serum glucose levels.[15] Symptoms of "true" hyponatremia include abdominal cramping and hypotension.[20]

Hypernatremia may be the result of excessive water loss through diarrhea and/or vomiting (dehydration), the diuretic phase of acute tubular necrosis, and aggressive diuretic therapy without a sodium restriction. Symptoms of hypernatremia include flushed skin, dry tongue and mucous membranes, and thirst.[20]

Calcium

The majority of calcium in the body is found in the structural components of bones and teeth. A small percentage is also found in body fluids. The ionic calcium in these fluids regulates transport across cell membranes and is essential to neuromuscular irritability and blood coagulation.[21]

Patients who have CRF have decreased calcium absorption secondary to the altered metabolism of vitamin D as well as the inability to excrete excess phosphate. The results of decreased calcium absorption as well as hyperphosphatemia lead to decreased serum calcium levels. These decreased levels, in turn, contribute to hyperparathyroidism and renal osteodystrophy.[24]

It must be noted that when low serum calcium levels are apparent, the serum albumin level should be evaluated as well. A substantial portion of total calcium is protein bound; thus, a decrease in albumin results in a decrease in total serum calcium (without a change in ionized calcium). A helpful rule of thumb to "correct" the serum calcium level is to add 0.8 mg/dL to the laboratory value reported, for every gram per deciliter decrease in serum albumin from 4.0 g/dL.[15]

Example: If serum calcium level is reported by the laboratory as 8.5 mg/dL and serum albumin = 2.4 g/dL, 0.8×1.6 (difference in albumin from 4.0 g/dL) = 1.28 and 8.5 + 1.28 = a "corrected" calcium level of 9.78.

Symptoms of "true" hypocalcemia include tingling fingers, abdominal cramps, tetany, and seizures. Severe hypocalcemia can lead to respiratory or cardiac arrest.[20,24]

Hypercalcemia may also be present in the population with renal disease. It may often be caused by supplementation of calcium and 1, 25-dihydroxyvitamin D. When these medications are used, close monitoring of serum calcium and phosphorus levels is advised when they are initiated or changed.

Other causes of hypercalcemia may include primary hyperparathyroidism, some types of cancer including multiple myeloma, parathyroid tumors, bone metastasis, Hodgkin's disease and leukemia, Paget's disease, bone fractures combined with bed rest, prolonged immobilization, and aluminum deposition in the bone.[15]

Symptoms of hypercalcemia may include anorexia, nausea, vomiting, constipation, abdominal pain, ileus, muscle weakness, psychosis, and, if severe, stupor and coma.[25]

Phosphorus

Most of the total body phosphorus is combined with calcium in the skeletal structure. Plasma phosphate, essential for the metabolism of carbohydrate, protein, and fat, is a factor in the high-energy compound adenosine triphosphate, which is essential for all cell activity and is important for many enzyme systems.[26]

As already mentioned, elevated serum phosphate levels contribute to hypocalcemia and hyperparathyroidism. Restriction of dietary phosphorus intake and the use of phosphate-binding medications are used to help control these levels. Symptoms of high serum levels are itching and bone pain.[24]

Hypophosphatemia may also result from excessive phosphate-binding medication combined with decreased food intake, anabolism, and refeeding, especially with total parenteral nutrition if phosphate is not at least minimally supplemented in these solutions. Persistently low serum phosphate levels can progress to phosphorus depletion and osteomalacia.[24]

Calcium-Phosphorus Product

It is best to maintain the calcium-phosphorus product (the result of multiplying the serum values of both) below 60 to 70 to prevent metastatic calcification. Metastatic calcification is the development of calcium deposits in any soft tissue area, such as the conjunctivae of the eye, the heart and blood vessels, the lungs, and the extremities. The exact cause is not fully understood, but seems to be related to an increased calcium-phosphorus ratio, which often results from hyperphosphatemia.[24]

Alkaline Phosphatase

Alkaline phosphatase is an enzyme produced mainly in the liver, bones, and kidneys. Renal failure may disrupt normal skeletal metabolism, resulting in renal osteodystrophy. When this occurs, increased quantities of alkaline phophatase are secreted. This elevation may be used as an indicator of bone disease in the renal patient population.[27] It must be noted, however, that increasing serum levels of alkaline phosphatase in pediatric renal patients also may indicate bone growth.[15]

Liver abnormalities also may need to be investigated when serum alkaline phosphatase levels are elevated, and especially if other indices indicate liver dysfunction.

Magnesium

Magnesium is found primarily in the intracellular fluid. Its functions include enzyme activation in energy transport, regulation of body temperature, and neuromuscular contraction. Most magnesium is bound to protein, and serum levels may appear falsely low in protein deficiency. These levels, however, are often elevated in the renal population because of decreased excretion of this mineral.[15] For this reason, the use of antacids and laxatives containing magnesium is not usually recommended.

Glucose

Ideally, normal glucose levels should be maintained for renal patients with and without diabetes to prevent the complications of hypoglycemia and hyperglycemia. Abnormal carbohydrate metabolism has been noted in this population, especially in patients approaching ESRD. Patients with insulin-dependent diabetes may require a lower insulin dosage or discontinuation of insulin because of decreased insulin clearance by the kidneys.[28] Therefore, close monitoring of insulin and nutritional requirements is necessary, and both may need adjustment during the progression of renal disease.[29,30] On the other hand, glucose levels may be higher in nondiabetic patients approaching ESRD, because of abnormal glucose use as a result of altered insulin response and secretion.[28]

Glucose intolerance and unplanned weight gain may develop in patients undergoing peritoneal dialysis, because of glucose absorption from the dialysate. Thus, energy requirement determinations for peritoneal dialysis patients must take into consideration the glucose absorbed. Directions for calculating these kilocalories may be found in chapter 5, Nutrition Management of the Adult Peritoneal Dialysis Patient.

Iron Studies

Replacement therapy with recombinant human erythropoietin (rHuEPO) has been shown to be effective in reversing anemia associated with CRF.[31–38] Adequate iron stores are required to permit optimal erythropoiesis, however, and specific laboratory parameters must be evaluated on a regular basis to determine the need for and dosage of supplemental iron for patients undergoing this therapy. Percentage of transferrin saturation (iron/total iron binding capacity × 100) indicating bone marrow iron stores or "available" iron and serum ferritin levels indicating tissue iron stores must be closely monitored on a regular basis.[38] (See appendix C for a more complete discussion on the relationship between rHuEPO and iron therapy.)

Lipids

Disorders of lipid metabolism play an important role in the pathogenesis of cardiovascular complications. The primary abnormality in the population with renal disease seems to be a reduction in the catabolism of lipoproteins, unchanged or lowered hepatic synthesis, and the need for specific medications such as glucocorticoids.[40] Type IV hyperlipoproteinemia is associated with CRF, and after renal transplantation, the type II pattern may be seen (see chapter 13).[41] Research also suggests that hypercholesterolemia itself may contribute to the development of renal disease.[42]

It must be noted that low cholesterol levels are associated with malnutrition morbidity and mortality.[43] Hypocholesterolemia is frequently prevalent in the renal population, especially for those undergoing hemodialysis. Lowrie and Lew reported twice the risk for death in this population when serum cholesterol levels were less than 150 mg/dL.[44]

Urea Kinetic Modeling

Urea kinetic modeling was developed to assess the adequacy of dialysis and protein intake. It is greatly based on the work done by Sargent and Gotch, as derived from the National Cooperative Dialysis Study.[45] There are a variety of formulas that can be calculated manually or by using computer programs. The renal dietitian should be aware of the kinetic modeling practices in his or her facility.

The parameter Kt/V is used to assess the adequacy of dialysis. K is the dialyzer urea clearance in liters per minute combined with the urea removed by residual renal function, *t* is the dialysis time in minutes, and V is the volume of urea distribution in liters.[46] In National Cooperative Dialysis Study patients undergoing hemodialysis, K*t*/V value greater than 0.8 was shown to reduce the risk of morbidity and number of hospitalizations.[47] Most nephrologists, however, currently use a K*t*/V of 1 to 1.3 for three times per week treatments as a more appropriate goal for adequate dialysis.[48] An even higher K*t*/V is necessary for those patients undergoing hemodialysis treatments twice per week.

In urea kinetic modeling, the protein catabolic rate (PCR) is also used; this is a reflection of the amount of protein that is catabolized per kilogram of body weight in 24 hours. This PCR is equal to the dietary protein intake in the nutritionally stable patient.[49] Residual renal function must be considered when PCR is calculated.

A renal dietitian can use the PCR to monitor dietary protein intake without relying on patient food records, which may be much less accurate. Normal PCR values should be in the range of protein (grams per kilogram of body weight) prescribed for the patient. One must consider, however, that catabolized protein can be either endogenous or exogenous. Therefore, if the patient has an elevated PCR, food records could be compared with the PCR to indicate whether the catabolized protein is from muscle catabolism resulting from an inadequate protein and/or calorie intake or from excessive protein intake. On the other hand, low PCR can represent either inadequate protein intake or anabolism. The PCR can be used in conjunction with the patient's dry weight and serum albumin changes to prioritize diet counseling for patients who are nutritionally at risk. Use of the PCR may actually allow earlier detection of compromised protein intake.[50] Also, it is important to use the PCR in conjunction with the K*t*/V for patients undergoing dialysis. In fact, the dialysis prescription may not be adequate if the PCR is persistently low, implying that the patient needs even more dialysis for his or her appetite to improve.

The application of urea kinetics to peritoneal dialysis can be expressed by the relationship between the BUN level, protein intake, and nitrogen removal. Nitrogen removal occurs from a combination of exogenous losses, residual renal function, and the process of dialysis. Kinetic modeling for peritoneal dialysis provides a basis for calculating the amount of dialysis necessary to clear urea at specified levels of BUN and protein intake.[51,52] (See also chapter 5, Nutrition Management of the Adult Peritoneal Dialysis Patient.) As with hemodialysis, kinetic modeling may assist the dietitian in identification of patients who are at increased nutritional risk or those who need additional dietary counseling.

Prognostic Nutrition Index

Over the past several years, various parameters have been used to assess nutritional status in the population with CRF, as discussed in this chapter. Recently, Lowrie and Lew used logistic regression analysis in which a predictive model correlated singular individual nutritional-biochemical indices to mortality risk for hemodialysis patients.[44]

Many more comprehensive formulas, called prognostic nutrition indexes (PNIs), have been in existence for evaluation of a variety of patient types, including those with abdominal trauma or undergoing planned surgical procedures. These PNIs enable clinical specialists to identify high-risk patients, plan nutrition intervention, and evaluate outcomes.[53–57]

Unfortunately, the already existing PNIs use variables that are either directly or indirectly affected by renal failure or assessment techniques that are not practical for patients undergoing dialysis. Thus, current research has been aimed at determining whether a PNI exists for the hemodialysis population. A preliminary formula was developed by using statistical analysis of variables, including patient age, gender, length of time undergoing dialysis, hospitalization history, and monthly chemical values. This hemodialysis PNI is used to predict the likelihood of hospitalization as a result of infection.[58]

The preliminary formula will need to be tested in multicenter studies to establish its useful application. If validated, like existing PNIs, this PNI will help dietitians to identify patients at high risk and evaluate the effects of nutrition intervention.

References

1. Nelson EE. Anthropometry in the nutritional assessment of adults with end-stage renal disease. *J Renal Nutr.* 1991;1:164.

2. Schoenfield PY, Henry RR, Laird NM, et al. Assessment of nutritional status of the National Cooperative Dialysis Study Population. *Kidney Int.* 1983;23:(suppl 13)580–588.

3. Compher CW. Nutritional assessment in chronic renal failure. *Nutr Supp Serv.* 1985;5:18–21.

4. Frisancho R. New norms of upper limb fat and muscle areas for assessment of nutritional status. *Am J Clin Nutr.* 1981;34:2540–2545.

5. Grant JP, Custer PB, Thurlow J. Current techniques of nutritional assessment. *Surg Clin North Am.* 1981;61:437–460.

6. Wilkins K, Schiro KB, eds. *Suggested Guidelines for Nutrition Care in Renal Patients.* 2nd ed. Chicago, Ill: The American Dietetic Association; 1992.

7. Comty CM, Davis M. Nutritional assessment in end-stage renal disease. *Dial Transplant.* 1981;10:130–134.

8. Byham LD. News of note. *Renal Nutr Forum.* 1991;10:5.

9. Grant A, DeHoog S. Anthropometric assessment. In: *Nutritional Assessment and Support.* Seattle, Wash: Grant and DeHoog; 1991:9-86.

10. Blumenkrantz M, et al. Methods for assessing nutritional status of patients with renal failure. *Am J Clin Nutr.* 1980;33:1567–1585.

11. Hamwi G. Therapy: changing dietary concepts. In: Dunowski TS, ed. *Diabetes Mellitus: Diagnosis and Treatment.* New York, NY: American Diabetes Association; 1964;73–78.

12. Cooper A, Heird WC. Nutritional assessment of the pediatric patient, including the low birth weight infant. *Am J Clin Nutr.* 1982;35:1132–1141.

13. Kight MA. The nutrition physical examination. *CRN Q.* 1987;2:9–12.

14. HCFA adult medical review criteria screens. *CRN Q.* 1990;14:6–9.

15. Grant A, DeHoog S. Biochemical assessment. In: *Nutritional Assessment and Support.*

Seattle, Wash: Grant and DeHoog; 1991;99–152.

16. Coles GA, Peters DK, Jones JH. Albumin metabolism in chronic renal failure. *Clin Sci.* 1970;39:423–435.

17. Jacob V, et al. IGF-1: a marker of undernutrition in hemodialysis patients. *Am J Clin Nutr.* 1990;52:39–44.

18. Stark JL. BUN-creatinine—your key to kidney function. *Nursing 80.* 1981;33–38.

19. Kopple JD. Nutritional management of chronic renal failure. *Nutr MD.* 1980;6:1–2.

20. *Study of Renal Disease and Dietary Implications.* Hines, Ill: Hines Veterans Administration Hospital; 1975.

21. Blackburn G, et al. Nutritional and metabolic assessment of the hospitalized patient. *JPEN J Parenter Enter Nutr.* 1977;1:11–22.

22. Beto JA, Bansal VK. Hyperkalemia: evaluating dietary and nondietary etiology. *J Renal Nutr.* 1991;2:28–29.

23. Schneider HA, Anderson CE, Coursin DD, eds. *Nutritional Support of Medical Practice.* New York, NY: Harper & Row; 1977;367.

24. Schoolwerth AC, Engle JE. Calcium and phosphorus in diet therapy of uremia. *J Am Diet Assoc.* 1975;66:460–464.

25. McLaren DS. Clinical manifestations of nutritional disorders. In: Shils ME, Young VR, eds. *Modern Nutrition in Health and Disease.* Philadelphia, Pa: Lea & Febiger; 1988;154.

26. Anioli LV. Calcium and phosphorus. In: Shils ME, Young VR, eds. *Modern Nutrition in Health and Disease.* Philadelphia, Pa: Lea & Febiger; 1988:154.

27. Guyton A. *Textbook of Medical Physiology.* Philadelphia, Pa: WB Saunders; 1981:981.

28. Ekdoyan G. Effects of renal insufficiency on nutrient metabolism and endocrine function. In: Mitch WE, Klahr S, eds. *Nutrition and the Kidney.* Boston, Mass: Little, Brown, and Co; 1988:30.

29. DeFronzo RA, et al. Carbohydrate metabolism in uremia: a review. *Medicine.* 1973;52:469–481.

30. Frolich J, Schollmeyer P, Gerok W. Carbohydrate metabolism in renal failure. *Am J Clin Nutr.* 1978;31:1541–1546.

31. Winerals CG, et al. Effect of human erythropoietin derived from recombinant DNA on the anaemia of patients maintained by chronic hemodialysis. *Lancet.* 1986;2:1175–1177.

32. Eschbach JW, et al. Correction of the anemia of end stage renal disease with recombinant human erythropoietin: results of a combined phase I and II clinical trial. *N Engl J Med.* 1987;316:73–78.

33. Schaeffer RM, et al. Treatment of the anemia of hemodialysis patients with recombinant human erythropoietin. *Int J Artif Org.* 1988;11:249–254.

34. VanStone JC, Jones ME, Hires CI. A controlled study of recombinant erythropoietin (EPO) in chronic hemodialysis patients (abstr). *Kidney Int.* 1988;33:246.

35. Mayer G, et al. Working capacity is increased following recombinant human erythropoietin treatment. *Kidney Int.* 1988;34:525–528.

36. Lundin AP, et al. Recombinant human erythropoietin (rHuEPO) treatment enhances exercise tolerance in hemodialysis patients (HD) (abstr). *Kidney Int.* 1988;33:200.

37. Gibilaro SD, et al. Improved quality of life while receiving recombinant erythropoietin (abstr). *Kidney Int.* 1989;35:247.

38. Evans RW, et al. Correction of anemia with recombinant human erythropoietin enhances the quality of life of hemodialysis patients (abstr). *Kidney Int.* 1989;35:246.

39. VanWyck DB, et al. Iron status in patients receiving erythropoietin for dialysis associated anemia. *Kidney Int.* 1989;35:712–716.

40. Attman PO, Alaupovic P. Lipid abnormalities in chronic renal insufficiency. *Kidney Int.* 1991;39:(suppl 31):16–23.

41. Moorhead JF. Lipids and progressive kidney disease. *Kidney Int.* 1991;39:(suppl 31):35–40.

42. Kaysen GA, Don B, Schambelan M. Proteinuria, albumin synthesis and hyperlipidemia in the nephrotic syndrome. *Nephrol Dial Transplant.* 1991;6:141–149.

43. Rudman D, Mattson DE, Hoskote SN, et al. Prognostic significance of serum cholesterol in nursing home men. *JPEN J Parenter Enter Nutr.* 1988;12:155–158.

44. Lowrie EG, Lew NL. Death risk in hemodialysis patients: the predictive value of commonly measured variables and an evaluation of death rate differences between facilities. *Am J Kidney Dis.* 1990;15:458–482.

45. Sargent J, Gotch F. Mathematical modelling to dialysis therapy. *Kidney Int.* 1980;18(suppl 10):2.

46. Sargent J, Gotch F. Urea kinetics: a guide to nutritional management of renal failure. *Am J Clin Nutr.* 1978;31:1696.

47. Gotch F, Sargent J. A mechanistic analysis of the national cooperative dialysis study. *Kidney Int.* 1985;28:526.

48. Gotch F, Gee C. Urea kinetic modelling: a proven quantitative technique in dialysis therapy. *Nephrology News Issues.* September 1989.

49. Johnson J, Schniepp F. Comparison of urea kinetic modeling with other approaches to dietary prescription. *Dial Transplant.* 1981;10:280.

50. Goldstein D, Frederico C. The effects of urea kinetic modeling on the nutritional management of hemodialysis patients. *J Am Diet Assoc.* 1987;87:474.

51. Teehan B, Brown J, Schleifer C. Kinetic modelling in peritoneal dialysis. In: Nissenson A, Fine R, Gentile D, eds. *Clinical Dialysis.* Norwalk, Conn: Appleton and Lange; 1990:319–325.

52. Lysaght M, et al. The relevance of urea kinetic modeling to CAPD. *Trans Am Soc Artif Intern Org.* 1989;35:784–790.

53. Mullen JL, Waldman MT, Hobbs CL, et al. Prediction of operative morbidity and mortality by preoperative nutritional assessment. *Surg Forum.* 1979;30:80–82.

54. Harvey KB, Moldawer BS, Bistrain BR, et al. Biological measures for the formulation of a hospital prognostic index. *Am J Clin Nutr.* 1981;34:2013–2022.

55. Jones TJ, Moore EE, Van Way CW. Factors influencing nutritional assessment in abdominal trauma patients. *JPEN J Parenter Enter Nutr.* 1983;7:115–116.

56. Roy LB, Edwards PA, Barr LH. The value of nutritional assessment in the surgical patient. *JPEN J Parenter Enter Nutr.* 1985;9:170–172.

57. Hall J. Use of internal validity in the construct of an index of undernutrition. *JPEN J Parenter Enter Nutr.* 1990;14:582–587.

58. Kelly MP, Kight MA, Migliore V. A prognostic nutrition index: does one exist in hemodialysis patients? *Renal Nutr.* 1993;3:10–22.

3. Conservative Management— Dietary Treatment in Early Stages of Chronic Renal Failure

The goals for conservative dietary management in the early stages of CRF are to minimize uremic toxicity, delay the progression of renal disease, and prevent wasting and malnutrition. These goals can be accomplished by strict adherence to a diet that: (1) limits foods whose metabolic byproducts contribute to the buildup of toxic substances in the blood and also may cause more rapid deterioration of remaining kidney function; and (2) prescribes adequate calories to prevent body tissue catabolism. This diet is difficult to follow over a long period, and to be successful the patient must be highly motivated and encouraged regularly. With careful attention to diet and medication, dialysis often can be delayed.

Patients who are treated conservatively presently do not qualify for the federal ESRD Medicare program. The dietitian's services and prescribed oral nutrition supplements are not covered by Medicare or Medicaid programs in most states.

Research has been under way in the past few years to determine the effectiveness of conservative management, as well as its cost benefit. The National Institutes of Health sponsored a multicenter clinical trial in the United States called the Modification of Diet in Renal Disease study. This study was designed to determine if dietary protein and phosphorus affect the course of chronic progressive renal disease. Patients between the ages of 18 and 70 years with glomerular filtration rates (GFRs) in the range of 13 to 55 mL/min/1.73 m^2 were eligible to participate in this study. The study design included a baseline period (the first 3 months) during which participants underwent evaluation of their usual diet, general state of nutrition, and renal function. During the follow-up period, they were randomly assigned to one of three study diets with varying amounts of protein and phosphorus. The diet with the lowest protein and phosphorus content was supplemented with a mixture of keto acid analogs. Daily multivitamin and calcium supplements were provided in all study groups.

Because the results of the Modification of Diet in Renal Disease study were not published at the time of this Guide's publication, the following discussion will address the most current nutrition guidelines available for people with chronic progressive renal disease.

Typically, CRF progresses until treatment with dialysis or transplantation is required. This process usually occurs regardless of the underlying renal disease, even in cases in which the initial insult to the kidney is corrected or inactive. During the past 40 years, researchers

Portions of this chapter are reprinted, by permission, from the July 1984 edition of *Contemporary Dialysis* magazine, 6300 Variel Avenue, Suite 1, Woodland Hills, CA 91367.

have been investigating the cause for the chronic progression of kidney failure. Accumulating evidence from observations in both animals and human beings suggests that reductions in protein and/or phosphorus intake can slow or even halt the rate of progression of renal disease in experimental animals and probably in humans. The reports that dietary management can alter the rate of progression are exciting observations. The purpose of this chapter is to review available data regarding the following questions:

1. In a clinical setting, is a protein- and phosphorus-controlled diet effective in retarding the progression of renal disease?
2. At what level of GFR or serum creatinine concentration should diet therapy be initiated?
3. In view of current knowledge, what is the recommended dietary prescription for patients with CRF?

Approximately 45 years ago, Addis suggested that to reduce the "workload" of the surviving nephrons of diseased kidneys, protein intake should be restricted.[1] This premise was supported by studies conducted in the early 1900s in rats and dogs. Initial observations showed that renal mass increased when rats were fed high-protein diets for extended periods, while the GFR in dogs increased as much as 100% when their diets were changed from carbohydrate to protein.

Effectiveness of a Protein- and Phosphorus-Controlled Diet in Retarding Progression of Renal Disease

Since the work of Addis, numerous investigators have reported a deleterious effect of dietary protein on the course of experimentally induced nephritis and on the rate of progressive renal failure that occurs subsequent to the renal compensatory changes after subtotal renal ablation.[2] The mechanism by which this occurs is not yet clear. During the past few years the work of Brenner, Meyer, and Hostetter[1] has provided a physiologic explanation for the potential mechanisms by which dietary protein may affect the progression of renal disease.

Micropuncture studies demonstrated that the progressive azotemia, proteinuria, and glomerular sclerosis occurring after renal ablation is associated with sustained "adaptive" increases in glomerular pressure and flow. Thus, GFRs in uninephrectomized rats increase by about 40% in the remnant kidney. These "compensatory" changes in kidney function are the result of renal arteriolar vasodilation, which causes elevations in the flow and pressure in the capillaries of remnant glomeruli.[3] These changes also occur in other models of renal disease.

From their work, Brenner and associates concluded that the loss of functioning nephron mass in many renal diseases leads to increased glomerular capillary plasma flow, increased glomerular transcapillary hydraulic pressure, and increased single-nephron GFR in the remaining nephrons. These changes lead to a state of "intrarenal hypertension" resulting in proteinuria and structural alterations of epithelial cells. These investigators propose that the progression of CRF after loss of renal mass may be actively dependent on a final common pathway: glomerular hyperfiltration.

Further studies showed that feeding a low-protein diet to rats with remnant kidneys largely prevented the striking increase in glomerular plasma flow and capillary pressures that lead to hyperfiltration. With protein restrictions the glomerular hemodynamics of remaining nephrons were restored to near normal and were associated with preservation of glomerular structure. In experimental animals, the low-protein diet plays a major role in preserving kidney function.

The case in human beings, however, is not as clear. Some studies performed in the late 1930s and in the 1940s showed low-protein diets to be of some benefit in lessening symptoms of heart failure, hypertension, and severity of uremia. These diets were also low in sodium; the influence of the low-protein diet in renal failure could not be differentiated from other effects of these diets. With low-protein diets supplemented with essential amino aids and keto acids, Walser and coworkers[4] observed that the creatinine clearance stabilized or increased in some, but not all, chronically uremic patients. They suggested that the low phosphorus content of the keto acid diets and particularly the low serum calcium and phosphorus product might lower the rate of progression to ESRD.

Maschio and associates,[5] in a retrospective study of 75 patients with varying degrees of renal insufficiency, found that a diet moderately restricted in protein and phosphorus appeared to be effective in delaying progression of functional deterioration in early renal disease.

Barsotti and associates[6] observed that patients given a very low nitrogen diet supplemented with essential amino acids and keto acids experienced a significantly lower rate of progression of renal failure than did patients ingesting a more liberal intake of protein. Alvestrand and colleagues also showed a retardation in the rate of progression of renal failure in patients taking in low amounts of nitrogen by way of a newly formulated amino acid preparation. The rate of progression of renal insufficiency was measured by using a plot of the relationship between the reciprocal of serum creatinine concentration versus time.[7]

Various prospective studies in the past 5 to 10 years have shown significant slowing of the progression of CRF in human beings when a diet with 0.4 to 0.6 g of protein per kilogram body weight per day is used, but results were mixed in long-term effects on nutritional status.[8]

Other factors also may have a profound effect on GFR. Hypertension in particular can affect the rate of progression of renal disease. Brenner and associates suggested that treatment of systemic hypertension with angiotensin-converting enzyme inhibitors may be beneficial in delaying the progression of renal disease. This is a result of their vasodilatory effect on the efferent glomerular arteriole. At present, however, the unequivocal efficacy of these agents has not yet been demonstrated in human beings.[9]

Data are available to suggest that phosphorus restrictions may slow the rate of progression of renal disease in azotemic rats. However, it has been difficult to separate the effects of phosphorus restriction from other factors in the diet, such as protein restriction. The available data suggest that the effect on GFR was greatest when diets low in both phosphorus and protein were maintained.

GFR or Serum Creatinine Level and Initiation of Diet Therapy

At this time, clear guidelines do not exist to define the point at which diet therapy should commence. However, from the results of previously mentioned studies, it seems prudent to initiate dietary modifications as early as possible in the course of renal disease.

Larger-scale clinical trials (currently in progress) are indicated to determine the long-term effect of dietary restriction in patients with mild to moderate renal insufficiency. In view of current knowledge, however, it appears that dietary restriction of protein and phosphorus in mild to moderate renal failure should be a part of the treatment regimen. If dietary treatment is effective in delaying the need for dialysis or transplantation therapy, the long-term medical, social, and economic ramifications will be enormous.

Recommended Diet Prescription

Not only is additional research necessary to establish the factors involved in the progression of renal failure, but clearer guidelines and more information are needed to determine the safe limits for protein restrictions. At present, it is not clear as to what level of protein and phosphorus restriction should be recommended to obtain the maximum effect on the progression of renal disease without impairing the growth of children and/or producing long-term negative nitrogen balance and malnutrition.

Kopple and Coburn conducted a series of experiments comparing diets providing 20 g and 40 g of primarily high biological protein per day and 35 kcal/kg. Nitrogen balance was more positive with 40 g of protein, a quantity close to the minimal requirement of healthy subjects.[10] Mitch, in a review of diet therapy in CRF, stressed that the essential amino acids must be supplied if daily protein intake is restricted to less than 40 g, or negative nitrogen balance will occur.[11]

In reviewing these studies, as well as more recent papers, it appears that the protein prescription for nutritionally stable patients with CRF should be at least 0.6 g/kg/d (on the basis of "ideal" or adjusted ideal body weight), incorporating approximately 65% high biological value protein.[12] A more liberal restriction of 0.8 g/kg/d may be prescribed, especially for those who are malnourished and/or diabetic, or 1 g of high biological value protein for each gram of proteinuria may be added to the lower range of protein restriction.[13,14] Currently, 0.8 to 1 g/kg/d is recommended for patients with nephrotic syndrome.[15] In some medical centers a very low protein diet providing approximately 0.28 g/kg/d is used in conjunction with a mixture of essential amino acids and/or keto acids. The essential amino acid mixture contains the nine essential amino acids (including histidine), while the keto acids are hydroxy-analogs of amino acids that contain a keto- or hydroxy- group in place of an amino group. Keto acids are currently available only for clinical studies in the United States, and amino acids, though available, are costly.

The energy requirements for patients with CRF are not well established. Neutral or positive nitrogen balance has been observed with approximately 35 kcal/kg.[16] This level of caloric intake is similar to the Recommended Dietary Allowances for the healthy adult population. Obese subjects and diabetic patients may require lower calorie levels. Patients who are more active or severely underweight may need more calories. It is generally recommended that patients with CRF eat a diet that is high in carbohydrates (approximately 50% to 60% of total calories) and high in monounsaturated and polyunsaturated fats (approximately 30% to 40% of total calories). The use of monounsaturated and polyunsaturated fats should be recommended because of the increased risk of hyperlipidemia in patients with diabetes and CRF.[12]

Vitamin requirements of patients with CRF are not well defined, and many investigators recommend that these patients take vitamin supplements daily. Vitamin preparations should contain the minimum daily requirements of the water-soluble vitamins, including folic acid. There is biochemical evidence of pyridoxine deficiency in CRF, and for this reason a supplement of pyridoxine containing at least 5 mg/d is recommended. There is also evidence that vitamin A stores are increased in uremia, and therefore vitamin A should be avoided.[12] (See *Table 3.1* for overall vitamin recommendations for patients with CRF and not undergoing dialysis.)

Table 3.1
Suggested Nutrient Requirements for Patients With Chronic Renal Failure and Not Undergoing Dialysis

Nutrient	Requirement
Protein	0.6–0.8 g/kg/d (65% high biological value); 0.8–1.0 g/kg/d (nephrotic syndrome); or 0.28 g/kg/d (high or low biological value supplemented with essential amino acids or keto acids)
Calories	≥ 35 kcal/kg/d; fat: 30%–40% of total kilocalories (polyunsaturated-to-saturated fatty acid ratio of 1:1); carbohydrate: remainder of nonprotein kilocalories
Minerals	
Sodium	1–3 g/d if sodium or fluid retention is present
Potassium	≤70 mEq/d if serum level is elevated
Calcium	1200–1600 mg/d (elemental; including supplements)
Phosphorus	8–12 mg/kg/d*
Iron	Approximately 100 mg/d (elemental) if supplementation is needed
Vitamins	
Niacin	20 mg NE[†] per day
Thiamin (B$_1$)	2 mg/d
Riboflavin (B$_2$)	2 mg/d
Pantothenic acid (B$_3$)	10 mg/d
Pyridoxine (B$_6$)	5 mg/d
Biotin	200 µg/d
Folic acid	0.8–1 mg/d
Vitamin B$_{12}$	3 µg/d
Vitamin C	60 mg/d
Vitamin D	See text
Vitamin K	None (supplement with 10 mg every other day if patient is receiving antibiotics and not eating)

* For phosphorus, 5–10 mg/kg is recommended in the literature, but 8–12 mg/kg frequently is used as a more practical restriction.

[†] NE, niacin equivalents.

Because high serum phosphorus levels have been linked to progression of renal failure as well as to secondary hyperparathyroidism and because diets low in phosphorus appear to be effective in delaying this progression, a phosphorus-restricted diet is recommended. Generally, the diet should contain approximately 5 to 10 mg of phosphorus per kilogram daily,[12] but only diets with keto or essential amino acids will be able to attain the lower end of this range. Frequently, 8 to 12 mg/kg is a more practical restriction. As renal failure progresses, the use of phosphate-binding medications in addition to dietary phosphorus restriction may be necessary to maintain normal serum phosphorus levels.

Several studies have demonstrated that intestinal calcium absorption is decreased early in the course of CRF. Protein- and phosphorus-restricted diets are also generally low in calcium content, and calcium supplementation is therefore required. To provide additional elemental calcium, supplements of calcium carbonate or calcium acetate should be prescribed for patients with CRF.[16] These calcium preparations also are used currently as the phosphate binders of choice when given with meals. Phosphate binders containing aluminum are used only temporarily or in small doses in conjunction with these calcium preparations because of the potential for aluminum toxicosis in the renal disease population.

Data suggest that altered vitamin D metabolism contributes to the abnormal calcium homeostasis in CRF. Some studies have shown that serum $1,25(OH)_2 D_3$ levels may be normal in patients with mild to moderate renal failure (GFR greater than 40 mL/min). However, as renal failure progresses, the synthesis of this most active vitamin D metabolite is impaired, and supplemental $1,25(OH)_2D_3$ (calcitriol) may be of benefit.[13]

Supplementation of iron is necessary for some patients with CRF during the predialysis phase, especially in conjunction with erythropoietin therapy.[12] Body iron stores and/or available iron are measured by ferritin and percentage transferrin saturation rates, respectively (see appendix C).

Because restricted diets are prescribed for patients with CRF on a long-term basis, careful follow-up is necessary to monitor adherence to the diet and to assess the patient's nutritional status. To assess compliance with the protein prescription, the urea nitrogen appearance or protein catabolic rate may be checked routinely.[17] To evaluate nutritional status, diet intake records, body weight, skinfold measurements, and serial plasma protein levels (keeping urinary protein losses in mind) should also be monitored serially in conjunction with these parameters. A comprehensive nutrition care plan should be developed and maintained for each patient.

Conclusion

Evidence is now sufficient that dietary manipulation can benefit patients with CRF, even early in the course of their disease. It appears that reducing protein and phosphorus intake to the minimum requirement can slow the progression of renal insufficiency. Current suggested guidelines for the overall diet prescription in long-term treatment of CRF before initiation of dialysis are provided in Table 3.1. It must be noted again that careful attention is required to maintain adequate nutritional status and to monitor adherence to the diet. As mentioned previously, further study is being conducted to determine the most appropriate form of diet therapy.

References

1. Brenner BM, Meyer TW, Hostetter TH. Dietary protein intake and the progressive nature of kidney disease: the role of hemodynamically mediated glomerular injury in the pathogenesis of progressive glomerular sclerosis in aging, renal ablation, and intrinsic disease. *N Engl J Med.* 1982;307:652–659.

2. Adler SG, Kopple JD. Factors influencing the progression of renal insufficiency. *Semin Nephrol.* 1983;3:335–343.

3. Olson JK, Hostetter TH, Rennke HG, Brenner BM, Venkatachalam MA. Altered glomerular permselectivity and progressive sclerosis following extreme ablation of renal mass. *Kidney Int.* 1982;22:112–126.

4. Walser M, Mitch WE, Collier VU. Essential amino acids and their nitrogen-free analogues in the treatment of chronic renal failure. In: Schreiner G, ed. *Controversies in Nephrology.* Washington, DC: Georgetown University Division of Nephrology; 1979.

5. Maschio G, Oldrizzi L, Tessitore N, et al. Effects of dietary protein and phosphorus restriction on the progression of early renal failure. *Kidney Int.* 1982;22:371–376.

6. Barsotti G, Guidricci A, Ciardella F, Giavannetti S. Effects on renal function of low-nitrogen diet supplemented with essential amino acids and ketoanalogues and of hemodialysis and free protein supply in patients with chronic renal failure. *Nephron.* 1981;29:113–117.

7. Alvestrand A, Ahlberg M, Furst P, Bergstrom J. Clinical results of long-term treatment with a low protein diet and a new amino acid preparation in patients with chronic uremia. *Clin Nephrol.* 1983;19:67–73.

8. Mitch WE. Rationale and prospects for nutritional therapy in renal failure. In: *Renal Nutrition, Report of the Eleventh Ross Roundtable on Medical Issues.* Columbus, Ohio: Ross Laboratories; 1991:1–10.

9. Badalamenti J, DuBose TD. Chronic renal failure. In: Levine D, ed. *Care of the Renal Patient.* Philadelphia, Pa: WB Saunders; 1991:139–154.

10. Kopple JD, Coburn JW, Metabolic studies of low protein diets in uremia. 1. Nitrogen and potassium. *Medicine.* 1983;52:583–595.

11. Mitch WE. Conservative management of chronic renal failure, In: Brenner BM, Stein JH, eds. *Contemporary Issues in Nephrology, Chronic Renal Failure.* New York, NY: Churchill Livingstone; 1981;7:116–152.

12. Hirschberg RR, Kopple JD. Nutritional therapy in patients with renal failure. In: Levine D, ed. *Care of the Renal Patient.* Philadelphia, Pa: WB Saunders; 1991:169–180.

13. Tuttle KR, DeFonzo RA, Stein JH. Treatment of diabetic nephropathy: a rational approach based on its pathophysiology. *Semin Nephrol.* 1991;2:220–235.

14. Zeller K, Whittaker E, Sullivan L, Raskin P, Jacobson HR. Effect of restricting dietary protein on the progression of renal failure in patients with insulin-dependent diabetes mellitus. *N Engl J Med.* 1991;324:78–84.

15. Kaysen GA. Nutritional management of nephrotic syndrome. *J Renal Nutr.* 1992;2:50–58.

16. Coburn JW, Goodman WG, Salsby IB. Renal bone diseases and aluminum toxicity in renal patients. In: Levine D, ed. *Care of the Renal Patient.* Philadelphia, Pa: WB Saunders; 1991:155–168.

17. Mitch W. Dietary protein restriction in patients with chronic renal failure. *Kidney Int.* 1991;40:326–341.

4. Nutrition Management of the Adult Hemodialysis Patient

Hemodialysis is a process in which an artificial kidney (*hemodialyzer*) is used to cleanse the blood. Hemodialysis can return the body to a more normal state by removing excess fluid and waste products, but it does not replace the endocrine functions of the kidney. The average treatment lasts 2 to 4 hours, depending on the method of hemodialysis chosen and individual patient requirements; it is usually required three times per week.

Presently, there are three methods of hemodialysis: conventional or standard hemodialysis; rapid high efficiency hemodialysis; and high flux hemodialysis. Conventional dialysis involves types of machines that have been in use for more than two decades. In rapid high efficiency dialysis, these machines are also used, but with variations in the components of the dialysis process. These variations include bicarbonate dialysate, ultrafiltration control, high blood flow rates, and high efficiency dialyzers.[1] In high flux dialysis, on the other hand, new machines and newly developed hemodialyzers are used.

Artificial Kidneys and the Dialysate Bath

Artificial kidneys fall into two fundamental categories: plate and hollow fiber devices. The hollow fiber is perhaps the most popular type used today. The fibers are made from a variety of materials, including cellulose acetate, cuprophan, polycarbonate, and polysulfone materials.

The artificial kidney contains two compartments—one for blood and one for the cleansing solution or dialysate bath—that are separated by a semipermeable membrane. Excess fluid and waste products can pass through this semipermeable membrane into the dialysate bath. Membranes of differing thickness and surface areas are used, depending on the amount of fluid and waste products to be removed. Large molecules such as albumin and red blood cells are unable to pass through this semipermeable membrane, while smaller molecules such as urea, glucose, sodium, and potassium are able to do so. To prevent transfer of unwanted chemicals into the blood, deionized water is used as the base for the dialysate bath. The concentration of electrolytes and minerals found in the dialysate bath can be varied. The lesser the concentration in the dialysate, the more electrolyte or mineral will be lost during the dialysis process.

Dialysis works on the principles of *osmosis* and *diffusion*. Osmosis is the movement of fluid through a semipermeable membrane from an area of lesser concentration to an area of greater concentration. Diffusion is the movement of particles through a semipermeable membrane from a solution of greater concentration to an area of lesser concentration. The patient begins dialysis with a higher concentration of waste products present in his or her blood; when these wastes pass through the semipermeable membrane to the dialysate bath, the movement is from a greater to a lesser concentration.

Many variations are available in dialysate baths. First, there are two types of *buffers* used in these solutions: *acetate* and *bicarbonate*. (A buffer is a substance that, in solution, tends to maintain a constant hydrogen ion concentration or pH with the addition of either acid or base.[2]) Bicarbonate solutions are not chemically stable and must be prepared shortly before each clinical use. Acetate solutions, in contrast, are chemically stable and can be prepared far in advance of the dialysis treatment. At the present time, acetate solutions are no longer routinely used in most dialysis centers.

Next, there is a glucose-free dialysate or dialysate with 200 mg/dL glucose. When glucose-free dialysate is used in normoglycemic patients, about 20 to 50 g of glucose are lost with each hemodialysis treatment. It is suggested that the removal of glucose during hemodialysis with glucose-free dialysate may promote glycogenolysis and gluconeogenesis.[3] Therefore, dialysate containing glucose is the currently used standard of practice.

The potassium content of dialysate may be 1, 2, or 3 mEq/L. The amount of calcium generally ranges from 2.5 to 3.5 mEq/L. Sodium content may be 135 to 150 mEq/L, and the magnesium content usually ranges from 0.5 to 1.0 mEq/L.

Hemodialysis Accesses

Before beginning hemodialysis, access to the patient's blood is necessary. The access is the route through which the patient's blood can be removed, sent through the hemodialyzer, cleaned, and then returned. Different types of accesses exist; all require a minor surgical procedure.

An arteriovenous (AV) *fistula* is an internal connection of an artery and a vein; with time, the vein eventually becomes enlarged or "arterialized." In adults, the fistula is usually located in the arm. During dialysis, two needles are inserted into this enlarged vein, one to send blood to the hemodialyzer and one to return the blood to the patient.

A *graft* is a tubelike device made of special material that connects an artery and vein. It is used in the same way as an AV fistula and is also located under the skin, meaning venipuncture is required.

The use of a graft or fistula allows normal activity and provides a durable, long-term access. They both require some time to develop or heal before they can be used. Conservative dietary management may be necessary during this development phase if no other access is available for dialysis.

A *shunt* (cannula) consists of two small tubes that are inserted in an artery and a vein, again, usually in the arm. The junction of these two tubes is located on the outside of the skin. During dialysis, one tube is connected to the hemodialyzer and the other tube returns blood from the hemodialyzer to the patient. When the patient is not undergoing dialysis, the tubes are joined together, and the blood is shunted from the artery to the vein. This access currently is rarely used.

A *femoral* or *subclavian catheter* is a single narrow tube inserted into a large vein in the groin (femoral) or neck (subclavian). By using an adaptive apparatus or special needle, blood can be removed from the body, cleansed, and returned into the single tube or catheter.

Both the shunt and catheter are intended for immediate but temporary use when a permanent access is not available. Because they open to the outside of the body, they are susceptible to infections and clotting. Catheters are more popular than shunts because the site used will not be needed later for a permanent fistula or graft.

Settings for Hemodialysis

Once a permanent access has been established, hemodialysis can be performed in a variety of settings.

Home hemodialysis is a treatment setting that allows the patient the greatest flexibility in treatment schedules and enables him or her to maintain an independent life-style. A machine is installed in the home. A helper such as a spouse, family member, friend, or a paid aide is required.

Self-care hemodialysis is performed in a dialysis unit. Patients are taught to perform their own dialysis in the unit, with staff available to assist when necessary.

In-center or *staff-assisted hemodialysis* also is performed in a dialysis unit. The staff performs the treatment, and the setting allows for the least personal choice in time and treatment scheduling, but the most medical supervision.

Nutrition Considerations

The nephrologist selects the artificial kidney, dialysate components, rate of blood flow through the artificial kidney, and duration of dialysis on the basis of the medical needs of the patient. The type of access needed by the patient and the type of setting for dialysis must also be selected. These factors, in addition to the patient's residual kidney function, determine each individualized diet prescription. *Table 4.1* summarizes the recommendations for the daily nutrient requirements for patients undergoing maintenance hemodialysis.

A team approach to dietary management is critical to dietary adherence. The dietitian should design meal plans to suit individual disease states, as well as tastes, eating patterns, and socioeconomic situations. Family participation should be encouraged during diet instruction. Routine follow-up is extremely important. Positive reinforcement is an ongoing responsibility of the renal dietitian and medical team.

The nutrition needs of the patient vary as the residual renal function decreases. The patient who still has urine output has a distinct advantage over the anuric patient. A more liberal diet is possible because of the ability to eliminate some of the metabolic wastes, electrolytes, and water via the urinary tract. The diet should be periodically reevaluated as the patient progresses to anuria.

Protein

On the basis of a literature review, 1.1 to 1.2 g of protein per kilogram per day should be the initial prescription for hemodialysis patients.[4] Some researchers, however, including Alvestrand, Silberman, Feinstein, and Blumenkrantz, now suggest that the requirement may reach 1.4 g/kg/d.[5-9] These recommendations should be adjusted for normalized body weight. Normalized body weight is the average body weight of healthy persons of the same age, height, and sex as the patient.[10] (See chapter 2, Nutrition Assessment in Chronic Renal Failure.)

During a single hemodialysis treatment, approximately 5 to 8 g of free amino acids are

Table 4.1
Daily Nutrient Requirements for Hemodialysis Patients[4,7,44]

Nutrient	Amount
Protein*	1.1–1.4 g/kg
Calories*	30–35 kcal/kg/d (maintenance)
Fat	30%–40%, polyunsaturated to saturated fatty acid ratio 1:1
Carbohydrate	Rest of nonprotein calories
Vitamins	
A	No additional
K[†]	None
Folic acid	0.8–1 mg
Pyridoxine hydrochloride	10 mg
Riboflavin	1.8–2.0 mg
Niacin	20 mg
Ascorbic acid	60 mg
Thiamin	1.5–2.0 mg
Pantothenic acid	10 mg
B_{12}	3–6 μg
Biotin	200–300 μg
E	10 IU
Minerals	
Sodium	2–3 g
Potassium	1.5–3 g
Calcium	1400–1600 mg
Phosphorus[‡]	12–17 mg/kg
Zinc	15 mg
Iron[§]	Approximately 100 mg (elemental)
Fluid	700–1000 mL + urine output in 24 h
Fiber	20–25 g (promotes bowel regularity)

*Based on ideal body weight.

[†]Vitamin K should be given every other day to patients who are being treated with antibiotics and who are not eating.

[‡]Although ≤12 mg/kg is cited in the literature, 12–17 mg/kg is believed to be most practical to meet the protein needs of the patient undergoing hemodialysis.

[§]Patients receiving erythropoietin usually require oral or intravenous iron supplementation.

lost into the dialysate, of which about one third consists of essential amino acids. In addition, 4 to 5 g of peptide-bound amino acids are lost per dialysis. Thus, the total amount of amino acids lost is about 10 to 13 g per treatment.[7] In fasting patients, the loss of amino acids decreased when glucose was added to the dialysate,[3,11] but in nonfasting patients, addition of glucose to the dialysate did not reduce the loss of free amino acids during routine hemodialysis.[12] About 30% to 40% of the amino acids lost during hemodialysis are essential.[13] Therefore, the need for high biological value protein containing all nine essential amino acids (including histidine) is increased. Because human beings cannot synthesize these amino acids, high biological value protein should represent at least 50% of the total protein content of the diet.[7,14]

In assessment of protein status, it is advisable to keep in mind the volume status of the patient. Extracellular volume depletion (dehydration) may cause overestimation of serum albumin concentration, while volume expansion (fluid overload) may cause underestimation.[15] For the somatic protein evaluation of the patient, anthropometric measurements should always be made after dialysis, because fluid volume status influences these as well.

For nutritionally stable patients, it is possible to determine the amount of protein the patient is actually consuming from the protein catabolic rate. This is the amount (in grams) of protein that the patient turns over in 24 hours. (See Chapter 2, Nutrition Assessment in Chronic Renal Failure.)

Kilocalories

Energy requirements for patients undergoing maintenance hemodialysis are currently not well defined. The minimum daily intake for the adult patient probably should be approximately 35 kcal/kg/d, unless the patient's relative body weight is greater than 120% or unwanted weight is gained.[4,9] Many patients, however, are unable to ingest sufficient kilocalories, and they should be encouraged to supplement their diets accordingly. Generally, increasing or decreasing dietary intake by 500 kcal/d will result in a 0.5-kg (1-lb) weight gain or loss per week.

Suggested kilocalorie guidelines (based on ideal weight):[16]
- 30–35 kcal/kg/d for weight maintenance
- 20–30 kcal/kg/d for weight loss (monitor nutrient adequacy)
- 35–50 kcal/kg/d for weight gain

Energy supply, along with protein intake, determines whether the diet will produce positive or negative nitrogen balance. Unless there are sufficient calories from carbohydrates and fats, protein will be used for energy production.[17]

To prevent the wasting syndrome that often accompanies hemodialysis, adequate intake of carbohydrates and fats is encouraged. Complex carbohydrates providing extra fiber are also stressed whenever possible, since constipation is a frequent problem in uremic patients. A high-fiber diet may aid in the control of serum lipid concentration.[18] A diet containing from 20 to 25 g of fiber is recommended, but this amount may be contraindicated because of the potassium and phosphorus content of foods that are rich in fiber.[4,10] A fiber supplement may also be necessary.

Patients with CRF frequently have a type of hyperlipidemia associated with an increase in low density and very low density lipoproteins. Total cholesterol level is generally normal, but the distribution is abnormal, with a decreased amount of high density lipoproteins.[7] Inclusion of monounsaturated and polyunsaturated fats as a good proportion of the total fat intake and encouragement of programmed aerobic exercise in addition to a high-fiber diet, may help reduce or avoid these lipid abnormalities.[19] The percentage of kilocalories from fat should be from 30% to 40% of total energy intake, with a polyunsaturated-to-saturated fatty acid ratio of 1:1.[4] Some physicians also prefer to prescribe medications now available to lower the cholesterol level, but it is not yet known whether the long-term outcome of this therapy is beneficial or whether it may promote unwanted side effects.

Sodium and Fluid

The sodium allowance for a patient undergoing hemodialysis can vary from 2 to 3 g/d (85 to 129 mEq) and depends largely on urine output. The more urine the patient produces, the more sodium may be eliminated in the urine.

Under steady-state conditions, urinary output usually provides a good guide for the fluid intake. Patients undergoing maintenance hemodialysis are generally restricted to intake of 700 to 1000 mL of fluid per day plus the volume of urine produced in 24 hours.[4] Excessive interdialytic weight gains, increased thirst, and edema are indications that the patient needs to reduce sodium and fluid intake. Persistent hypertension may require more aggressive ultrafiltration and/or antihypertensive medication. Hypotension and little or no weight gain between treatments may indicate that the patient could increase sodium and fluid intake. If antihypertensive medications are prescribed, however, they may need to be tapered or discontinued as a first step in the management process.

The usual diet contains about 500 mL water that is contributed by food and not included in the patient's fluid allowance. Fruits and vegetables contain about 90% water, while meat, fish, and poultry contain about 50% water. Foods that are liquid at room temperature, such as ice, gelatin, soup, and ice cream, as well as fluids taken with medications, are all part of the total daily fluid allowance. Generally, the goal of sodium and fluid control is to achieve a fluid weight gain of 1 to 2 lb a day between treatments.

Potassium

The failing kidney has a reduced capability to excrete potassium. Two mechanisms, however, act to prevent excessive accumulation of this mineral. The kidney becomes more efficient at excreting potassium relative to the remaining kidney function, and fecal excretion of potassium increases. Thus, hyperkalemia usually does not develop in renal patients who have urine outputs of at least 1000 mL/d even without dietary limitation.[13]

When hyperkalemia occurs in CRF, it is usually due to oliguria or reduced urine output; excessive potassium intake; acidosis; the catabolic stress of infection, surgery, or trauma; and hypoaldosteronism.[13] Generally, patients undergoing maintenance hemodialysis manage to achieve serum potassium levels between 3.5 and 5.5 mEq/L with diets containing 1.5 to 3 g of potassium per day (38 to 75 mEq).[4]

High-potassium foods such as potatoes, bananas, apricots, orange juice, dried fruit, nuts, tomato sauce, avocados, split peas, dried beans, melons, spinach, prune juice, and chocolate are usually limited or avoided. The potassium content of potatoes and some other vegetables can be reduced if they are peeled, cut, and soaked in water for several hours. This is referred to as *leaching* or *dialyzing*.

The potassium content of the dialysate bath is important because of its influence on the serum potassium level of the patient. The patient who is undergoing dialysis with a 1.0 mEq/L potassium dialysate bath will lose more potassium during the treatment than the patient undergoing dialysis with a dialysate bath of 2.5 mEq/L or higher.

Hyperkalemia (serum potassium of 6 mEq/L or greater) should be appropriately treated.[20] If it is not feasible to alter the diet further in potassium content, the physician can prescribe a dialysate solution with low potassium content and/or an oral exchange resin called Kayexalate, which can be given together with a sorbitol solution in divided doses. Sorbitol is not absorbed by the intestine and helps propel the resin through the gut.[20] However, since Kayexalate exchanges 1 mEq of potassium for 1 mEq of sodium, this medication is not regularly recommended because it causes sodium accumulation. The patient should be advised to control serum potassium levels with dietary restrictions whenever possible. The consequences of hyperkalemia should be conveyed to the patient as well, since potassium intoxication causes death by inducing arrhythmias.[21] Hyperkalemia most often occurs after the longest interdialytic period.

Patients who have persistent anorexia, nausea, or vomiting may present with a low predialysis serum potassium level. This is of concern for those prescribed digitalis or digoxin. If the dialysate bath is standardized and cannot be modified to minimize the potassium loss, the risk of hypokalemia is great. The patient's diet should include adequate potassium to prevent hypokalemia if he or she is eating at all, and serum potassium levels should be followed regularly.

Phosphorus, Calcium, and Vitamin D₃

Renal bone disease develops in the early stages of CRF, during loss of excretory kidney function. Hyperphosphatemia usually develops when the glomerular filtration rate (GFR) falls below 25 mL/min.[22]

Phosphorus is routinely restricted for hemodialysis patients, because hyperphosphatemia contributes to secondary hyperparathyroidism and raises the calcium-phosphorus product in the plasma. Long-term follow-up of patients who have advanced renal insufficiency and have been undergoing hemodialysis has demonstrated that control of the concentration of serum phosphate ameliorates secondary hyperparathyroidism, provided that there is adequate supplemental calcium.[23] A calcium-phosphorus product greater than 60 to 70 increases the likelihood of calcium phosphate deposition in soft tissues, that is, the skin, lungs, eyes, heart, and blood vessels.[24] Precipitation of calcium in the skin may be responsible in part for pruritus, which is usually seen in patients with advanced uremia. Other clinical consequences of hyperphosphatemia include metabolic bone disease and vascular calcification.

The phosphate restriction is recommended to be 12 mg/kg/d for the hemodialysis patient,[4] although most practitioners would agree that this restriction must often be liberalized to meet protein needs. High-phosphorus foods such as milk, milk products, cheese, beef liver, chocolate, nuts, and legumes are usually limited or avoided.

Control of the serum phosphorus level is usually not possible with diet alone, however. Calcium carbonate or calcium acetate are the medications of choice for phosphate control. Aluminum hydroxide was the most common agent used for binding ingested phosphate in the gut; however, large amounts of aluminum given to patients over a long duration may contribute to buildup of aluminum, resulting in aluminum toxicosis.[25,26] Investigators such as Alfrey, et al have shown that this toxicosis may be deleterious to bone metabolism or brain tissue.[26] The use of aluminum hydroxide binders is often discontinued when the serum phosphorus level is normalized and calcium carbonate or calcium acetate is added.[27,28] Whichever binder is used, it is given at mealtime to bind phosphate in food. The prescribed amount should be individualized according to the amount of phosphate present in a meal.[29] The goal of therapy is to achieve and maintain serum phosphate levels at approximately 4.5 to 6.0 mg/dL.[30]

Calcium supplementation is prescribed for several reasons. Intestinal absorption of calcium is impaired in uremia because of the lack of the active form of vitamin D, known as calcitriol. Also, diets prescribed for patients with CRF tend to be low in calcium because of the restriction of dairy products. Calcium supplements frequently are needed for hemodialysis patients to maintain positive calcium balance. Approximately 1400 to 1600 mg of supplemental elemental calcium is needed.[4,31,32] Calcium carbonate is 40% elemental calcium, and calcium acetate is 25% elemental calcium. The goal of therapy is frequently to achieve serum calcium levels between 10.5 and 11.0 mg/dL.[29,33,34] Close monitoring of serum calcium is needed to avoid hypercalcemia. It is sometimes necessary to reduce the calcium in the dialysate to 2.5 mEq/L or less to prevent hypercalcemia when large doses of calcium binders and calcitriol are administered.[28,32,33]

The failure of the endocrine function of the kidneys in producing calcitriol (1,25-dihydroxycholecalciferol) plays a major role in the bone disease seen in patients with renal insufficiency. The relative or absolute deficiency of 1,25-dihydroxycholecalciferol results in secondary hyperparathyroidism early in renal failure.[35–37] This deficiency leads to disorders of calcium, phosphorus, magnesium, and bone and muscle metabolism.[13]

Many forms of vitamin D are available for clinical use, but it is the active form that helps prevent bone disease. The active form of vitamin D is available in an oral form (Rocaltrol) and in an intravenous form (Calcijex). Treatment with calcitriol may help raise serum calcium and suppress secondary hyperparathyroidism.[32] A major advantage of 1,25-dihydroxycholecalciferol over other forms of vitamin D is the shorter half-life, should hypercalcemia develop. The intravenous form of calcitriol offers additional advantages over the oral form: (1) It is ensured that the patient receives it, since it is given during the hemodialysis treatment, and (2) studies indicate that calcitriol given intravenously results in a greater delivery of the active metabolite to peripheral tissues and effects direct suppression of parathyroid hormone.[36,37]

Alternative approaches such as "pulse therapy," with high doses of oral calcitriol given twice weekly at the end of dialysis, have been shown to be efficient in decreasing hyperparathyroidism, with less hypercalcemia.[38,39] This was introduced in Japan, where the nurses administer 4 µg of the oral calcitriol twice weekly in the clinic, to ensure patient compliance. The goal is to approximate what normal, functioning kidneys produce (1 to 1.5 µg of calcitriol daily).

Clinical trials for a newer oral form of vitamin D called OCT (22-oxacalcitriol) are under way.[40] The advantage of using this noncalcemic analog of vitamin D is that it does not produce the hypercalcemic effect that is sometimes manifested in patients receiving the other oral form of calcitriol.[40]

It must be noted that vitamin D therapy should not be initiated until the serum phosphate level is at or near normal level.[13,32] Indications of a response to vitamin D include radiographic evidence of improvement of bone disease, decrease in the blood levels of parathyroid hormone and alkaline phosphatase, an increase in the concentration of calcium or phosphorus, and a decrease in myopathy (muscle weakness) and bone pain.[16]

Magnesium

The kidney is the main organ responsible for the normal maintenance of serum magnesium.[41] Most patients with uremia should avoid the use of laxatives, enemas, or phosphate binders containing magnesium.[4] Hypermagnesemia may occur when tap water used to prepare dialysate contains excessive amounts of magnesium. The dialysate should not contain more than 0.5 to 1.0 mEq of magnesium per liter.[41] The magnesium requirement in CRF is about 200 mg/d. This is usually achieved or surpassed with a patient's dietary intake.[4]

Iron

One of the clinical consequences of CRF is anemia. This anemia is caused primarily by decreased production of the hormone erythropoeitin, which is normally produced by the healthy kidneys. The function of this hormone is to stimulate the bone marrow to produce red blood cells. Erythropoeisis requires an adequate available iron supply.

In the past, the usual treatment for anemia in patients undergoing hemodialysis was androgen therapy and/or blood transfusions. Patients receiving frequent transfusions receive approximately 200 mg of iron with each unit of blood.[42] One problem with excessive transfusions has been iron overload or hemosiderosis. This condition of iron overload has been treated with deferoxamine (an iron chelating substance) during dialysis when it has occurred.[34] The use of deferoxamine therapy is now limited, however, because of a serious fungal infection, known as *mucormycosis,* that may result from its use.[43]

With the advent of recombinant human erythropoietin (Epoetin alfa), the approach to the treatment of anemia has completely changed. Epoetin alfa may be given to hemodialysis patients intravenously during dialysis or subcutaneously just after dialysis treatment . Before initiation of erythropoietin therapy, however, the patient's iron status must be assessed. Plasma ferritin levels may be used to estimate iron stores. Most patients receiving regular erythropoietin therapy will require oral or intravenous iron supplementation with time, even if they do not require it before beginning therapy, because iron stores are depleted when erythropoiesis takes place.[4] The route of iron supplementation is usually oral at first, but many patients do not consistently take the supplements because of gastrointestinal intolerance or other reasons. Intravenous iron therapy often is given during dialysis as well.

Zinc

Patients undergoing maintenance hemodialysis are known to have decreased levels of zinc in serum, hair, and the kidneys. Researchers suggest that zinc supplementation in the amount of 15 mg/d may improve dysgeusia (loss of taste) and may be helpful for the management of impotence in male hemodialysis patients.[4]

Vitamins

In a recent review of current research, Makoff suggests that the food intake of persons with renal disease is altered and often substandard with regard to water-soluble vitamins, because dietary restrictions limit foods that are high in sodium and potassium, which also tend to be high in B and C vitamins.[44] Also, there may be an inability on the part of the patient, spouse, or care facility to prepare the "renal diet" properly. There may be losses or a breakdown of vitamins from cooking procedures such as boiling. Furthermore, since patients with renal disease often have a loss of appetite, intake of some vitamins may be suboptimal.

Makoff also states that many persons with renal disease require medications specific for this disease and often additional medication for related diseases. The required drugs may interfere with the absorption or action of specific vitamins. Folic acid and cobalamin (B_{12})

are two vitamins for which specific drugs are known to interfere with proper utilization.[44] Additionally, kidney failure causes vitamins to be treated differently due to changes of absorption, retention, and excretion of metabolic products, and dialysis promotes water-soluble vitamin removal. Some vitamins may build up to high levels due to inappropriate diet and lack of excretion. This is particularly important in regard to the fat-soluble vitamins.[45–47]

Because serum retinol-binding protein and vitamin A are elevated in uremia, the routine use of supplemental vitamin A (Retinol) is not recommended. Even relatively small doses of vitamin A (ie, 7500 to 15,000 IU per day) may cause bone toxicity.[48] Supplements of vitamin K are usually not necessary; however, approximately 10 mg of vitamin K should be given every other day to patients who are treated with antibiotics and who are not eating food.[4] Ten international units of vitamin E per day is recommended.[4]

Newer research has revealed that no more than 60 mg/d of vitamin C (the RDA) is advised because ascorbic acid can be metabolized to oxalate. Large doses of ascorbic acid have been associated with increased plasma and tissue oxalate levels in renal failure patients.[49–52] Thiamin, riboflavin, biotin, pantothenic acid, and niacin should be supplemented at the RDA level, and pyridoxine (vitamin B_6) should be supplemented at 10 mg daily.[4,44] Vitamin B_{12} deficits may occur, because it is unclear how the protein-bound form of vitamin B_{12} is affected by the dialysis procedure. Therefore, Hirschberg and Kopple[4] and Makoff[44] suggest from 3 to 6 µg of vitamin B_{12} daily for patients with renal failure.

Research indicates possible improvement in patients suffering from encephalopathy and peripheral neuropathy when 10 mg of biotin is given each day.[53] The dietary restriction routinely imposed by the renal diet decreases the intake of biotin, while the various supplementary vitamin regimens given dialysis patients often are completely biotin-free. Biotin is a substance of low molecular weight that is loosely bound to serum proteins. Therefore, it may be lost from the blood to the dialysate during hemodialysis.[53]

References

1. Keshaviah P, Davis-Pollack R, Luhring D, Lee P. *A Practical Guide to Rapid High Efficiency Dialysis.* Minneapolis, Minn: Regional Kidney Disease Program, Minneapolis Medical Research Foundation;1987:2.

2. Gutch CF, Stoner MH. *Review of Hemodialysis for Nurses and Dialysis Personnel.* 4th ed. St. Louis, Mo: CV Mosby; 1983:18.

3. Wathen RL, et al. The metabolic effects of hemodialysis with and without glucose in the dialysate. *Am J Clin Nutr.* 1978;31:1870.

4. Hirschberg RR, Kopple JD. Nutritional therapy in patients with renal failure. In: Levine DZ, ed. *Care of the Renal Patient.* Philadelphia, Pa: WB Saunders; 1991:169–180.

5. Silberman H. Nutritional therapy: clinical applications. In: *Parenteral and Enteral Nutrition.* 2nd ed. Norwalk, Conn: Appleton and Lange; 1989:392.

6. Blumenkrantz M, Salehmoghaddam S, Boken R, et al. An integrated approach to the treatment of patients with multiple organ system failure requiring intensive nutritional support and hemodialysis. *Trans Am Soc Artif Intern Org.* 1984; 30:468–472.

7. Alvestrand A. Nutritional requirements of hemodialysis patients. In: Mitch WE, Klahr S, eds. *Nutrition and the Kidney.* Boston, Mass: Little, Brown, and Co; 1988:180–197.

8. Feinstein EI, Massry SG. Nutritional therapy in acute renal failure. In: Mitch WE, Klahr S, eds. *Nutrition and the Kidney.* Boston, Mass: Little, Brown and Co; 1988:80–103.

9. Kopple JD. Nutrition, diet and the kidney. In: Shils ME, Young VR, eds. *Modern Nutrition in Health and Disease.* 7th ed. Philadelphia, Pa: Lea & Febiger; 1988:1230–1268.

10. Kopple JD, Blumenkrantz M. Nutrition in adults on continuous ambulatory peritoneal dialysis. *Perspectives Peritoneal Dialysis.* 1984;2.

11. Kopple JD, et al. The free and bound amino acids removed by hemodialysis. *Trans Am Soc Artif Intern Org.* 1973;19:309.

12. Ono K, Sasaki T, Waki Y. Glucose in the

dialysate does not reduce free amino acid loss during routine hemodialysis of non fasting patients. *Clin Nephrol.* 1984;21:106.

13. Massry S, Kopple J. *Dietary Therapy in Renal Failure, Quick Reference to Clinical Nutrition.* Lippincott, Conn: Saunders Press;1979:223–231.

14. Kopple J. Nutritional management. In: Massry S, Glassock R, eds. *Textbook of Nephrology.* Baltimore, Md: Williams & Wilkins, 1983;2: 8.3–8.12.

15. Foulks CJ. Nutritional evaluation of patients on maintenance dialysis therapy. *Am Nephrol Nurses Assoc J.* 1988;15:13–17.

16. Grant A, DeHoog S. *Nutrient Requirements in Nutritional Assessment and Support.* Seattle, Wash: Grant and DeHoog; 1991:232.

17. Giordano C. The role of diet in renal disease. *Hosp Pract.* 1977;12:113-119.

18. Anderson J. Fiber and health: an overview. *Am J Gastroenterol.* 1986;81:894.

19. Goldberg A, Hagberg JM, Delmez JA, et al. The benefits of exercise in hemodialysis patients (abstr). *Clin Res.* 1979;27:415A.

20. Kurokawa K. Management of sodium, potassium, and water in chronic renal failure. In: *Nutritional Support for the Hospitalized Patient, Nutritional Support in a Major Organ System Failure: Renal Failure.* Los Angeles, Calif: American Society of Parenteral and Enteral Nutrition; 1979.

21. Forland, M. *Nephrology: A Review of Clinical Nephrology.* New York, NY: Medical Examination Publishing; 1977:153.

22. Hruska KA. Requirements for calcium, phosphorus, and vitamin D. In: Mitch WE, Klahr S, eds. *Nutrition and the Kidney.* Boston, Mass: Little, Brown, and Co; 1988:104.

23. Slatopolsky E. Hyperphosphatemia. In: Massry S, Glassock R, eds. *Textbook of Nephrology.* Baltimore, Md: Williams & Wilkins; 1983: 3.99–3.102.

24. Coburn J, Slatopolsky E. Presentation at the Council on Renal Nutrition Annual Meeting, National Kidney Foundation, Washington, DC; 1984.

25. Moriniere P, Sebert J, Gregoire I, et al. Control of hyperparathyroidism, hyperphosphatemia, and hyperaluminemia in hemodialysis patients in high doses of calcium carbonate (abstr). Madrid, Spain: 19th Congress of the European Dialysis and Transplant Association; 1982:101.

26. Alfrey AC, LeGendre GR, et al. The dialysis encephalopathy syndrome, possible aluminum intoxication. *N Engl J Med.* 1976;294:184.

27. Fournier A, et al. 20th Congress of the European Dialysis and Transplant Association;

London, England; 1983:44.

28. Slatopolsky E, et al. Long-term effects of calcium carbonate and 2.5 mEq/L Ca dialysate on mineral metabolism in hemodialysis patients. *Kidney Int.* 1989;35:264.

29. Norris KC, Coburn JW. Rocaltrol, guidelines for management. *Dial Transplant.* 1985; 14(suppl):1.

30. Coburn J, Salusky I. Control of serum phosphorus in uremia. *N Engl J Med.* 1989;320:1140.

31. Bergstrom J. Nutritional problems in chronic renal failure. *EDTNA/ERCA.* 1990;13.

32. Delmez JA, Slatopolsky E. Renal osteodystrophy: pathogenesis and treatment. *Kidney.* 1990;22:5.

33. Slatopolsky E. Calcium carbonate as a phosphate binder in patients with chronic renal failure undergoing dialysis. *N Engl J Med.* 1985; 315:157.

34. What are the most common errors in the management of renal osteodystrophy? *Semin Dial.* 1989;2:145–157.

35. Malluche HH, Faugere MC. Effects of $1,25(OH)_2D_3$ administration on bone in patients with renal failure. *Kidney Int.* 1990;38 (suppl 29): S48–S53.

36. Slatopolsky E, Weerts C, Thielan J, et al. Marked suppression of secondary hyperparathyroidism by intravenous administration of 1,25-dihydroxycholecalciferol in uremic patients. *J Clin Invest.* 1984;74:2136–2143.

37. Delmez JA, Tindira C, Grooms P, et al. Parathyroid hormone suppression by intravenous 1,25-dihydroxyvitamin D: a role for increased sensitivity to calcium. *J Clin Invest.* 1989;83:1349–1355.

38. Tsukamoto Y. Oral $1,25(OH)_2D_3$ pulse therapy. *JBMM.* 1991;9:54–57.

39. Tsukamoto Y, Nomura M, Naorumo F. Medicamentous parathyroidectomy by oral $1,25(OH)_2D_3$ pulse therapy. *Nephron.* 1989;51: 130–131.

40. Brown AJ, Ritter CS, Finch JL, et al. The noncalcemic analogue of vitamin D, 22-oxacalcitriol, suppresses parathyroid hormone synthesis and secretion. *J Clin Invest.* 1989;84:728–732.

41. Coburn JW. Management of calcium, phosphorus, magnesium and vitamin D in chronic renal failure. In: *Nutritional Support for the Hospitalized Patient, Nutritional Support in a Major Organ System Failure: Renal Failure.* Los Angeles, Calif: American Society of Enteral and Parenteral Nutrition; 1979.

42. Harter H, Klahr S, Slatopolsky E. Prevention of renal osteodystrophy. *ASAIO J.* 1979;2:136.

43. Boelaert JR, Fenves AZ, Coburn JW. Deferoxamine therapy and mucormycosis in dialysis patients. Report of an International Registry *Am J Kidney Dis.* 1991;18:660–667.

44. Makoff R. Water-soluble vitamin status in persons with renal disease treated with hemodialysis or peritoneal dialysis. *J Renal Nutr.* 1991;1:56–73.

45. Farrington K, et al. Vitamin A toxicity and hypercalcemia in chronic renal failure. *Br Med J.* 1981;282:1999.

46. Werb R, Clark WF, Lindsay RM, et al. Serum vitamin A levels and associated abnormalities in patients on regular dialysis treatment. *Clin Nephrol.* 1979;12:63.

47. Shmunes E. Hypervitaminosis A in a patient with alopecia receiving renal dialysis. *Arch Dermatol.* 1979;115:882.

48. Yatzidis H, Digenis P, et al. Hypervitaminosis accompanying advanced chronic renal failure. *Br Med J.* 1975;2:352–353.

49. Pru C, Eaton J, Kjellstrand C. Vitamin C intoxication and hyperoxalemia in chronic hemodialysis patients. *Nephron.* 1985;39:112.

50. Thompson CS, Weinman EJ. The secondary oxalosis of renal failure. *Semin Dial.* 1988;1:94.

51. Ono K. Secondary hyperoxalemia caused by vitamin C supplementation in regular hemodialysis patients. *Clin Nephrol.* 1986;26:239.

52. Ono K. The effect of vitamin C supplementation and withdrawal on the mortality and morbidity of regular hemodialysis patients. *Clin Nephrol.* 1989;31:31.

53. Yatzidis H, Koutsicos D, Agroyannis B, et al. Biotin in the management of uremic neurologic disorders. *Nephron.* 1984;36:183–186.

5. Nutrition Management of the Adult Peritoneal Dialysis Patient

Peritoneal dialysis (PD) involves the removal of body waste products and water within the peritoneal cavity by using the peritoneal membrane as a filter. Since the early 1970s, PD has gained increased acceptance as a form of renal replacement therapy. The development of a silicone elastomer (Tenckhoff) catheter provided a permanent access into the peritoneal cavity, and the replacement of glass bottles with plastic bags for the dialysis solutions increased the convenience of this therapy. Improvements in catheters and connection devices have also enhanced the safety of peritoneal dialysis and decreased the incidence of peritonitis.[1–4] Approximately 13% of the dialysis population worldwide and 17% of the dialysis population in the United States undergoes PD.[1,4]

Medical and psychological reasons for favoring PD over hemodialysis are varied. For the home patient, PD can be learned more easily. The routines are less complex, allowing the patient to travel, work, and manage his or her own dialysis. PD offers continuous dialysis that promotes steady-state chemistries and fluid balance with fewer dietary restrictions. The potential for hypotensive crisis is also reduced, since there is no direct compromise of the vascular volume during dialysis. PD also may be favored for senior citizens, children, and patients who have advanced cardiovascular disease or diabetes. It is also appropriate for those who are unable to maintain reliable access to blood circulation for hemodialysis and those awaiting kidney transplantation.[3,5–7]

It has also been reported that residual renal function may decline more slowly with PD than with hemodialysis.[8] Nutrition-related advantages of PD include good metabolic and fluid control with corresponding steady-state chemistries, effective removal of middle molecules, improved control of metabolic acidosis, and avoidance of intradialytic catabolism.[6,9]

PD is performed by instilling the dialysis solution (dialysate) through the peritoneal catheter into the peritoneal cavity or peritoneum. The many blood vessels and capillaries throughout the peritoneum are separated from the peritoneal cavity by a layer of mesothelium. The uremic toxins cross the membrane by passive movement from the peritoneal capillaries into the dialysate in the peritoneal cavity. The dextrose contained in the dialysate increases the osmolality of the solution and results in the removal of fluid. The fluid moves from the vascular space into the peritoneal cavity to equilibrate the osmolality of the solutions. The toxins and excess fluids are then drained from the body through the peritoneal catheter and discarded.[6]

There are three methods of peritoneal dialysis: intermittent peritoneal dialysis, continuous ambulatory peritoneal dialysis (CAPD), and automated or "cycler" peritoneal dialysis (APD).

Intermittent peritoneal dialysis is not commonly used as a long-term therapy today because it requires 36 to 40 hours of dialysis each week. The total dialysate volume is approximately 40 L, and each cycle contains up to 3 L, with two cycles performed each hour. This procedure can be performed manually or automatically with a machine.[6] The term "intermittent" has also been applied to newer forms of cycler therapy, wherein the dialysis fluid is left out of the peritoneal cavity for a significant period, such as in cyclic intermittent peritoneal dialysis, in which the patient has a dry day.[10]

In CAPD, a technique is used whereby the continuous presence of dialysis solution in the peritoneal cavity is interrupted intermittently for drainage and instillation of fresh dialysate. The exchanges are usually performed at least four times per day, with only a 30- to 35-minute interruption of daily activity for each exchange. The fluid is instilled, left to dwell for approximately 3.5 to 4 hours, and drained. The dialysate dwells in the peritoneal cavity for approximately 8 to 10 hours at night. The quantity of dialysis can be manipulated by varying the number of exchanges and/or the volume of each exchange. Dialysate is available in varying volumes, from 1 to 3 L per bag, so that the regimen can be optimized for individual patient needs.[6,10]

The APD process is facilitated by a machine (cycler) that cycles the dialysate into and out of the peritoneal cavity at more rapid intervals than with CAPD. This regimen is a reversal of the CAPD exchange schedule and is performed at night, which allows for more daytime freedom and fewer catheter connections (two per day). The patient may leave 1 to 2 L of dialysate in the peritoneal cavity during the day (continuous cyclic peritoneal dialysis [CCPD]), or may have a dry (no fluid) cavity during the day (cyclic intermittent PD or nightly peritoneal dialysis). The type of PD chosen depends on the patient's dialysis needs, activity level, and life-style.[10,11]

Tidal PD is a regimen that decreases the actual time spent instilling and draining dialysate. With tidal PD, a reserve volume of dialysate (usually 50% of the total volume) is always in contact with the peritoneum, and fresh dialysate cycles in on a regular basis, just as the name implies. Not only does tidal PD increase the time that the dialysate solutions are in contact with the blood, it also ensures that fresh dialysate is always available to maintain the concentration gradient for solute and fluid removal. Potential benefits include obtaining adequate clearances in less time and obtaining better clearances than with CCPD.[9–11] The additional dialysate volume, however, adds to the cost of the treatment.

Recent developments in PD technology have arisen out of the recognition that not all peritoneums perform alike, and that dialysis must be individualized to meet the needs of the specific patient. A number of patient variables such as body size, gender, urine output, nutritional status, food intake, life-style, blood chemistries, and characteristics of the peritoneal membrane should be considered when determining which PD regimen to use.[10] The success of PD depends primarily on providing enough dialysis to allow the patient to be clinically free of uremic symptoms, fluid imbalance, and the negative impacts of renal failure.[12,13]

Inadequate dialysis can be the result of large patient size, uncontrolled eating and drinking, loss of residual renal function (RRF), change in membrane transport characteristics, poor catheter function, lack of patient compliance, or insufficient fluid exchange. There is still some controversy about which of the clinical tools can best be used to assess PD patients for adequacy of dialysis.[12,13] Some of those tools include the protein catabolic rate, peritoneal equilibration test (PET), dialysis index, Kt/V (dialyzer urea clearance in liters per minute combined with the urea removed by RRF × minutes of dialysis time/volume of urea distribution in liters), total creatinine clearance in liters per week (dialysate and RRF), and standard

BUN and creatinine measurements.[12–17]

The use of urea kinetic modeling to assess adequacy of treatment in hemodialysis has been commonplace since the results of the National Dialysis Cooperative Study were published in 1983.[18] While there has been no such large-scale prospective trial for kinetic modeling with PD, some guidelines for monitoring the adequacy of dialysis have been formulated from individual dialysis centers or small study group results.[12,13] Currently, the Health Care Financing Administration requires that the adequacy of PD be assessed every 6 months by using Kt/V or liters of creatinine clearance per week.

Although Kt/V for CAPD can be calculated easily, the clinical significance of the calculated Kt/V has not been well defined, and optimal target values have not been established.[13,14] If the Kt/V for PD is standardized to that with hemodialysis, a weekly Kt/V of 1.67 in PD would be approximately equal to a weekly Kt/V of 2.4 (0.8 per day) with hemodialysis. It must be remembered that a Kt/V of 1.67 in PD would be equivalent to a minimal hemodialysis level, below which patients begin to have a higher incidence of morbidity.[13] Because the continuous nature of PD provides a more steady level of urea in the blood, it is postulated that a Kt/V lower than required for hemodialysis may be adequate for PD. Inversely, a higher Kt/V is needed for hemodialysis, because of the peak concentrations of urea that develop between dialysis runs. In PD, Kt/V values can be improved by increasing the number of exchanges or cycles, increasing the volume of exchanges, altering dwell time, or changing the PD method.[12,13]

The protein catabolic rate (PCR) provides a measurable estimate of dietary protein intake in patients with stable weight, on the bases of urea generation and nitrogen removal. When the patient is catabolic, anabolic, or has peritonitis, the protein catabolic rate value will not correctly reflect the patient's dietary protein intake.[13] A number of studies have identified a correlation between Kt/V and PCR, indicating that better clearance of solutes can improve intake of protein.[15,16]

The transport and ultrafiltration characteristics of the peritoneal membrane can be assessed by performing a PET and comparing results to standard PET curves. The PET results help predict dialysis needs and determine which regimen(s) will meet those needs. The PET results can also be used in calculating total creatinine clearance liters per week and Kt/V to assess the adequacy of dialysis delivered.[10,13]

The dialysis index is the dialysate volume (DV) needed to remove enough nitrogen to maintain a BUN concentration of 70 mg/dL, considered to be an appropriate level for a PD patient eating sufficient protein. The ratio of the calculated drainage volume to the measured volume serves as an index of the amount of clearance a patient is getting compared with what is needed (dialysis index = actual DV/prescribed DV). With a stable protein intake, a dialysis index of 1 is expected. A value above or below 1 suggests over- or underdialysis.[13,17]

Total creatinine clearance per week is dependent on the volume of dialysate drained in a specific time, the cumulative dwell time of dialysis, and the plasma creatinine concentration. The daily creatinine clearance can be measured from the total daily dialysate drain volume and the urine creatinine clearance. The weekly creatinine clearance can be extrapolated from the PET data, the dialysate volume per day, dwell time, and the number of dialysis days per week. The extrapolated data approximate the directly measured data, except with the use of the cycler.[13,17] The goal of therapy is thought to be 40 to 50 L of creatinine clearance per week.

More extensive evaluation and validation of the clinical tools for the assessment of PD adequacy are needed.[13,14] The collective use of the above parameters, however, with attention to patient symptoms, should help clinicians provide dialysis therapy that promotes longevity and enhances the quality of life for the PD patient.[13]

When used for long-term management of ESRD patients, PD has been associated with wasting and malnutrition. A number of factors contribute to those states, including anorexia (resulting from inadequate dialysis, superimposed illnesses, discomfort or fullness from dialysate fluids, absorption of dextrose); dietary restrictions; reactions to medications; losses of protein, amino acids, and vitamins to the dialysate; or peritonitis that can lead to catabolism.[9,19–21] It has been suggested that protein-energy malnutrition is a major determinant in PD patient morbidity and mortality.[22] A multicenter study of PD patients found that 32.6% of patients studied were mildly to moderately malnourished and 8% were severely malnourished.[20] It has been suggested that PD patients show a greater degree of protein malnutrition rather than energy malnutrition.[13,20]

Because of the relationship between nutritional status and morbidity and mortality, the renal dietitian must play a key role in the care of PD patients.[23] It is important to assess thoroughly the nutritional status and needs of all patients beginning treatment with PD. Regular, ongoing evaluation, including a review of dietary intake and laboratory values together with adequacy markers, is also crucial to the success of PD.[19,20] Because PD patients may only visit the clinic on a monthly basis, a questionnaire (*Figure 5.1*) is provided to help assess patient progress or problems. The questionnaire can be completed by the patient, the dietitian, or the nurse. Information on the completed questionnaire can be used to evaluate abnormal chemical values, medication compliance, and dietary intake. Nutrition care can then be prioritized and delivered in a timely fashion.

Nutrition Considerations

Nutritional goals can be found in *Table 5.1*. Most of the recommendations for PD (*Table 5.2*) are based on CAPD studies and are calculated with a realistic ideal body weight (IBW) or IBW with the patient's usual body weight considered. While there are differences in the dialysis properties of various forms of PD, these differences have not yet been shown to effect changes in nutrient recommendations. Nutrient losses and nutrition recommendations within this chapter are for all forms of PD unless otherwise noted. Many of the original nutrient recommendations are based on the work of Blumenkrantz and colleagues and are still appropriate. Their work included balance studies that quantified protein losses, absorption of calories, and the exchange of other nutrients between blood and dialysate in the peritoneal cavity.[21]

Protein

Because of the losses of amino acids and albumin to the dialysate through the peritoneal membrane, ingestion of adequate protein is extremely important for patients being treated with PD. Protein losses vary tenfold from patient to patient but are fairly consistent within an individual patient.[19,23–25] The most rapid loss is in the first 2 hours of the exchange, and the total amount of protein lost increases in long-dwell exchanges.[25] Of the 4 to 15 g (average 9 g) of protein lost, 50% to 80% is as albumin.[19,25,26] Protein losses in CCPD are thought to approximate those with CAPD,[27] except for potential differences in the loss of large molecular weight proteins.[28] Losses are affected by the size and molecular weight of the protein, the composition of dialysate, and the permeability of the peritoneal membrane, as well as the clinical status and serum protein levels of the patient.[21,23,25,29] Protein losses

Figure 5.1
Nutrition Questionnaire

Please complete the following questions. This will help me as I review the results of your blood work that is drawn each month. You can complete this form during your clinic visit or return it to me by mail.

1. What is your weight today?_____Has it changed?_____Yes_____No
   _____Increased _____Decreased   How much have you gained/lost?_____
   Do you have any signs of fluid overload?_____Shortness of breath
   _____Swelling (ankles, eyelids, hands, and/or fingers) _____High blood pressure

2. Rate your appetite. _____Good _____Poor _____Fair _____Excellent

3. Has your food intake changed recently?____Eating more _____Eating less. How long
   has it been different? _____ 1 day _____A few days _____A week_____ 2 or more weeks

4. Please estimate "average" amounts of each of the following:
   How many cups of milk are you drinking or using each day? _____cups
   How many ounces of meat, fish, and poultry are you eating each day?
       (palm of hand = approximately 4 oz) _____oz
   How many eggs do you eat each week? _____
   How many ounces of cheese do you eat each week? (1 slice = 1 oz)_____oz
   How many tablespoons of peanut butter do you eat each week?_____tbsp

5. Which phosphate binders do you take?_____Calcium acetate (PhosLo)
   ____Calcium carbonate (Tums, CalciChew, NephroCalci, generic brand)
   ____Alucaps____Dialume____Alternagel____Basaljel____Other____None
   How many binders do you take with____Breakfast____Lunch____Dinner____Snacks
   Have you changed the number of binders you are taking this month?
   ____Yes ____No Increased by_____ Decreased by_____

6. What exchange concentrations are you using on a normal day?
   How many _____1.5% _____2.5% _____4.25% exchanges
   How many _____1.5 L _____2 L _____ 2.5 L _____3 L

7. Please list everything you ate yesterday. Please estimate the amounts in cups, ounces, tablespoons, etc.

Breakfast	Lunch	Dinner	Snacks

8. Was this a typical day for you? _____Yes ____No If no, explain why it was not usual for you (ie, went out to dinner, skipped lunch, was sick, etc).
   _____

9. Do you have any concerns regarding your diet at this time?_____
   _____

Table 5.1
Guidelines for Nutrition Therapy in Peritoneal Dialysis

1. Recover or maintain normal nutritional status, including desirable body weight/body mass index and normal visceral and somatic protein stores
2. Replace protein losses without generating toxic levels of protein waste products
3. Replace abnormal losses of vitamins and minerals
4. Maintain acceptable electrolyte levels
5. Modify diet and/or manipulate dialysate concentrations to restore and/or maintain sodium fluid balance
6. Monitor patient for signs of inadequate dialysis (anorexia, nausea, vomiting, lethargy, neuropathy, pruritis) and collaborate with the medical team to provide adequate dialysis
7. Maintain calcium-phosphorus balance to control parathyroid hormone and prevent bone disease and metastatic calcification
8. Encourage the patient to eat well-balanced, regular meals by using a variety of foods, with planning for ethnic favorites

Table 5.2
Daily Dietary Recommendations for Adult PD Patients

Nutrient	Goal	Intermittent PD	CAPD or APD
Protein (g/kg)*	>50% high biological value		
Maintenance	Stable LBM, albumin	1.2–1.3	1.2–1.3
Repletion	Increased LBM, albumin	1.5	1.5
Reduction	Stable LBM, decreased fat mass	1.2	1.2
Diabetes	Stable LBM, albumin	1.2–1.5	1.2–1.5
Calories (kcal/kg)*†			
Maintenance	Stable dry weight	35	25–35
Repletion	Increased dry weight, LBM	35–50	35–50
Reduction	Decreased fat mass, stable LBM	20–25	20–25
Diabetes	Maintain IBW, stable blood sugar	35	35
Sodium	Maintain blood pressure control, sodium-fluid balance	2 g/d (individualize)	3–4 g/d (individualize)
Potassium	Normal serum levels (3.5–6.0 mEq/L)	2–2.5 g/d (individualize)	3–4 g/d (unrestricted unless serum level is increased or decreased)
Phosphorus	Serum level 4.5–6.5 mg/dL	15 mg per g protein	15 mg per g protein
Calcium	High normal serum levels; Ca-PO$_4$ product <70	1000–1500 mg/d‡	1000–1500 mg/d‡
Fluids	Fluid balance, absence of edema and shortness of breath	Output plus 2–3 cups	Unrestricted if weight, blood pressure, and lipids are controlled and RRF = 2–3 L/d
Vitamins and trace minerals			
Ascorbic acid	No signs of deficiency	60–100 mg/d	
Folate	or toxicosis, replace	0.4–1.0 mg	
Pyridoxine	reported losses, no aggravation	5–10 mg	
Other water-soluble vitamins	or creation of other negative conditions	RDA	
Iron		Maintain serum ferritin >100 ng/mL and transferrin saturation >20%	
Vitamin D		Individualize based on Ca, PTH, alkaline phosphatase levels	
Zinc		10–50 mg/d if deficient	

LBM, lean body mass; IBW, ideal body weight; RRF, residual renal function; PTH, parathyroid hormone.
*Based on IBW.
†An estimation of dialysate calories should be determined and subtracted from the total calories to determine oral calorie allowance. Values presented include calories from dialysate.
‡Includes calcium from supplements, dialysate, and diet.

have been reported to be higher in diabetic patients than in nondiabetic patients.[30] Amino acid losses approximate those found with use of hemodialysis and can usually be replaced with normal dietary intake.[29] Losses of amino acids, which are similar in molecular weight to creatinine, are affected by the concentration in the plasma and the volume of outflow.[29]

With insufficient protein intake, muscle wasting, decreased serum protein (albumin) levels, the potential for increased susceptibility to infection, and delayed wound healing will develop.[31] Blumenkrantz and colleagues found that a minimum of 1.1 g of protein per kilogram per day, along with adequate calories, was necessary for clinically stable CAPD patients to maintain nitrogen balance.[21,32] While others have found neutral or positive nitrogen balance at lower levels of protein intake for short periods, these findings have not been validated in long-term studies.[19,26,33]

Some studies have shown that protein intake of patients being treated with CAPD decreases over time.[34] It is therefore important for the renal care team to monitor and encourage protein intake continually.[9,34] Patients who are unable to ingest adequate dietary protein should be encouraged to take a supplement.[9] Supplements that provide protein without excessive carbohydrate or fat calories may be most appropriate, especially in a patient who has difficulty with undesired weight gain or hyperlipidemia.

The use of dialysate containing amino acids has been reported to be beneficial in patients who are malnourished and are unable to ingest adequate amounts of protein.[35–38] Bernard[35] reported preliminary results from a multicenter study that showed improvement in nitrogen balance and nutritional state in malnourished PD patients who used these solutions. Amino acid solutions have also been shown to facilitate adequate removal of wastes and fluid,[39–44] but may increase the BUN concentration and the occurrence of acidosis, requiring the buffering capacity of the dialysate to be increased.[38–40,45] To date, the cost and instability of these solutions and lack of Medicare or insurance coverage have limited their use.[45]

Calories

The use of dextrose as an osmotic agent in PD fluids must be considered when the caloric needs of PD patients are calculated. The total calories recommended in *Table 5.2* should include both the oral and the dialysate calories. Dextrose has been widely used as an osmotic agent because it is inexpensive, effective, and safe. Disadvantages of use of dextrose as an osmotic agent include the undesirable absorption of calories; anorexia; rapid loss of untrafiltration; and metabolic abnormalities such as hyperglycemia, hyperinsulinemia, hyperlipidemia, and obesity.[42,44–47] Because dextrose is absorbed from the dialysate, oral calories may need to be decreased to prevent weight gain and obesity.[44] Reports of average weight gains in patients treated with PD have ranged from 0 to 5 kg per year.[47–49] As much as 60% to 80% (100 to 250 g) of the dialysate dextrose can be absorbed.[44,50] It has been reported that many patients stabilize near ideal body weight, except those who are already overweight.[51] Glucose absorption varies in each patient, because of individual peritoneal membrane permeability as well as the dextrose concentration, dwell time, and number and volume of exchanges.[9,19,50] Fewer calories may be absorbed with APD, since the dwell times are shortened and equilibration does not take place.[11,52] There are several ways to estimate the calories absorbed from the dialysate.[9,50] One of them can be found in *Table 5.3*. Calorie absorption can also be determined by comparing the dextrose level of the fresh dialysate to that in the resulting effluent.[53] Some CAPD patients have been shown to absorb more than 800 kcal per day from dialysate.[46] The calories absorbed from dialysate could account for more than one third of the patient's daily caloric needs.[50] If the dietary calories are not mod-

Table 5.3
Estimated Glucose Absorption from Peritoneal Dialysate

Concentration of Solution*	Dextrose (g) per				
	1 L	*1.5 L*	*2 L*	*2.5 L*	*3 L*
1.5%	15.0	22.5	30.0	37.5	45.0
2.5%	25.0	37.5	50.0	50.0	75.0
4.25%	42.5	63.8	85.0	106.3	127.5

1. Calculate total grams of dextrose in each exchange
   Example: patient uses 1 2-L exchange of 4.25% solution (85 g of dextrose) and 3 2-L exchanges of 1.5% solution (90 g of dextrose) for a total of 175 g of dextrose
2. Multiply total grams of dextrose by 3.4 kcal/g (monohydrous dextrose)
   $175 \times 3.4 = 595$ kcal
3. Multiply total kilocalories by estimated absorption rate of 70%
   $595 \times 0.70 = 416.5$ kcal
4. Estimate total calories gained from dialysate. Absorption of glucose varies from patient to patient. Excessive weight gain and/or hypertriglyceridemia may indicate increased absorption rate.
   Patient using above exchanges is estimated to absorb 417 kcal/d.

*Solutions used outside the United States may be composed of anhydrous dextrose. These contain: 1.36% (13.6 g dextrose/L); 2.27% (22.7 g/L); and 3.86% (38.6 g/L). The conversion factor is 3.7 kcal/g of dextrose.

ified and physical activity is not encouraged, undesired weight gain and hypertriglyceridemia can result.[46]

In the nutritionally compromised patient, it was initially hoped that the absorption of PD calories might improve nutritional status and allow patients to regain desired weight. However, many patients spontaneously decrease their oral carbohydrate intake in response to the dextrose load, which precludes weight gain and reversal of malnutrition.[54]

Restriction of calories for weight reduction or weight maintenance in PD patients is difficult because of the calories absorbed from dialysate and the calories necessitated by protein requirements. Restricting calories significantly will affect palatability of the diet by forcing patients to "spend" most of their calories on protein food sources. After the initial estimation of dialysate calories absorbed, the patient's intake, dry weight, and lipid levels must be monitored and dietary calories adjusted accordingly.

Sodium

Sodium balance and blood pressure can be well controlled in patients being treated with PD. Moncrief has reported that as much as 5700 mg/d of sodium can be removed with CAPD.[55] Most patients clear between 3 and 4 g of sodium per day, depending on their dialysis regimen.[56] As much as 6 to 8 g of sodium can be tolerated by some patients, if they are able to use hypertonic exchanges without adversely affecting their weight or triglyceride level.[32] Each patient must be aware of the need for sodium and fluid balance and be trained to alter his or her dialysis regimen to maintain that balance. Sodium requirements must be individually determined by using parameters such as weight, blood pressure, shortness of breath, edema, and other signs of volume status. Most patients require little or no restriction of sodium; however, patients with excessive weight gain, hypertriglyceridemia, or overhydration may need to modify their sodium intake.[19,55]

Fluid

Fluid is not generally restricted with PD because most patients ultrafilter 2 L or more per day.[19,55] Many patients can tolerate an intake of 3 L or more of fluid per day, especially if they have residual urine output. Variation in drainage volumes between patients is great because fluid balance is maintained by manipulating the quantity or strength of dialysate solutions and the frequency of exchanges.[16] The maximum ultrafiltration occurs during the first 2 hours of dwell time in an exchange.[57] Thus, APD (frequent exchanges and shorter dwell times) allows for greater fluid removal.[57] Patients must monitor their blood pressure and weight to determine the appropriate dialysis regimen necessary. As with sodium, it may be prudent to modify fluid intake in fluid overload, excessive weight gain, and/or hypertriglyceridemia.

Potassium

Potassium intake must be individualized to patient tolerance for maintainance of normal serum potassium levels. As much as 19 mEq of potassium per day or about 30% of intake can be lost in the stool of dialysis patients.[19,21] The other 70% must be cleared in urine and dialysate. Weekly clearances of potassium are greater with PD than with hemodialysis because of the continuous nature of the therapy.[19,21] PD patients may not require potassium restriction, but it is prudent to recommend that the potassium ingested should be distributed throughout the day, not eaten at one time. Some patients become hypokalemic when treated with PD, especially in response to poor dietary intake, diarrhea, or vomiting. Correction of the hypokalemia may require intraperitoneal or oral potassium supplementation as well as the encouragement to ingest foods that are high in potassium. Correction of hyperkalemia requires restriction of dietary potassium, the use of an ion exchange resin, and/or increased dialysis. Other causes of hyperkalemia (acidosis, constipation, gastrointestinal bleeding, medications) should be investigated when no obvious dietary cause is identified in a hyperkalemic patient.[58]

Phosphorus

Clearance of phosphorus by PD is less than was originally predicted. The shape and electrical charge of the molecule prevent it from being cleared freely.[57] Dietary phosphorus should be moderately restricted. It is difficult to restrict phosphorus intake to less than 1000 to 1200 mg/d and provide recommended protein levels. Phosphate binders are still required by most patients, although some researchers report phosphorus control with lower levels of binders.[6,59,60]

The recognition of problems precipitated by the long-term use of aluminum-based phosphate binders has necessitated a change to other binder sources for prevention of hyperphosphatemia. Calcium-based binders (calcium carbonate, calcium acetate) have gained popularity since they have been shown to be effective.[61] Some patients, however, may require aluminum hydroxide or a combination of calcium and aluminum binders to control phosphorus.[62] Calcium citrate should be avoided because of the potential for increased aluminum absorption.[61-65] Because a portion of the calcium is absorbed from these binders, potential for hypercalcemia exists.[10,59,61,66] Dialysate solutions with a lower concentration of calcium are available for patients who are at risk for hypercalcemia.[10,59,61,66] An initial binder prescription can be calculated by using *Table 5.4*.[21,61–63,65,67] Because this prescription is based on the in vitro binding power of calcium carbonate and estimates of the phosphorus absorption, the binder prescription must be monitored and adjusted with consideration for binder tolerance, serum chemistry values (phosphorus, calcium, parathyroid hormone, alkaline phosphatase), changes in RRF, and the use of active vitamin D.

Calcium

There is some controversy concerning the transperitoneal calcium balance, but most research indicates that calcium is absorbed from all but hypertonic and low calcium solutions.[21,65,67,68] Absorption of calcium is inversely proportional to the patient's serum calcium level and is affected by the tonicity (strength) of the solutions and the ultrafiltration volume.[21,66,68] When determining the calcium needs of a patient, one must consider the amount absorbed from dialysate and binders as well as the dietary and supplemental intake. Absorption from binders can be up to 25% of the total calcium in the binder,[69] and dialysate can contribute from 80 to 300 mg/d.[21] Calcium-based products taken with meals will act as

Table 5.4
Steps to Determine an Initial Prescription of $CaCO_3$ for Phosphate Binding

Steps	Example	Results
Assign recommended amount of dietary phosphorus	1200 mg	Phosphorus taken in diet
Multiply by 50% absorption	1200 × 0.50 = 600 mg	Phosphorus absorbed
Subtract average PD clearance (300 mg/d)	600 mg − 300 mg = 300 mg	Phosphorus to be bound [75]
Divide remaining phosphorus by estimated binding power of $CaCO_3$ (1 g $CaCO_3$ binds approximately 40–60 mg phosphorus in vitro [62])	300 ÷ 60 = 5 g	$CaCO_3$ needed to bind remaining phosphorus
		The initial binder prescription for an anuric patient is 5 g $CaCO_3$ divided according to the phosphorus content and size of the meal.*

*Calcium acetate (after meals) binds approximately 39 mg of phosphorus per gram.[94]
Liquid aluminum hydroxide binds approximately 22.3 mg of phosphorus per 5 mL.[63]
Solid aluminum hydroxide binds approximately 15.3 mg of phosphorus per tablet.[63]
Note—The goal of phosphate binder therapy is to control serum phosphorus and prevent hypercalcemia. The dose of phosphate binders is usually established by trial and error. The method above will only give an estimated beginning dose, which must be refined as individual patient response is assessed. Phosphate binding needs can be altered by type and timing of the binder, the patient's absorption rate for calcium and phosphorus, the phosphorus content of the meal, and interactions with other medications and/or nutrients.

binders, with less absorption of calcium. Those taken between meals will serve as calcium supplements, since more of the calcium will be absorbed.[69] Instructions to the patient should reflect the intended use of the products prescribed. Most patients will need a supplement of at least 500 to 600 mg of elemental calcium per day to reach recommended levels.

Fiber

Kopple and Blumenkrantz recommend at least 20 to 25 g of fiber per day for PD patients.[32] While PD allows more dietary freedom (potassium and fluid) for a high-fiber diet, it may still be difficult to reach this level without fiber supplements.

Vitamins and Minerals

Vitamin depletion can occur in PD patients because of the loss of both water-soluble and protein-bound vitamins to the dialysate.[19,70] Renal failure and drug therapy can interfere with vitamin and mineral metabolism as well.[19,70–72] While few studies have regarded the need for vitamin supplementation in PD patients, some low blood levels of water-soluble vitamins have been found.[71,72] Experts agree that vitamin supplementation as outlined in *Table 5.1* is not harmful and may prevent mild deficiencies. Prophylactic supplementation of vitamins A, E, and K is not recommended.[73]

Vitamin D therapy in PD must be individualized to help the patient maintain calcium-phosphorus balance and control serum parathyroid hormone levels. Research to determine the most efficient method to administer calcitriol in PD patients is ongoing. While intraperitoneal administration of active vitamin D has been shown to help suppress the parathyroid hormone through increased calcium absorption,[74–76] there is a potential for adherence (35% to 40%) of the calcitriol to the tubing and the bags, necessitating increased dosages for efficacy.[77]

While routine zinc supplementation may not be appropriate, PD patients should be monitored, and supplements should be recommended if signs of zinc deficiency are present.[78]

Iron stores in PD patients should be regularly assessed. Oral or intravenous supplements must be administered to maintain serum ferritin levels of more than 100 ng/dL and transferrin saturation rate of 20% or more. This is especially important for patients receiving recombinant human erythropoietin.[79]

Cholesterol and Triglycerides

Blood lipid elevations have been associated with the risk of heart disease. The typical pattern in PD patients includes a normal cholesterol level, high triglyceride levels, and a low high density lipoprotein level.[9,51,80–82] The elevated triglyceride levels are thought to be partly due to dextrose absorption from the dialysate.[49] Protein losses into the peritoneal dialysate also contribute to impaired triglyceride clearance.[80] Lindholm and Norbeck[80] suggest that the initial increase in triglycerides is transitory and that an adaptation to the peritoneal dextrose load allows triglyceride levels to return to baseline in about 1 year.[47,81] Other investigators have seen sustained high triglyceride levels in as many as 25% of the patients.[51,83]

Because many ESRD patients die of heart disease, the possible role of diet should be addressed.[17] Serum triglyceride levels may be lowered through weight control in overweight patients and through exercise, drug therapy, increased fiber intake, and limitation of dietary and dialysate carbohydrate and total fat in the diet.[19,82] Use of amino acid dialysate may also help in reducing the incidence of hypertriglyceridemia.[39,40]

Diabetes

The benefits of PD therapy for diabetic patients include maintenance of steady-state chemical values, well controlled fluid balance and blood pressure, lack of vascular compromise, intraperitoneal insulin administration, simplicity of techniques, ability to dialyze without blood heparinization, and independence.

Some of the drawbacks include: absorption of dialysate dextrose that may hinder control of the blood sugar level, aggravate hyperlipidemia, and increase thirst; neuropathy and retinopathy, which may make self-care difficult; increased protein loss, which can lead to a greater incidence of protein malnutrition and ultimately a decreased immune response; and fluid in the abdomen, which can aggravate gastrointestinal distress and gastroparesis.[5,19,84–86] Nutrition care may require frequent small meals with a higher protein content, careful monitoring and manipulation of insulin, increased insulin dosages, and aggressive support during acute illness.[19,84–86]

Exercise

Exercise has both metabolic and psychosocial benefits for dialysis patients and can indirectly affect nutritional status.[19,87] Exercise can help control weight gain and may reduce hypertriglyceridemia. Patients who exercise regularly report having more energy, better appetite, less insomnia, and an improved sense of well being.[19,87] Exercise must be initiated only with a physician's approval, taking into consideration the individual tolerance and capabilities of each patient. Walking has been shown to be well tolerated by PD patients.[88]

Peritonitis

One of the major areas of concern in PD is the incidence of peritonitis. Nutrition needs change during episodes of peritonitis, in part because of changes in the permeability of the peritoneal membrane.[19,89,90] There is an increase in glucose absorption, which causes a decrease in osmotic force and less extracellular water and sodium removal.[89–92] These alterations make it difficult for the patient to maintain fluid balance. Absorption of insulin may also increase in diabetic patients, necessitating dose changes during peritonitis.[90] There are increased clearances of creatinine and protein,[23] and albumin is the main protein lost.[24,93] The increased protein losses continue for several days after antibiotics are administered and the clinical signs of peritonitis subside.[24,94] These losses, coupled with increased protein needs due to infection or fever, put the patient at risk for protein malnutrition. Patients who are nutritionally compromised may also be more susceptible to peritonitis and have a more severe course of infection.[91] Pain and gastrointestinal distress may also compromise oral nutrient intake.[89] Special encouragement to maintain an adequate intake (especially of protein) is important, and most patients must take supplements to meet nutrient needs during episodes of peritonitis.

A number of nutrition problems may arise with the use of PD as a long-term form of renal replacement therapy. The problems, their actual or postulated causes, and possible solutions are listed in *Table 5.5*.

It has become increasingly clear that good nutrition care is essential for the success of peritoneal dialysis. The quality of life as well as morbidity and mortality are affected by nutritional status. The renal dietitian must work with the entire patient care team to provide ongoing, individualized nutritional assessment and care to allow each patient the best chance for success with PD.

Table 5.5
Common Problems Affecting Nutrition in Patients Treated with PD

Problem	Actual or Postulated Cause	Possible Solutions
Weight gain	Absorption of dialysate calories	Limit sodium and fluid to decrease glucose concentration of exchanges
	Feeling of well being, increased appetite	Limit dietary calories, decrease sugars and fats
		Increase exercise
		Use alternate osmotic agent such as amino acids (experimental, expensive)
Hypertrigly-ceridemia	Conversion of excess glucose to triglycerides by liver	Limit sodium and fluid to decrease glucose concentration of exchanges
	Reduction of metabolic clearance of VLDL or degradation of lipoprotein lipase	Limit dietary simple sugars, sweets, and alcohol
		Increase exercise
		Supplement with omega-3 fatty acids, carnitine, niacin; use lipid-lowering medications
		Use alternate osmotic agent (varied experimental results; expensive)
Satiety or full feeling	Pressure from fluid in peritoneal cavity	Encourage patient to eat while draining, leave effluent out for 30 minutes before instilling next bag
		Use more frequent, smaller-volume bags
		Save fluids until between meals to minimize stomach distention
		Use more frequent, smaller meals; build up tolerance slowly
	Constant glucose load	Use lower-concentration exchanges to minimize glucose load
Protein losses	Permeability of peritoneal membrane allows loss of whole protein (mostly albumin) as well as amino acids	Educate patient regarding need for protein, how to achieve optimum levels
	Peritonitis	Encourage easy-to-eat protein (cheese, cottage cheese, eggs, seafood, peanut butter, casseroles)

Problems	Actual or Postulated Cause	Possible Solutions
		Encourage patient to eat more protein at hungriest time and eat protein first in the meal
		Plan frequent small protein snacks and add protein to other foods (ie, cheese on potato)
		Allow added salt to enhance flavors and encourage patient to choose favorite foods
		Educate about protein supplements and provide them (high protein, low carbohydrate may be best)
Malnutrition or wasting	Losses of protein, vitamins, and minerals Inability to eat, fullness Inadequate dialysis Drug-nutrient interactions Gastrointestinal dysfunction Frequent peritonitis Overly restricted meal pattern Constant glucose load: anorexia	Increase salt allowance to enhance flavor, encourage patient to eat favorite foods Protein supplements, especially during acute peritonitis; use of amino acids solutions Individualize nutritional goals and therapy, educate regarding needs Constant, regular follow-up; encouragement by all team members Medications for gastrointestinal dysfunction, frequent small meals Evaluate drug-nutrient interactions, discontinue or change medications affecting nutrition Assess adequacy of dialysis, switch modalities, or increase volume or number of exchanges Minimize dietary restrictions
Hypokalemia	Excessive clearance or loss in stool Inadequate intake	When serum potassium is 3.2–3.5 mEq/L, encourage dietary intake of fresh fruits and vegetables, milk, and peanut butter When serum potassium is ≤3.2 mEq/L, supplement orally or intraperitoneally
Hyperkalemia	Excessive intake, constipation Inadequate dialysis	Limit high-potassium foods Assess adequacy of dialysis, increase number of exchanges or volume

(Continued)

Table 5.5—continued
Common Problems Affecting Nutrition in Patients Treated with PD

Problem	Actual or Postulated Cause	Possible Solutions
Hypotension	Overuse of hypertonic exchanges Fluid and salt overly restricted Vasodilation Overmedication	Decrease use of hypertonic exchanges Increase use of salt and fluid Limit use of alcohol Adjust medications if appropriate
Constipation	Fluid pressure from dialysate Excess fiber, inadequate fluids	Smaller exchange volumes Encourage adequate fluid and high-fiber foods as allowed Stool softeners, change in binders

References

1. Nolph KD. Continuous ambulatory peritoneal dialysis as long-term treatment for end stage renal disease. *Am J Kidney Dis*. 1991;17:154–156.

2. Nolph KD. Open forum: peritoneal dialysis—what's ahead? *Dial Transplant*. 1980; 11:663,667,670.

3. Nolph KD. Continuous ambulatory peritoneal dialysis. *Am J Nephrol*. 1981;1:1–10.

4. Nolph KD, Cutler SJ, Steinberg SM, et al. Factors associated with morbidity and mortality among patients on CAPD. *Trans Am Soc Artif Org*. 1987;33:57–650.

5. Gokal R. Continuous ambulatory peritoneal dialysis. In: Maher JF, ed. *Replacement of Renal Function by Dialysis*. 3rd ed. Boston, Mass: Kluwer Academic Press; 1989.

6. Popovich RP, Moncrief JW, Nolph KD, et al. Continuous ambulatory peritoneal dialysis. *Ann Intern Med*. 1978;88:449–456.

7. Jenkins-Ross C, Rutsky EA. Dialysis modality selection in the elderly patient with end-stage renal disease: advantages and disadvantages of peritoneal dialysis—peritoneal dialysis in the geriatric patient. *Adv Periton Dial*. 1990;6:11–17.

8. Nolph KD. Is residual renal function preserved better with CAPD than with hemodialysis? *AKF Professional Newsletter*. 1990;7:1–4.

9. Lindholm B, Bergstrom J. Nutritional management of patients undergoing peritoneal dialysis. In: Nolph RD, ed. *Peritoneal Dialysis*. Boston, Mass: Kluwer Academic Publishers, 1989:230–260.

10. *Peritoneal Dialysis Today, The Science and the Art*. Deerfield, Ill: Baxter Healthcare Renal Division; 1991.

11. Diaz-Buxo JA. Current status of continuous cyclic peritoneal dialysis (CCPD). *Periton Dial Int*. 1989;9:9–14.

12. Digenis GE, Dombros N, Oreopoulos DG. Peritoneal dialysis: how much is enough? *Semin Dial*. 1988;1:72–73.

13. Schreiber MJ Jr. Clinical tools for assessing the adequacy of peritoneal dialysis/nephrology update. *Cleveland Clinic Foundation*. 1990;1–4.

14. Hallett MD, Charlton B, Farrell PC. Adequacy of peritoneal dialysis. *Semin Dial*. 1990;3:230–236.

15. Lindsay RM, Spanner E. A hypothesis: the protein catabolic rate is dependent upon the type and amount of treatment in dialyzed uremic patients. *Am J Kidney Dis*. 1989;13:382–389.

16. Keshaviah PR, Nolph KD, Prowant B, et al. Defining adequacy of CAPD with urea kinetics. *Adv Periton Dial*. 1990;6:173–177.

17. Teehan BP, Brown JM, Schleifer CR. Urea kinetic modeling in CAPD for course on dialysis. Presented at 36th Annual Meeting of ASAIO, April 1990.

18. Parker TF, Laird NM, Lowrie EG. Comparison of the study groups in the National Cooperative Dialysis Study and a description of morbidity, mortality, and patient withdrawal. *Kidney Int*. 1983;23(suppl 13):S42–S49.

19. Blumenkrantz MJ. Nutritional aspects of peritoneal dialysis. In: Diamond L, Benis J, Deane N, eds. *Proceedings of the Renal Physicians Association: Northeastern Meeting, New York*. 1979;3:9–29.

20. Young GA, Kopple JD, Lindholm B, et

al. Nutritional assessment of continuous ambulatory peritoneal dialysis patients: an international study. *Am J Kidney Dis.* 1991;17:462–471.

21. Blumenkrantz MJ, Kopple JD, Moran JK, Coburn JW. Metabolic balance studies and dietary protein requirements in patients undergoing continuous ambulatory peritoneal dialysis. *Kidney Int.* 1982;21:849–861.

22. Fenton SA, Johnston N, Delmore T, et al. Nutritional assessment of continuous ambulatory peritoneal dialysis patients. *Trans Am Soc Artif Org.* 1987;23:650–653.

23. Dulaney JT, Hatch FE Jr. Peritoneal dialysis and loss of proteins: a review. *Kidney Int.* 1984;26:253–262.

24. Blumenkrantz MJ, Gahl GM, Kopple JD, et al. Protein losses during peritoneal dialysis. *Kidney Int.* 1981;19:593–602.

25. Lindholm B, Bergstrom J. Protein and amino acid metabolism in patients undergoing continuous ambulatory peritoneal dialysis (CAPD). *Clin Nephrol.* 1988;30(suppl 1):S59–S63.

26. Young GA, Brownjohn AM, Parsons FM. Protein losses in patients receiving continuous ambulatory peritoneal dialysis. *Nephrol.* 1987;45:196–201.

27. Diaz-Buxo J, Walker P, Farmer C, et al. Continuous cyclic peritoneal dialysis (CCPD). *Kidney Int.* 1981;19:145.

28. Kagan A, Bar-Khayim Y, Schafer Z, Fainaru M. Kinetics of peritoneal protein loss during CAPD. 1. Different characteristics for low and high molecular weight proteins. *Kidney Int.* 1990; 37:971–979.

29. Kopple JD, Blumenkrantz MJ, Jones MR, et al. Plasma amino acid levels and amino acid losses during continuous ambulatory peritoneal dialysis. *Am J Clin Nutr.* 1982;36:395–402.

30. Krediet RT, Zuyderhoudt FMJ, Boeschoten EW, Arisz L. Peritoneal permeability to proteins in diabetic and non-diabetic continuous ambulatory peritoneal dialysis. *Nephron.* 1986;42:133–140.

31. Blumenkrantz MJ, Kopple JD, Gutman RA, et al. Methods for assessing nutritional status of patients with renal failure. *Am J Clin Nutr.* 1980;33:1567–1585.

32. Kopple JD, Blumenkrantz MJ. Nutritional requirements for patients undergoing continuous ambulatory peritoneal dialysis. *Kidney Int.* 1983;24(suppl 16):S295–S302.

33. Ginsberg NS, Lynn RI. Nitrogen balance in patients on CAPD eating their usual diets. *CRN Q.* 1988;12:12–14.

34. Heide B, Pierratos A, Khanna R, et al. Nutritional status of patients undergoing continuous ambulatory peritoneal dialysis (CAPD). *Perit Dial Bull.* July–September 1983.

35. Bernard D. International Congress, Harrogate (in press).

36. Khanna R, et al. Use of amino acid containing solutions on CAPD patients. *Perit Dial Bull.* July–September (suppl) 1984.

37. Hutchison AJ, Gokal R. Peritoneal dialysis fluids for the future: do we have the solution? *Dial Transplant.* 1992;21:57–61.

38. Arfeen S, et al. The nutritional, metabolic, and hormonal effects of 8 weeks of continuous ambulatory peritoneal dialysis with a 1% amino acid solution. *Clin Nephrol.* 1990;33:192–199.

39. Lindholm B, Werynski A, Bergstrom J. Peritoneal dialysis with amino acid solutions: fluid and solute transport kinetics. *Artif Org.* 1988;12:2–10.

40. Oreopolos D, Marliss E, Anderson HG, et al. Nutritional aspects of CAPD and the potential use of amino acid containing dialysis solutions. *Perit Dial Bull.* 1983 (suppl);3:S10–S12.

41. Williams P, Marliss E, Anderson HG, et al. Amino acid absorption following intraperitoneal administration in CAPD patients. *Perit Dial Bull.* 1982;2:124–129.

42. Oren A, Wu G, Anderson GH, et al. Effective use of amino acid dialysate over four weeks in CAPD patients. *Perit Dial Bull.* 1983;3:66–73.

43. Pederson F, Dragsholt C, Laier E, et al. Alternate uses of amino acid and glucose solutions in CAPD. *Perit Dial Bull.* 1985;5:215–218.

44. Hanning R, Balfe JW, Zlotkins S. Effectiveness and nutritional consequences of amino acids vs glucose-based dialysis solutions in infants and children receiving CAPD. *Am J Clin Nutr.* 1987;46:22–30.

45. Mistry CD, Gokal R. New osmotic agents for peritoneal dialysis: where we are and where we're going. *Semin Dial.* 1990;4:9–12.

46. DeSantos NG, Capodicasa G, Senatore T, et al. Glucose utilization from dialysate in patients on continuous ambulatory peritoneal dialysis (CAPD). *Int J Artif Org.* 1979;2:119–124.

47. Bouma S, Dwyer JT. Glucose absorption and weight change in 18 months of continuous ambulatory peritoneal dialysis. *J Am Diet Assoc.* 1984;84:194–197.

48. Oreopoulos DG, Khanna R, McCready W, et al. Continuous ambulatory peritoneal dialysis in Canada. *Dial Transplant.* 1980;9:224–226.

49. Traneous A, Heimburger O, Lindholm B, Bergstrom J. Six years' experience of CAPD at one centre: a survey of major findings. *Periton Dial Int.* 1988;8:31–41.

50. Grodstein GP, Blumenkrantz MJ, Kopple JD, et al. Glucose absorption during continuous ambulatory peritoneal dialysis. *Kidney Int.* 1983;1;19:564–567.

51. Boeschoten EW, Zyunderhoudt FMJ, Krediet RT, Arisz L. Changes in weight and lipid concentrations during CAPD treatment. *Periton Dial Int.* 1988;8:19–24.

52. Holley JL, Piraino BM. Complications of peritoneal dialysis: diagnosis and management. *Semin Dial.* 1990;3:245–248.

53. Ginsberg NS, Lynn RI. Glucose absorption in patients on continuous ambulatory peritoneal dialysis. *CRN Q.* 1989;13:10–11.

54. Von Baeyer H, Gahl GM, Riedinger H, et al. Adaptation of CAPD patients to continuous peritoneal energy uptake. *Kidney Int.* 1983;23:29–34.

55. Moncrief JW. Continuous ambulatory peritoneal dialysis. *Dial Transplant.* 1979;8:1077.

56. Nolph KD, Sorkin MI, Moore H. Autoregulation of sodium and potassium removal during continuous ambulatory peritoneal dialysis. *Artific Intern Org.* 1980;26:334–338.

57. Diaz-Buxo JA, Burgess WP. Comparison of kinetics: CAPD and CCPD. *Perspect Periton Dial.* 1985;3:378–441.

58. Beto JA, Bansal VK. Hyperkalemia: evaluating dietary and nondietary etiology. *J Renal Nutr.* 1992;2:28–29.

59. Weinreich T, Rambausek M, Ritz E. Is control of secondary hyperparathyroidism optimal with the currently used calcium concentrations in the CAPD fluid? *Nephrol Dial Transplant.* 1991;6:843–845.

60. Cannata JB, Briggs JD, Fell GS, Junor BJR. Comparison of control of serum phosphorus levels during continuous ambulatory peritoneal dialysis and during hemodialysis. *Perit Dial Bull.* 1983;3:97–98.

61. Morton AR, Hercz G, Coburn JW. Control of hyperphosphatemia in chronic renal failure. *Semin Dial.* 1990;3:219–223.

62. Slatopolsky E, Weerts C, Lopez S, et al. Calcium carbonate as an effective phosphorus binder in dialysis patients. *Kidney Int.* 1985;27:173.

63. Balasa RW, Murray RL, Kondelis NP, Bischel MD. Phosphate-binding properties and electrolyte content of aluminum hydroxide antiacids. *Nephron.* 1987;45:16–21.

64. Mischel M, Salusky IB, Goodman WC, et al. Calcium citrate markedly augments aluminum absorption in man (abstr). *Kidney Int.* 1989;35:399.

65. Slatopolsky E, Weerts C, Lopez-Hilkas S, et al. Calcium carbonate as a phosphorus binder in patients with chronic renal failure undergoing dialy-

sis. *N Engl J Med.* 1986;315:157–161.

66. Martis L, Serkes KD, Nolph KD. Calcium carbonate as a phosphate binder: is there a need to adjust peritoneal dialysate calcium concentrations for patients using CaCO$_3$? *Periton Dial Int.* 1989;9:325–328.

67. Delmez JA, Slatopolsky E, Martin KJ, et al. Minerals, vitamin D and parathyroid hormone in continuous ambulatory peritoneal dialysis. *Kidney Int.* 1982;21:862–867.

68. Parker A, Nolph KD. Calcium mass transfer during continuous ambulatory peritoneal dialysis. *Trans Am Soc Artif Intern Org.* 1980;26:194–196.

69. Schiller LR, Sheikh MS, et al. Effect of time of administration on calcium acetate phosphate binding. *N Engl J Med.* 1989;320:1110–1113.

70. Mydlik M, Derzsiova K, Valek A, et al. Vitamins and continuous ambulatory peritoneal dialysis (CAPD). *Int Urol Nephrol.* 1985;17:281–286.

71. Blumberg A, Hanck A, Sander G. Vitamin nutrition in patients on continuous ambulatory peritoneal dialysis (CAPD). *Clin Nephrol.* 1983;30:244–250.

72. Boeschoten EW, Schrijven J, Krediet RT, et al. Deficiencies of vitamins in CAPD patients: the effects of supplementation. *Nephrol Dial Transplant.* 1988;3:187–193.

73. Digenis G, Dombros N, Charytan C, Oreopoulos D. Supplements for the CAPD patient (vitamins, folic acid, zinc, iron, anabolic steroids). *Periton Dial Bull.* 1987;7:219–223.

74. Rapoport J, Shany S, Chaimovitz C. Continuous ambulatory peritoneal dialysis and vitamin D. *Nephron.* 1988;48:1–3.

75. Gokal R. Renal osteodystrophy and aluminum bone disease in CAPD patients. *Clin Nephrol.* 1988;1(suppl):S64–S67.

76. Delmer JA, Dougan CS, Gearing BK, et al. The effects of intraperitoneal calcitriol on calcium and parathyroid hormone. *Kidney Int.* 1987;31:795–799.

77. Salusky IB, Adams JS, Horst R, et al. Enhanced calcitriol delivery after intraperitoneal administration (abstr). *Kidney Int.* 1989;35:276.

78. Mahajan SK. Zinc requirements in uremia. In: *Ross Report of the Eleventh Ross Roundtable on Medical Issues.* Columbus, Ohio: Ross Laboratories; 1991:72–75.

79. Van Wyke DB. The challenge of iron deficiency during r-HuEP therapy. *Semin Dial.* 1989;2:135–136.

80. Lindholm B, Norbeck HE. Serum lipids and lipoproteins during continuous ambulatory peritoneal dialysis. *Acta Med Scand.* 1986;220:143–152.

81. Young GA, Hobson SM, Young SM, et al.

Adverse effects of hypertonic dialysis fluid during CAPD. *Lancet.* 1983;2:1421.

82. Pagenkemper JJ. Attaining nutritional goals for hyperlipidemic and obese renal patients. In: *Ross Report on the Eleventh Roundtable on Medical Issues.* Columbus, Ohio: Ross Laboratories; 1991.

83. Lamiere N, Matthys D, Matthys E, Beheydt R. Effects of long-term CAPD on carbohydrate and lipid metabolism. *Clin Nephrol.* 1988;30(suppl):S53–S58.

84. Khanna R. Peritoneal dialysis in diabetic end stage renal disease patients. In: Twardowski ZJ, Nolph KD, Khanna R, eds. *Peritoneal Dialysis: New Concepts and Applications.* New York, NY: Churchill Livingstone; 1990;211–229.

85. Rottenbourg J. Clinical aspects of continuous ambulatory and continuous cyclic peritoneal dialysis in diabetic patients. *Periton Dial Int.* 1989;9:289–294.

86. Flynn CT. CAPD and the diabetic patient. In: Catto GRD, ed. *Continuous Ambulatory Peritoneal Dialysis.* Boston, Mass: Kluwer Academic Publishers; 1988.

87. Boone JL. Exercise and the hemodialysis patient. *Dial Transplant.* 1987;16:243.

88. Painter PL, Messer D, Widener C, Zimmerman SW. Response to graded exercise testing in patients treated with CAPD. *Periton Dial Bull.* 1984;4(suppl):S94–S97.

89. Bannister DK, Acchiardo SDR, Moore LW, Krause AP Jr. Nutritional effects of peritonitis in continuous ambulatory peritoneal dialysis (CAPD) patients. *J Am Diet Assoc.* 1987;87:53–56.

90. McIntosh ME, Smith WGJ, Junor BJR, et al. Increased peritoneal permeability in patients with peritonitis undergoing continuous ambulatory peritoneal dialysis. *Eur J Clin Pharmacol.* 1985;28: 187–191.

91. Young GA, Young JB, Young SM, et al. Nutrition and delayed hypersensitivity during continuous ambulatory peritoneal dialysis in relation to peritonitis. *Nephron.* 1986;43:177–186.

92. Rubin J, Ray R, Barnes T, Bower J. Peritoneal abnormalities during infectious episodes of continuous ambulatory peritoneal dialysis. *Nephron.* 1981;29:124–127.

93. Rubin J, Deraps G, Walsh D, et al. Protein losses and tobramycin absorption in peritonitis treated by hourly peritoneal dialysis. *Am J Kidney Dis.* 1986;8:124–127.

94. Schiller L, Santa Ana C, Mudassir B, et al. Effect of the time of administration of calcium acetate on phosphorus binding. *N Engl J Med.* 1989;320:1110–1113.

6. Nutrition Management of the Adult Renal Transplant Patient

Renal transplantation is the preferred method of treatment for many ESRD patients. Recipients enjoy a decreased hospitalization rate with an increased survival rate compared with groups receiving dialytic therapy. Approximately 8900 renal transplantations are performed each year, with the waiting list growing to more than 13 000 candidates. Insufficient organ donation accounts for the discrepancy between the number of recipients and candidates. Kidney transplantation is also economically advantageous, costing less than long-term dialytic support, an important factor in today's health care economy.[1]

Nutrition care of the renal transplant recipient is a dynamic process. It involves the integration of knowledge of the patient's complex medical condition related to chronic renal disease and the impact of ongoing therapeutic interventions on the patient's nutritional status. Continual reassessment of the nutritional goals and efficacy of therapy allow for the adjustment of nutrition priorities during different phases of care.

Three phases of care have been identified for organ transplant recipients: pretransplantation, the acute posttransplantation phase, and the chronic posttransplantation phase.[2] In the pretransplantation period, the goal is to optimize the patient's nutritional status to decrease surgical risk, postsurgical complications, and length of hospital stay. In the acute posttransplantation period (up to 8 weeks after transplantation), the goal is to support the increased metabolic demands of surgery and immunosuppressive therapy. A plan for nutritional rehabilitation is formulated and initiated. During the chronic posttransplantation period, nutritional rehabilitation can be realized. Also of concern is the nutritional management of complications related to long-term immunosuppressive therapy.

The Pretransplantation Period

A complete evaluation of the patient's nutritional status before transplantation is imperative to identify deficits, and when possible, to correct them before surgery. The dietitian must keep in mind that the transplantation candidate has been subjected to the deleterious effects of organ failure and chronic disease and that not all deficiencies identified can be corrected without organ replacement. The baseline data gathered during initial assessment are used to begin developing a plan of care for that candidate. Assessment of the patient with ESRD has been discussed in previous chapters. The pretransplantation evaluation should include a medical history, dietary history, anthropometric data, biochemical indices of nutritional status, evaluation of gastrointestinal abnormalities, nutritional supplement and vitamin and/or mineral use, social history, medication usage, and information regarding present renal replacement therapy.[3]

An assessment of nutrition needs is then performed, and recommendations are formulated. For the severely malnourished patient, specialized nutrition support before surgery may be warranted.

Presurgical malnutrition can involve undernutrition or overnutrition and has been associated with an increased risk for postsurgical complications.[4–6] Although the clinical relevance of specific nutritional indices in the ESRD population related to posttransplantation complication has not been extensively investigated, obesity is one index that has been studied. Holley et al[7] studied the relationship between obesity and the incidence of posttransplantation complications. Obesity was defined as a body mass index greater than or equal to 30. It was found that obese patients receiving cadaveric renal transplants had a significantly higher mortality rate, lower immediate graft function and 1-year graft survival rates, and an increased incidence of wound complications. Obese recipients experienced more frequent intensive care unit admissions, reintubations, and an increased incidence of development of posttransplantation diabetes mellitus. It is suggested that aggressive attempts at pretransplantation weight reduction be made for the obese candidate.[7]

The Acute Posttransplantation Period

Immunosuppressive Therapy

Pharmacologic immunosuppression is used to halt the body's rejection response to the transplanted kidney, thus enhancing long-term graft survival. The goal of immunosuppression is to inhibit selectively this adaptive immune response while allowing nonspecific immune functions to remain intact.[8,9] Unfortunately, this therapy has yet to be perfected. Immunosuppressive agents also have nonimmunologic side effects. The common use of multidrug regimens is an attempt to use lower doses of individual agents to minimize associated side effects. Cyclosporine, azathioprine, and corticosteroids are the most common agents in use today.

CYCLOSPORINE

Cyclosporine is a cyclic polypeptide extracted from the fungus *Tolypocladum inflatum gams*. It is lipophilic, with the intravenous preparation stabilized in castor oil and the oral preparation stabilized in olive or corn oil. Cyclosporine selectively inhibits adaptive immune responses but also has some nonimmunologic side effects, which include gingival hyperplasia, gastrointestinal disturbances, hyperglycemia, gynecomastia, hepatotoxicity, and nephrotoxicity. Cyclosporine is absorbed in the upper small intestine and is dependent on bile availability. Its absorption is adversely affected by cholestasis, biliary diversion, cholestyramine therapy, slow gastric emptying (as in gastroparesis), increased gastrointestinal motility, and steatorrhea. Absorption is enhanced by normal low density lipoprotein serum levels, coadministration with food, and prolonged therapy.[8,10]

AZATHIOPRINE

Azathioprine is thought to be a nonspecific immunosuppressant whose mode of action is the inhibition of proliferation of immunocompetent cells. It is typically used in multidrug therapy and may be administered intravenously or orally.[9]

CORTICOSTEROIDS

Corticosteroids have anti-inflammatory properties and inhibit the production of lymphokines. Associated side effects are believed to be dose-dependent and include impaired wound healing, avascular necrosis of long bones, upper gastrointestinal ulceration, protein catabolism, hypertension, steroid-induced diabetes mellitus, cataract formation, and stimulation of appetite.[9]

OTHER AGENTS

Monoclonal antibodies and antilymphocyte globulin are examples of immunosuppressants used as adjunctive agents in the treatment of rejection episodes. These agents may cause gastrointestinal distress and flulike symptoms, and appropriate adjustments in nutritional therapy should be made.[9]

New immunosuppressive agents continue to be researched and some are now in clinical trials. It is a challenge for dietitians to identify and report nutrition-related side effects and their management.

Table 6.1 lists known adverse effects and nutrition implications of the common immunosuppressive agents.

Nutrition Requirements

Nutrition recommendations for adult renal transplant patients are shown in *Table 6.2*.

PROTEIN

The acceleration of the transplant recipient's protein catabolic rate (PCR) is related to the administration of supraphysiologic doses of corticosteroids, as well as postoperative stress.[11] This increase in PCR appears to persist at least through the third postoperative week and may further increase during rejection therapy. Maintenance of protein balance during this period is a formidable task, and negative protein balance will ensue if the intake of protein does not equal the PCR. The present recommendation for protein intake is 1.3 to 2.0 g/kg of normalized body weight (NBW) and is based on the assumption that the corticosteroid dose is approximately 1 mg/kg of NBW. Normalized body weight is defined as dry weight when the patient is within normal limits of weight for height or an adjusted weight if the person is obese.[12] The administration of 2.0 to 4.0 mg of corticosteroid per kilogram of NBW during periods of rejection may increase protein needs to 2.0 to 2.5 g/kg of NBW per day.[11,13–16]

CARBOHYDRATE

Carbohydrate intolerance related to corticosteroid therapy[17] and hyperglycemia associated with decreased hepatic glycogen synthesis during cyclosporine therapy[8] may necessitate restricting simple carbohydrates. A high-protein, low-carbohydrate dietary regimen has also been shown to ameliorate the cushingoid side effects associated with high-dose cortocosteroids.[17] Carbohydrates are often limited to provide less than 50% of total calories and are sometimes restricted to 1 to 1.5 g/kg of NBW, though the latter approach may not be practical for many patients.[16,18]

FAT

During the acute postoperative period, fat is used to supply the remainder of the total calories after calculating the amount provided by protein and carbohydrate. The amount of

Table 6.1
Adverse Effects of Immunosuppressants With Nutritional Implications

Agent	Adverse Effect	Nutritional Implication
Cyclosporine	Hyperkalemia	Restrict potassium intake
	Hyperglycemia	Restrict simple carbohydrate intake
	Gingival hyperplasia	Good oral hygiene
	Hypertension	Restrict sodium intake
	Gastrointestinal distress	Alter vehicle for drug: use chocolate milk, juice, or root beer; use gelatin capsules
Azathioprine	Infection	Increased nutrient demands
	Mouth ulcers	Diet texture modifications
	Folate deficiency	Folate supplementation
Corticosteroids	Cushingoid appearance	Restrict simple carbohydrate and increase protein intake
		Restrict sodium intake
	Sodium retention	Restrict sodium intake
	Enhanced appetite	Low-calorie snacks
	Hyperlipidemia	Restrict cholesterol and simple carbohydrate intake
	Hyperglycemia	Utilize diabetic diet guidelines
	Protein catabolism	Increase protein provision
	Gastrointestinal ulceration	Small, frequent feedings; Caffeine restriction
Monoclonal Antibodies	Congestive heart failure, pulmonary edema	Administer when patient is euvolemic
	Nausea, vomiting, diarrhea, and other flulike symptoms	Clear fluids, oral nutritional supplements; if prolonged symptoms, parenteral nutrition may be needed
Antilymphocyte Globulin	Nausea, vomiting	Clear fluids, oral nutritional supplements; if prolonged symptoms, parenteral nutrition support

fat is only limited by the appropriate calorie level and often provides more than 30% of the total calories. Emphasis is placed on the provision of polyunsaturated and monounsaturated fat sources while limiting saturated fat.[16,18] Hyperlipidemia is of considerable concern but is not aggressively treated until the chronic posttransplantation period. Nutrition education in the acute period, however, should introduce the importance of "heart healthy" dietary habits.

SODIUM

Dietary sodium intake is often limited to 2 to 4 g/d in the acute posttransplant period. This limitation is an attempt to control the sodium and concomitant fluid retention experi-

Table 6.2
Nutrition Recommendations for the Adult Renal Transplant Recipient

Nutrient	Daily Recommendation Acute Period	Chronic Period
Protein	1.3–2.0 g/kg NBW*	RDA[†]; limit with chronic rejection
Calories	30–35 kcal/kg NBW or BEE × 1.3 May increase with postoperative complications	Maintain desirable body weight
Carbohydrate	Limit simple carbohydrate intake if intolerance is apparent	Emphasize complex carbohydrate intake
Fat	Remainder of calories Emphasize PUFA and MUFA*	Emphasize PUFA and MUFA
Sodium	2–4 g	2–4 g with hypertension
Potassium	2–4 g if hyperkalemic	Unrestricted
Calcium	800–1500 mg	800–1500 mg
Phosphorus	RDA[†]; may need supplementation to normalize serum levels	RDA[†]
Other vitamins	RDA[†]	RDA[†]
Other minerals	RDA[†]	RDA[†]
Trace elements	RDA[†]	RDA[†]
Fluid	Limited only by graft function	Limited only by graft function; generally unrestricted

*NBW, the dry weight when the patient is within normal limits of weight for height, or an adjusted weight if the person is obese; PUFA, polyunsaturated fatty acids; MUFA, monounsaturated fatty acids.

[†]Due to lack of research, no specific recommendations are available for this population. Currently, the RDA is used as a guideline.

enced with corticosteroid administration. Posttransplantation hypertension may be sodium-sensitive, further indicating a need for dietary restriction.[16,18]

POTASSIUM

A moderate dietary potassium restriction is indicated if serum potassium levels are elevated. Poor graft function as well as impaired potassium excretion associated with cyclosporine immunosuppression may contribute to hyperkalemia.[8,19]

VITAMINS AND OTHER MINERALS

Little research has been undertaken regarding the vitamin and mineral needs of the renal transplant recipient in the acute postoperative period. Dietitians must therefore take a diagnostic approach to identifying vitamin and mineral deficiencies when determining requirements. Existing literature will be discussed in the chronic posttransplantation section.

TRACE ELEMENTS

Information regarding the effect of renal transplantation on trace element nutriture is scarce, with the exception of the effects on zinc. Because uremic patients have abnormal zinc metabolism, it is one of the trace elements most likely to become deficient in patients with ESRD.[20,21] Candidates presenting for renal transplantation may therefore be zinc-deficient. In a study by Mahajan and colleagues, patients with subnormal plasma and hair zinc levels as well as abnormal taste detection and recognition thresholds during the pretransplantation period did not show normalization of these parameters until 1 year after transplantation. These patients showed a persistence of zinc depletion, despite correction of uremia. The suboptimal zinc nutriture appeared to be related to increased urinary zinc losses. The mechanism underlying hyperzincuria and the clinical significance of zinc depletion after renal transplantation has not yet been determined; therefore, no specific recommendations have been made for this population.[22] When faced with wound complications, however, the dietitian should consider zinc status and use supplements if zinc intake is insufficient.

Common Postsurgical Problems

HYPOPHOSPHATEMIA

Abnormalities of renal phosphate handling occur even with stable, functioning allografts. The actual incidence of postoperative hypophosphatemia has not been recently reported, nor has the pathogenesis of the tubular phosphate leak been clearly elucidated.[23] Other factors that may contribute to the development of hypophosphatemia in the acute postoperative period include (1) the use of aluminum-containing antacids, (2) intracellular phosphorus shifts associated with high levels of dextrose provision and aggressive refeeding, and (3) inadequate phosphorus intake, which is often seen with lactose-intolerant patients. It may be necessary to use phosphorus supplements to normalize serum levels. These supplements, however, contain significant amounts of potassium. Even those with lower levels of potassium can contribute a significant load, requiring close monitoring of serum potassium levels. With persistent hyperkalemia, a change to a sodium phosphate preparation for phosphorus supplementation may be suggested. Doses should be less than that which would effect a laxative response. Sodium phosphate preparation should be given in juice or other flavored liquids because it is unpalatable.

HYPERKALEMIA

Postsurgical hyperkalemia is associated with poor graft function, cyclosporine therapy, and cell lysis related to the catabolic effect of both surgery and corticosteroid administration. Dietary interventions include the restriction of potassium intake and the provision of adequate calories and protein to minimize catabolism of endogenous tissue.[8,24]

INCREASED APPETITE

Many patients experience great increases in appetite and intake related to corticosteroid therapy. The nutritional concern lies with rapid weight gain. Nutrition intervention may include the use of low-calorie between-meal snacks to assist with curbing the appetite. A gradual increase in exercise can also assist with controlling weight gain.

Specialized Nutrition Support Considerations

Typically, transplant recipients are able to meet their nutrition needs with an oral diet. Liquid nutritional supplements may be used to assist patients experiencing difficulty with adequate intake.

If a patient is unable to meet his or her metabolic demands orally or the gastrointestinal tract is nonfunctional, specialized nutrition support is administered to prevent nutritional compromise. The aforementioned guidelines for determining nutrition requirements should be used, with consideration of the patient's level of renal function. Use of nutrient-dense enteral formulas such as those with 2 kcal/mL will assist with reducing the volume needed to meet nutrition requirements if fluid provision must be restricted. Parenterally, 10% to 15% amino acids, 70% dextrose, and 20% lipid solutions may be used to concentrate the intravenous formula.

Standard monitoring protocols should be observed and usually include serum lipid, glucose, phosphorus, magnesium, copper, zinc, and electrolyte levels. Nutrition assessment parameters such as weight, circulating protein status, and nitrogen balance studies may be used to evaluate the adequacy of nutrient provision.

The Chronic Posttransplantation Period

Nutrition rehabilitation of patients with ESRD can be realized following successful renal transplantation. Miller and Levine[25,26] have reported significant improvements in body weight, weight for height, and serum albumin level from the pretransplantation to the posttransplantation periods. These improvements were evident in recipients with and without diabetes mellitus.[25,26] Long-term nutrition management is complicated, however, by the adverse effect of chronic immunosuppressive therapy.

Nutrition Requirements

Once maintenance levels of immunosuppressive agents have been reached, renal transplant recipients without complicating factors can enjoy a dietary regimen consistent with guidelines for the healthy population. These include a moderately low sodium and fat intake. It is prudent to have a protein intake of 0.8 to 1.0 g/kg of NBW. If renal insufficiency or chronic rejection is evident, a protein restriction similar to that recommended by predialysis guidelines may be needed to control azotemia. Evidence supporting protein restriction for the specific purpose of prolonging graft function is not conclusive.

CALCIUM

Long-term corticosteroid therapy with resultant inhibition of bone formation and the stimulation of bone resorption can lead to osteoporosis.[27] Corticosteroids also decrease the intestinal absorption of elemental calcium to 42% of that ingested, compared with 61% for people not being treated with corticosteroids. The amount of calcium excreted in the urine is also increased with corticosteroid therapy.[28] For these reasons, it has been suggested that the renal transplant recipient requires a higher level of calcium intake to absorb the amount equal to that expected to be provided by the RDA.[29] Because no definitive study has been reported, the actual requirement remains speculative. Calcium supplementation, however, is not always used because of concern for renal stone formation. If supplementation is initiated, counseling regarding adequate fluid intake is warranted.[29]

VITAMIN A

It is known that serum vitamin A levels are elevated in patients with ESRD. In 1976, Yatzidis et al reported three cases of renal transplant recipients in which normalization of serum vitamin A concentrations was not realized until 2 years after transplantation.[30] This delayed restoration was believed to indicate a whole-body hypervitaminosis A.[31] Kelleher and colleagues studied the changes in serum vitamin A levels after renal transplantation.[32] Preoperative levels of vitamin A were significantly higher in the patients with ESRD than in the control group of healthy subjects. Although vitamin A levels decreased after surgery in patients with transplants, they remained significantly higher than in the control group at all times during the subsequent 22 days. The mean serum vitamin A level in an additional group of patients with transplants (mean time from renal transplantation, 26.5 months) also remained significantly higher than in the control group.[32] Because transplant recipients follow relatively unrestricted diets, an intake equal to that of the RDA should be sufficient, and supplementation should be avoided unless a deficiency is demonstrated.

OTHER VITAMINS

Lacour et al measured plasma B_6 levels in 116 nonuremic kidney transplant recipients being treated with azathioprine-prednisone immunosuppressive therapy at various time intervals after transplantation.[33] Sixty-five percent of the patients showed a marked deficit in B_6 levels, but some may have been deficient before surgery. Oral supplementation was used to normalize serum levels. The maintenance of a B_6 deficit or newly developed deficiency, despite an unrestricted diet, may be related to the azathioprine-prednisone therapy.[33]

Diminished serum folic acid levels in 29% of 52 renal recipients being treated with azathioprine-prednisone therapy with unrestricted diets were observed by Zazgornik and colleagues.[34] The folic acid depletion was unrelated to the length of time following transplantation. Serum B_{12} levels were within normal range. The cause of decreased folic acid levels was thought to be related to either an abnormality of intestinal absorption due to mucosal damage associated with long-term immunosuppressive therapy and/or drug interference with folic acid metabolism.[34]

It must be noted that most of the studies just described were performed before the use of cyclosporine and lower corticosteroid doses.

Nutrition Management of Long-Term Complications

CARDIOVASCULAR DISEASE

Many factors contribute to the development of cardiovascular disease in renal patients. By recognizing these factors as risks, attempts to eliminate or minimize them can commence. Nutrition-related factors associated with the greatest risks for disease in the general population include elevated plasma cholesterol level, elevated blood pressure, diabetes mellitus, and obesity.[35] These same risk factors are prevalent in the renal transplantation population.

The incidence of hypercholesterolemia has been reported to be as high as 37.6% in patients treated with cyclosporine and prednisone and 42.4% in those treated with azathioprine and prednisone.[36,37] Hypertriglyceridemia and combined hyperlipidemia is multifactorial. Contributing factors identified include corticosteroid-induced glucose intolerance with basal hyperinsulinemia, renal dysfunction, obesity, diuretic and/or antihypertensive drug therapy, increasing age, diabetes mellitus, proteinuria, increased hepatic lipoprotein synthesis, and a decrease in plasma lipoprotein clearance. Hypertriglyceridemia has been strongly correlated with the patient's degree of obesity.[36,37] The treatment of hyperlipidemia after transplantation has not been without problems and has been reported with varying degrees of success. Dietary intervention can be used safely in this population and is considered initial therapy, despite the fact that the optimal lipid-lowering diet has yet to be identified.[38]

Moore and colleagues[39] reported a decrease in total cholesterol levels without significant change in high density and low density lipoprotein levels along with a mean weight loss of 2 lb after patients followed the American Heart Association Step One diet for 8 weeks.[40] A significant decrease in total cholesterol and triglyceride levels with an improvement in high density lipoprotein levels and an average weight loss of 2.8 lb was reported by Shen and associates[40] after patients subscribed to a diet containing 500 mg or less of cholesterol, 35% of the total calories as fat, and less than 50% of the total calories as carbohydrate for 3 months. Another study followed patients for 1 year after diets were modified by restricting cholesterol intake to 300 mg or less, increasing polyunsaturated fat intake, restricting simple sugars, and discouraging the consumption of alcohol. These patients experienced significant decreases in total cholesterol levels and body weight and a substantial decrease in triglyceride levels.[41] A 3-week study conducted in a metabolic research unit reported significant decreases in cholesterol and triglyceride levels after 15 days of treatment with an experimental diet containing less than 300 mg of cholesterol.[42]

The efficacy of omega-3 fatty acids given at a dose of 3 g daily was investigated in a group of 31 renal transplant recipients. Patients experienced a significant reduction in serum triglyceride and very low density lipoprotein levels. No significant reductions in total cholesterol or other lipid fractions were evident. Pagenkemper and colleagues concluded that omega-3 fatty acids could be used at this dose for the reduction of serum triglycerides when reduction is not amenable to dietary intervention.[43]

Pharmacologic intervention for hyperlipidemia in renal transplant recipients may be considered when dietary therapy with increased exercise is unsuccessful. Several lipid-lowering agents are being investigated to determine the degree of interaction with immunosuppressive agents, incidence of complicating side effects, and overall efficacy in this population. Lipid-lowering dietary regimens are usually used in conjunction with pharmacologic agents.[30]

POSTTRANSPLANTATION DIABETES MELLITUS

The development of posttransplantation diabetes mellitus (PTDM) is a recognized long-term complication of renal transplantation. Boudreaux et al[44] reported the development of PTDM in 19% of 173 previously nondiabetic recipients. The incidence was greater in patients older than 45 years and heavier than 70 kg, and who were recipients of cadaveric donor kidneys.[44] These findings were confirmed by Sumrani and colleagues,[45] who studied their 5-year experience of 337 cyclosporine-treated recipients to identify the incidence of PTDM and the characteristics associated with its development. PTDM was diagnosed in 11.6% of the population, with onset appearing between the third and twelfth month after transplantation. The incidence was higher in black and hispanic recipients and was more likely to develop with cadaveric transplants and in older recipients. Patients with PTDM experienced more infection-related complications, and PTDM was associated with poorer patient and graft survival. In this study the incidence of PTDM was found to be independent of weight gain after transplantation; the degree of obesity, however, was not evaluated.[45] While studying obesity as a risk factor after cadaveric renal transplantation, Holley et al found the onset of PTDM to be significantly higher (12%) in the obese group of recipients than in the nonobese group (0%).[7]

Nutrition intervention for the patient with PTDM should comply with the most current medical literature. Specific nutrition concerns related to transplantation should be integrated into the overall care plan.

Pregnancy and Lactation

Along with the restoration of kidney function after successful renal transplantation comes the return of fertility. For many patients the possibility of pregnancy becomes a reality.[46] There have been more frequent reports of successful pregnancy outcomes after transplantation, even in patients with insulin-dependent diabetes mellitus.[47–50] General guidelines have been suggested for the transplant recipient desiring to conceive, to improve the possibility of a successful outcome. The patient should be in good general health and have adequate kidney function approximately 2 years after transplantation and minimal or no hypertension or proteinuria.[46,48] Once pregnancy has been confirmed, the patient should be monitored as a high-risk pregnancy. Preterm deliveries are reported in 45% to 60% of gestations, and intrauterine growth retardation is reported in at least 20% of gestations after renal transplantation.[46,48] Despite the high-risk status assigned to these patients, there is little or no mention of maternal nutritional status, weight gain, or differences in nutritional requirements (if there are any) in comparison with pregnancies in women without renal transplants.

Because immunosuppressive agents are secreted in breast milk and no definitive data exist regarding their effects on the infant, breast-feeding is presently discouraged.[46,48]

References

1. *U.S. Renal Data System 1990 Annual Data Report*. Bethesda, Md: National Institute of Diabetes and Digestive and Kidney Diseases, National Institutes of Health; August 1990.

2. Kumar MR, Coulston AM. Nutritional management of the cardiac transplant patient. *J Am Diet Assoc*. 1983;83:463–465.

3. Camel SP, Lawson KM. Nutrition education needs identified in the pretransplant evaluation. *CRN Q*. 1990;14:13–14.

4. Butterworth CE. Malnutrition in hospital patients: assessment and treatment. In: Goodhart RS,

Shils ME, eds. *Modern Nutrition in Health and Disease*. Philadelphia, Pa: Lea & Febiger; 1980.

5. Warnold I, Lundholm K. Clinical significance of preoperative nutritional status in 215 non-cancer patients. *Ann Surg*. 1984;199:299–305.

6. Windsor JA, Hill GL. Depleted protein stores lead to an increased complication rate after major surgery. *Aust NZ J Surg*. 1987;57:259.

7. Holley JL, Shapiro R, Lopatin WB, et al. Obesity as a risk factor following cadaveric renal transplantation. *Transplantation*. 1990;49:387–389.

8. Kahan BD. Cyclosporine. *N Engl J Med*. 1989;321:1725–1738.

9. Henry JL, Ferguson RM. Immunosuppression. In: Toled-Pereyra LH, ed. *Kidney Transplantation*. Philadelphia, Pa: FA Davis; 1988:187.

10. *Sandimmune Practical Guide*. East Hanover, NJ: Sandoz Pharmaceuticals Corp; 1988;SDI-104.

11. Seagraves A, Moore EE, Moore FA, et al. Net protein catabolic rate after kidney transplantation: impact of corticosteroid immunosuppression. *J Parenter Enter Nutr*. 1986;10:453–455.

12. Jequler E. Energy, obesity and body weight standards. *Am J Clin Nutr*. 1987;45:1035.

13. Cogan MG, Sargent JA, Yarbrough SG, et al. Prevention of prednisone induced negative nitrogen balance. *Ann Intern Med*. 1981;95:158.

14. Hoy WE, Sargent JA, Freeman RB, et al. The influence of glucocorticoid dose on protein catabolism after renal transplantation. *Am J Med Sci*. 1986;291:241–247.

15. Hoy WE, Sargent JA, Hall D, et al. Protein catabolism during the postoperative course after renal transplantation. *Am J Kidney Dis*. 1985;5:186.

16. Gammarino M. Renal transplant diet: recommendations for the acute phase. *Dial Transplant*. 1987;16:497,500–502.

17. Whittier FC, Evans DH, Dutton S, et al. Nutrition in renal transplantation. *Am J Kidney Dis*. 1985;6:405–411.

18. Edwards MS, Doster S. Renal transplant diet recommendations: results of a survey of renal dietitians in the United States. *J Am Diet Assoc*. 1990;90:843–846.

19. Rosenberg ME. Nutrition and transplantation. *Kidney*. 1986;18:19.

20. Mahajan SK, Prasad AS, Rabbani P, et al. Zinc deficiency: a reversible complication of uremia. *Am J Clin Nutr*. 1982;36:1177–1183.

21. Sandstead HH. Trace elements in uremia and hemodialysis. *Am J Clin Nutr*. 1980;33:1501–1508.

22. Mahajan SK, Abraham J, Migdal SD, et al. Effect of renal transplantation on zinc metabolism and taste acuity in uremia. *Transplantation*. 1984;38:599.

23. Ulmann A, Chkoff N, Lacour B. Disorders of calcium phosphorous metabolism after successful kidney transplantation. *Adv Nephrol*. 1983;12:331–340.

24. Beto J, Bansal VK. Hyperkalemia: evaluating dietary and nondietary etiology. *J Renal Nutr*. 1992;2:28–29.

25. Miller DG, Levine SE, D'Elia JA, et al. Nutritional status of diabetic and non-diabetic patients after renal transplantation. *Am J Clin Nutr*. 1986;44:66–69.

26. Levine SE. Determining changes in nutritional status following renal transplantation. *CRN Q*. 1987;11:15.

27. Reid IR, Ibbertson HK. Calcium supplements in the prevention of steroid-induced osteoporosis. *Am J Clin Nutr*. 1986;44:287–290.

28. Hahn TJ, Halstead LR, Buran DT. Effects of short term glucocorticoid administration on intestinal calcium absorption and circulating vitamin D metabolite concentrations. *Trans J Clin Endocrinol Metab*. 1981;2(suppl):111.

29. Morehouse ML, Marr CM, Paylinac JM, et al. Preliminary recommendations for calcium intake after renal transplantation: a pilot study. *CRN Q*. 1989;13:9.

30. Yatzidis H, Digenis P, Koutsicos D. Hypervitaminosis A in chronic renal failure after transplantation. *Br Med J*. 1976;1076:1675.

31. Yatzidis H, Digenis P, Fountas P. Hypervitaminosis A accompanying advanced renal failure. *Br Med J*. 1975;1075:352.

32. Kelleher J, Humphrey CS, Homer D, et al. Vitamin A and its transplant proteins in patients with chronic renal failure receiving maintenance haemodialysis and after renal transplantation. *Clin Sci*. 1983;65:619–626.

33. Lacour B, Parry C, Drueke T, et al. Pydrioxal 5-phosphate deficiency in uremic undialyzed, hemodialyzed, and non-uremic kidney transplant patients. *Clin Chem Acta*. 1983;127:205–215.

34. Zazgornik J, Druml W, Balcke P, et al. Diminished serum folic acid levels in renal transplant recipients. *Clin Nephrol*. 1982;18:306–310.

35. Kritchevsky D. Atherosclerosis: diet and risk factors. *Transplant Proc*. 1987;19(suppl 5):53–56.

36. Vathsala A, Weinberg RB, Schoenberg L, et al. Lipid abnormalities in cyclosporine-prednisone treated renal transplant recipients. *Transplantation*. 1989;48:37–43.

37. Bittar AE, Ratcliffe PJ, Richardson AJ.

The prevalence of hyperlipidemia in renal transplant recipients. *Transplantation*. 1990;50:987–992.

38. Kight RJ, Vathsala A, Schoenberg L, et al. Treatment of hyperlipidemia in renal transplant patients with gemfibrozil and dietary modification. *Transplantation*. 1992;53:224–225.

39. Moore RA, Callahan MF, Cody M, et al. The effect of the American Heart Association Step One diet on hyperlipidemia following renal transplantation. *Transplantation*. 1990;49:60–62.

40. Shen SY, Lukens CW, Alongi SV, et al. Patient profile and effect of dietary therapy on post-transplant hyperlipidemia. *Kidney Int*. 1983;24(suppl 16):147–152.

41. Disler PB, Goldberg RB, Kuhn L, et al. The role of diet in the pathogenesis and control of hyperlipidemia after renal transplantation. *Clin Nephrol*. 1981;16:29–34.

42. Nelson J, Beauregard MG, St Louis G, et al. Rapid improvement of hyperlipidemia in kidney transplant patients with multifactorial hypolipidemia diet. *Transplant Proc*. 1988;20:1264–1270.

43. Pagenkemper JJ, DiMarco NM, Hull AR. The management of hyperglyceridemia and hypercholesterolemia by omega-3 fatty acids in renal transplant patients. *CRN Q*. 1989;13:9.

44. Boudreaux JP, McHugh L, Canafax DM, et al. Cyclosporine, combination immunosuppression in posttransplant diabetes mellitus. *Transplant Proc*. 1987;19:1811–1813.

45. Sumrani NB, Delaney V, Ding Z, et al. Diabetes mellitus after renal transplantation in the cyclosporine era—an analysis of risk factors. *Transplantation*. 1991;51:343–347.

46. Gaudier FL, Santiago-Delphin E, Rivera J, et al. Pregnancy after renal transplantation. *Surg Gynecol Obstet*. 1988;167:533.

47. Hadi HA, Stafford CR, Williamson JR, et al. Pregnancy outcome in renal transplant recipients: experience at the Medical College of Georgia and review of literature. *South Med J*. 1986;79:959.

48. Davison JM. Renal transplantation and pregnancy. *Am J Dis*. 1987;9:374.

49. Vinicor F, Golichowski A, Filo R, et al. Pregnancy following renal transplantation in a patient with insulin-dependent diabetes mellitus. *Diabet Care*. 1984;7:280.

50. Burrows DA, O'Neil TJ, Sorrells TL. Successful twin pregnancy after renal transplant maintained on cyclosporine A immunosuppression. *Obstet Gynecol*. 1988;72:459.

7. NUTRITION MANAGEMENT OF THE PATIENT WITH DIABETES AND RENAL DISEASE

Renal Insufficiency

Patients with newly diagnosed insulin-dependent (type 1) diabetes mellitus (IDDM) frequently demonstrate urinary albumin excretion and an increase in glomerular filtration rate (GFR). This phenomenon appears to be related to the extracellular volume expansion and altered levels of glucagon, growth hormone, and vasoactive hormones induced by hyperglycemia. In turn, hyperfiltration increases the transglomerular protein filtration and causes albuminuria. With the institution of insulin therapy, urinary albumin excretion ceases. The GFR, while decreasing to some extent, usually remains elevated.

Persistent microalbuminuria (urinary albumin excretion of 30 to 300 mg/d), which may appear 5 to 10 years after the onset of IDDM, is highly predictive for diabetic nephropathy and may be indicative of early renal damage.[1–3] The rate of increase in albumin excretion correlates with the degree of metabolic and blood pressure control.[3–5]

Overt or clinical proteinuria (excretion of more than 500 mg of protein per day) in conjunction with hypertension is indicative of significant renal damage and predictive of progressive loss of function. It is followed by a rise in serum creatinine and a decrease in GFR. After the onset of nephrotic range proteinuria (excretion of more than 3 g per day), progression to ESRD usually occurs within 1 to 3 years.[4] Although there is a wide variation in the rate of deterioration, the decrease in function is linear and proceeds at a steady rate.[5]

Daily urinary protein losses are typically 4 to 8 g but may be as high as 20 to 30 g per 24 hours and result in hypoalbuminemia. In the person with diabetes, significant fluid retention secondary to microvascular changes often occurs at serum albumin concentrations of 3.0 to 3.4 mg/dL.[4]

Attempts to slow the progression of renal insufficiency include control of hypertension and normalization of blood glucose.[2,3,5] Tight glycemic control (blood glucose of 70–140 mg/dL and glycosylated hemoglobin A_{1c} [HbA_{1c}] of less than 8%[2,4]) and early effective blood pressure control have been shown to reverse microalbuminuria in its early stages.[5,6] However, once proteinuria exceeds 0.5 g per 24 hours, these interventions will only slow, rather than reverse, the progression of diabetic nephropathy.[5]

More recently, low protein, low phosphorus diets (independent of blood glucose and blood pressure changes) have been shown to decrease albuminuria, improve serum lipid profiles, and slow the decline of renal function.[3,7–11]

Zeller and coworkers recently reported the results of a prospective randomized study comparing the effects of a low protein, low phosphorus diet (0.6 g protein per kilogram, 2 g

69

sodium and 500 to 1000 mg phosphorus) and a control diet (more than 1 g/kg protein, 2 g sodium, and more than 1000 mg phosphorus) on the progression of renal failure in patients with IDDM.[11] Blood pressure and glycemic control were maintained in both groups. Protein intakes were calculated from the urinary excretion of urea nitrogen, normalized for ideal body weight, and adjusted for additional nitrogen losses. Compliance was calculated to be within 11% of prescribed for a mean follow-up period of 37 months. The patients given the study diet had a fourfold reduction in the rate of progression of renal failure, compared with patients following the control diet. There were no significant changes in serum lipid profile and no evidence of decreased nutritional status in patients given the study diet.

Diet for Diabetic Nephropathy

The American Diabetes Association's 1986 position statement for nutrition management of people with diabetes states that goals are (1) to improve blood glucose and lipid levels; (2) to promote consistent nutrient intake in IDDM and weight management in non-insulin-dependent diabetes mellitus; and (3) to encourage healthful eating habits throughout life, including nutrient modification necessitated by coexistent medical conditions.[12]

Target levels for particular nutrients in the diet for diabetic patients are based on these goals. The diet recommendations for diabetic nephropathy, while similar for some nutrients, must be modified for others, as illustrated in *Table 7.1*.

Table 7.1
Nutritional Requirements for Diabetic Patients

Nutrient	Target Goals for People With Diabetes	Predialysis Modifications for Diabetic Nephropathy
Calories	Achieve or maintain desirable weight	No change
Protein	0.8 g/kg or 12%–20% of calories	0.6 g/kg + urinary losses (0.8–1.0 g/kg if nephrotic); 67% high biological value
Carbohydrate	55%–60% of calories	55%–65% of calories
	Individualized	No change
	Unrefined or high fiber	As possible within diet
	Refined in modest amounts	As needed to meet calorie requirement
Fat	<30% of calories	As needed to meet calorie requirement
	<300 mg cholesterol	No change
Fiber	25 g/1000 kcal	As possible within diet
Vitamins	Supplements not necessary	As needed to meet RDA for water-soluble vitamins
Minerals		
Sodium	≤1 g/1000 kcal	No change
Phosphorus	RDA	≤10 mg/kg (if practical)
Calcium	RDA	Supplement to 1200–1600 mg

CALORIES

Calories should be sufficient to reach and/or maintain a reasonable weight. Recent research indicates that some people who follow a low protein diet cannot maintain nitrogen equilibrium unless their calorie intake is at least 35 kcal/kg.[13]

The restriction of dietary protein necessitates a change in the relative proportion of calories contributed by carbohydrate and fat. All unrefined carbohydrates contain protein, which must be accounted for in a low protein diet. While it is still important to include unrefined carbohydrates containing fiber, many high-fiber foods (bran, dried beans and peas, whole grains) contain large quantities of phosphorus and a significant amount of protein. It is therefore usually necessary to use some refined carbohydrates and/or wheat starch products to provide calories. Wheat starch products are the logical first choice because of their satiety value and similarity to real food. They are expensive, however, and some patients may not be willing or able to use them.

CARBOHYDRATE

Significant amounts of sucrose and other refined carbohydrates can be incorporated into the diet of patients with IDDM without adversely affecting blood glucose or serum lipid levels.[9,11,14,15] For best results, the refined carbohydrates should be distributed throughout the day, in conjunction with other foods, and intake should be consistent.

FAT

Increased serum concentrations of very low density (VLDL) and low density lipoproteins, along with decreased levels of high density lipoproteins (HDL) are common in diabetic nephropathy. Because there is growing evidence that these disorders play a role in the progression of renal injury as well as in the development of cardiovascular morbidity,[16] maintaining serum lipids at a desirable level is a primary management goal. The limited amount of animal protein in the diet makes it relatively easy to substitute polyunsaturated and monounsaturated fats for saturated fat. It may not be possible, however, to keep the percentage of calories from fat below 30% and still meet caloric requirements. Researchers have demonstrated that a low protein diet in which the polyunsaturated to saturated fat ratio is 2:1 and cholesterol content no greater than 300 mg results in decreased VLDL and increased HDL levels, even with fat contributing more than 30% of the calories.[10,17–19]

PROTEIN

When dietary protein is restricted to approximately 0.6 to 0.8 g/kg, the rate of decline in renal function is blunted and urinary protein excretion diminished.[7,9,11] Thus, given the risk associated with hyperfiltration, protein content of the diet for diabetic patients should not exceed the RDA.[12]

Because insulin deficiency increases the rate of protein degradation and amino acid oxidation, the person with diabetes may be at greater risk for malnutrition while following a low protein diet.[20] Further, recent studies indicate that people with IDDM may be unable to preserve lean tissue mass and muscle function while following low protein diets. Preliminary data from one study showed that IDDM patients with early nephropathy and receiving 0.6 g/kg protein had persistently negative nitrogen balance, decreased muscle strength, and a reduction in lean to fat tissue ratio, while body weight, serum albumin, and transferrin levels remained unchanged.[20]

Currently, a protein intake of 0.6 to 0.8 g/kg[21,22] or 0.6 g/kg plus an amount equal to urinary losses[11] is recommended for the person with clinical proteinuria and evidence of progressive disease. Approximately two thirds of the protein should come from high-quality sources.

The patient with hypoalbuminemia secondary to nephrotic syndrome will require adequate protein and calories to facilitate albumin synthesis and replete the albumin pool. A protein intake of 0.8 to 1.0 g/kg should provide adequate amino acids for repletion yet still result in decreased urinary albumin excretion.[23,24]

SODIUM

Blood pressure control is an essential step in the management of the vascular complications associated with diabetic nephropathy. Because the hypertension associated with diabetes is usually related to volume expansion, a sodium restriction of 80 to 100 mEq is appropriate in most cases. If hyponatremia develops, a fluid restriction may also be required.

Follow-up

Because of metabolic derangements and urinary protein losses, negative nitrogen balance and nutrition problems can develop quickly. Frequent follow-up, including counseling and monitoring of nutritional status, is essential to identify problems before they become serious. It can be difficult for optimal calorie and protein levels to be maintained with a low protein diet. Ihle et al noted significant decreases in total lymphocyte count and serum transferrin levels in conjunction with an initial weight loss in patients treated with a low protein diet.[25] The problem was corrected and adequate intake was eventually achieved with additional education, diet adjustments, and/or supplementation.

Periodic assessment should include measurement of serum protein levels, urinary protein losses, weight, blood pressure, and glycemic control. Serial anthropometric measurements should also be obtained, since some patients on low protein diets have demonstrated substantial loss of muscle mass without a change in serum albumin level.[25-27] During periods of increased protein need (eg, infection, surgery) protein intake should be liberalized to meet the current nitrogen requirements of the patient.

Glycemic Control

The change in the fuel mix of the diet is likely to necessitate adjustment of insulin dosage and/or schedule. Blood glucose levels should be monitored and used to optimize insulin treatment. Because of glucose intolerance and a decrease in small peptide hormone catabolism by the diseased kidney, insulin requirements become inconsistent and may decrease significantly as the patient approaches end-stage disease. Blood sugar levels must be monitored closely and insulin adjusted as necessary to prevent hypoglycemia.

In the diabetic patient with advanced renal insufficiency, urine glucose testing is no longer accurate. The interpretation of HbA_{1c} levels can be complicated by anemia and by an elevated BUN concentration.[28] Therefore, comparing a single HbA_{1c} level with normal or desirable levels cannot be used as a method of determining the quality of glycemic control. Serial glycosylated hemoglobin values, however, can be useful in following trends in management. Uremic symptoms develop in patients with diabetic nephropathy at a higher level of function than in patients with other types of kidney failure. This may be at least partially from malnutrition, which results in decreased muscle mass and lower creatinine excretion. Dialysis is usually required when serum creatinine concentration is in the range of 5 to 10 mg/dL and GFR is approximately 10 mL/min.[4]

Hemodialysis

Diabetic nephropathy is the most prevalent and fastest growing cause of renal failure in the United States, accounting for 30% to 50% of patients entering chronic dialysis programs.[29] At initiation of dialysis, diabetic patients have more comorbid conditions, a higher incidence of complications, and are less well nourished in comparison with patients with other types of kidney disease.[30,31] Thus, they require more time of health professionals and demonstrate less rehabilitation potential than their nondiabetic counterparts. Survival, although greatly improved from the past, remains significantly lower in diabetic patients than in other patients treated with hemodialysis.

Nutritional requirements are similar to those of nondiabetic patients undergoing dialysis (see chapter 4). In addition, consistency in composition and timing of meals to control blood glucose levels is extremely important. In this patient population, blood glucose levels between 100 and 200 mg/dL indicate good management and are usually best achieved with a multiple mixed-dose insulin regimen. Slomowitz et al[32] reported that a minimum intake of 35 kcal/kg of desirable weight was required for patients undergoing hemodialysis to maintain nitrogen equilibrium. Because of suboptimal appetite and gastrointestinal problems, aggressive nutritional intervention is often required. Frequently, supplements are necessary to meet the calorie and protein needs of the patient.

Gastrointestinal Problems

Dialyzed diabetic patients are susceptible to gastrointestinal disorders including gastroparesis diabeticorum, an autonomic neuropathy associated with alternating bouts of diarrhea and constipation. Hyperglycemia, elevated BUN concentration, hemodialysis, and peritoneal dialysis have all been shown to impair gastric emptying.[4] Hyperosmolar solutions also may retard gastric emptying.[33] Early satiety and epigastric pain, as well as nausea and vomiting, are common symptoms. Undigested food remains in the stomach and may be vomited several hours after ingestion. The patient can actually experience an insulin reaction 1 to 2 hours after eating a meal.

It is important to monitor blood glucose levels closely and adjust insulin accordingly. Treatment with metaclopromide, which accelerates gastric motility and acts as an antiemetic, may ease symptoms in some patients. Small frequent feedings and liquids are usually best tolerated. Some patients with prolonged problems may require total parenteral nutrition or postpyloric tube feeding to maintain nutritional status.

Hypoglycemia

The usual methods of treating an insulin reaction may result in fluid overload and/or hyperkalemia in the oliguric diabetic patient. Jelly beans, pieces of hard candy, honey or jelly packets, and commercial glycemic agents are easy to carry and raise the blood glucose level without compromising the electrolyte and/or fluid status of the patient (*Table 7.2*).

Table 7.2
Glycemic Agents

Food	Amount to Equal 15 g Carbohydrate
Jelly beans	10
Roll (hard) candy	8 pieces
Honey or jelly	1 tbsp

Hyperglycemia

Glycemic control is a major factor in determining the length and quality of life in this patient population. Because of the absence of glycosuria, these patients are prone to rapid rises and wide fluctuations in blood sugar. Because there is no osmotic diuresis, with resulting dehydration and electrolyte losses, extremely high glucose levels may be present even though the patient may not appear symptomatic. Complications of hyperglycemia include thirst and fluid overload, hyperkalemia, hyperlipidemia, wasting, and deterioration of nutritional status.

THIRST AND FLUID OVERLOAD

Patients with diabetes have been shown to experience greater interdialytic weight gains than nondiabetic patients.[34] Thirst related to hyperglycemia can be severe, and fluid control is difficult. The resulting excess fluid intake can result in volume-dependent hypertension, pulmonary edema, and congestive heart failure. Further, fluid overload combined with hyperglycemia can cause osmotic shifts that contribute to hemodynamic instability and increase the risk of hypotensive episodes during dialysis.

HYPERKALEMIA

Because insulin is a major regulator of serum potassium concentration, hyperglycemia can produce life-threatening hyperkalemia by shifting fluid and potassium from intracellular to extracellular spaces.

HYPERLIPIDEMIA

After dialytic therapy is initiated, cholesterol levels tend to improve, but triglyceride levels worsen.[35] In the face of insulin deficiency, depressed levels of lipoprotein lipase reduce triglyceride clearance from the blood, further aggravating hyperlipidemia. Hyperglycemia, therefore, contributes to elevated serum triglyceride levels, which may increase the risk of a cardiovascular event.

MALNUTRITION AND LOSS OF NUTRIENTS

In the presence of hyperglycemia, dialysis can be a catabolic event. Glucose losses across the dialysis membrane can be considerable if the blood glucose concentration significantly exceeds that of the dialysate. Removal of glucose, while normalizing blood sugar levels, stimulates glucogenolysis and gluconeogenesis, resulting in protein catabolism and increased losses of amino acids across the dialysis membrane.

Peritoneal Dialysis

Continuous ambulatory peritoneal dialysis (CAPD) results in more steady-state chemical and fluid balance and provides better control of blood pressure and blood sugar than does hemodialysis.[36,37] In addition, residual renal function is better preserved,[37] allowing a more liberal diet and fluid regimen.

Hypertonic dextrose is the osmotic agent used to achieve fluid removal during CAPD. Absorption of glucose from the dialysate is significant and accounts for 15% to 30% of the daily calories.[38] This chronic absorption of dextrose may exacerbate hyperlipidemia, because cholesterol and triglyceride levels are higher in the CAPD population than in patients treated with hemodialysis.[35]

Despite glucose absorption from the dialysate, good blood sugar control, evidenced by near normal glycosylated hemoglobin levels, can be achieved.[36,37] Intraperitoneal insulin (added to the dialysate) is preferred, since it allows ongoing delivery of insulin to portal circulation.[37] If necessary, it can be supplemented with subcutaneous injections as indicated by blood glucose monitoring.

Patients treated with CAPD chronically lose 5 to 12 g of protein daily via the dialysate.[36,39] The amount of protein loss increases with the concentration of dextrose used,[39] and if peritonitis develops, these losses rise dramatically.[40] Protein needs are generally in the range of 1.2 to 1.5 g/kg of ideal body weight,[40] and good nutritional status can be difficult to achieve in the diabetic patient treated with this mode of dialysis. Satiety, anorexia, and nausea can be exacerbated by the presence of dialysate in the abdomen[37] and interfere with adequate intake. Frequent small meals and the use of metaclopromide may alleviate these symptoms.[37] However, because the combination of inadequate protein intake, gastrointestinal problems, and protein losses can quickly lead to malnutrition, supplements may be required to meet protein needs.

A patient who maintains optimum sodium and fluid intake is less likely to require frequent use of the higher dextrose concentrations, and therefore may have fewer problems with hyperglycemia, hyperlipidemia, malnutrition, and excess weight gain. Because of the impact of chronic dextrose absorption on nutritional status, other osmotic agents such as amino acids are being investigated.[41] Requirements for other nutrients are discussed in chapter 5.

Renal Transplantation

Because diabetic patients tend to be undernourished while being treated with dialysis, they are especially sensitive to the complications associated with high-dose steroid administration following transplantation. The lower steroid doses, made possible by the concurrent use of cyclosporine and antilymphocyte serum, have proved to lessen these complications and therefore are of great benefit to diabetic renal graft recipients.

Increased protein catabolic rate and negative nitrogen balance occur in the acute posttransplantation phase because of the combined effects of surgery and high-dose steroid treatment.[42,43] Evidence suggests that a high protein diet (1.3 to 2.0 g/kg) during this period may improve nitrogen balance,[42,44] thereby reducing the risk for poor wound healing, gastrointestinal ulceration, and infection. After approximately 1 month, a maintenance level of 1 g/kg of protein per day is recommended.[45]

Hyperlipidemia is exacerbated by steroid immunosuppression, and diabetic patients are likely to present with elevated levels of triglyceride and cholesterol in addition to depressed levels of HDL-C.[36] Altered glucose metabolism induced by glucocorticoids causes a sluggish response to insulin. Consequently, blood glucose levels can be difficult to control. Blood glucose monitoring and coordination of diet, insulin, and activity are necessary to attain optimal glycemic control.

Good blood sugar management in the posttransplantation patient with diabetes is of primary importance, since it appears that euglycemia can protect the transplanted kidney from recurrent diabetic glomerulopathy. Evidence for this includes a case in which glomerulosclerosis that developed in the graft of a diabetic transplant recipient reversed after pancreatic transplantation, with resultant normalization of blood glucose levels.[46] It has also been reported that glomerulosclerosis in a cadaver kidney (from a diabetic donor) reversed following transplantation into a nondiabetic recipient.[47]

Levine[48] examined nutrition parameters (height, weight, serum albumin and transferrin levels, triceps skinfold thickness, and midarm muscle circumference) in 45 patients before and 2 years after transplantation. She found that nutritional repletion, evidenced by increased visceral and somatic protein levels, occurred after transplantation. The diabetic renal transplant patients, however, tended to have significantly lower body weight and midarm muscle circumferences than nondiabetic patients, suggesting a definite need for more aggressive nutrition counseling in the population with diabetes.

Pretransplant nutritional status, lipid profile, and blood glucose control should all be taken into consideration when determining posttransplant nutrition priorities. Diet modification should be individualized with respect to clinical parameters and may include sodium restriction, lipid modification, and weight control. Guidelines for modification of nutrients are similar to those for nondiabetic patients and are covered in chapter 6.

References

1. Herman W, Hawthorne V, Hamman R, et al. Consensus statement: international workshop on preventing the kidney disease of diabetes mellitus. *Am J Kidney Dis.* 1989;13:2–6.

2. Mogensen CE. Prevention and treatment of renal disease in insulin-dependent diabetes mellitus. *Semin Nephrol.* 1990;10:260–273.

3. Viberti GC. Interventions based on microalbuminuria screening and low-protein diet in the treatment of kidney disease of diabetes mellitus. *Am J Kidney Dis.* 1989;13:41–44.

4. Markell MS, Friedman EA. Care of the diabetic patient with end-stage renal disease. *Semin Nephrol.* 1990;10:274–286.

5. Viberti G, Bending JJ. Preventive approach to diabetic kidney disease. *Controv Nephrol.* 1988;61:91–100.

6. Krolewski AS, Canessa M, Warram JH, et al. Predisposition to hypertension and susceptibility to renal disease in insulin-dependent diabetes mellitus. *N Engl J Med.* 1988;318:140–145.

7. Evanoff G, Thompson C, Brown J, Weinman E. Prolonged dietary protein restriction in diabetic nephropathy. *Arch Intern Med.* 1989;149:1129–1133.

8. Cohen D, Dodds R, Viberti G. Effect of protein restriction in insulin dependent diabetics at risk of nephropathy. *Br Med J.* 1987;294:795–798.

9. Walker JD, Dodds RA, Murrells TJ, et al. Restriction of dietary protein and progression of renal failure in diabetic nephropathy. *Lancet.* 1989;2:1411–1415.

10. Ciavarella A, DiMizio G, Stefoni S, Borgnino LC, Vannini P. Reduced albuminuria after dietary protein restriction in insulin-dependent diabetic patients with clinical nephropathy. *Diabetes Care.* 1987;10:407–413.

11. Zeller K, Whittaker E, Sullivan L, Raskin P, Jacobson HR. Effect of restricting dietary protein on the progression of renal failure in patients with insulin-dependent diabetes mellitus. *N Engl J Med.* 1991;324:78–84.

12. American Diabetes Association. Nutritional recommendations and principles for individuals with diabetes mellitus: 1986. *Diabetes Care.* 1987;10:126–132.

13. Kopple JD, Monteon RJ, Shaib JK. Effect of energy intake on nitrogen metabolism in nondia-

lyzed patients with chronic renal failure. *Kidney Int.* 1986;29:734–742.

14. Wise JE, Keim KS, Husinga JL, Willmann PA. Effect of sucrose-containing snacks on blood glucose control. *Diabetes Care.* 1989;12:423–426.

15. Bantle JP, Laine DC, Castle GW, Thomas JW, Hoogwerf BJ, Goetz FC. Postprandial glucose and insulin responses to meals containing different carbohydrates in normal and diabetic subjects. *N Engl J Med.* 1983;309:7–12.

16. Keane WF, Kasiske BL, O'Donnell MP. Hyperlipidemia and the progression of renal disease. *Am J Clin Nutr.* 1988;47:157–160.

17. Loschiavo C, Ferrari S, Panebianco R, et al. Effect of protein-restricted diet on serum lipids and atherosclerosis risk factors in patients with chronic renal failure. *Clin Nephrol.* 1988;29:113–118.

18. Sanfelippo ML, Swenson LS, Reaven GM. Response of plasma triglycerides to dietary changes in patients on hemodialysis. *Kidney Int.* 1978;14:180–186.

19. Loschiavo C, Ferrari S, Aprili F, Grigolini L, Faccini G, Maschio G. Modification of serum and membrane lipid composition induced by diet in patients with chronic renal failure. *Clin Nephrol.* 1990;34:267–271.

20. Brodsky IG. Nutritional therapy for patients with diabetic nephropathy. In: Anderson P, Snetselaar L, eds. *Renal Nutrition: Report of the Eleventh Ross Roundtable on Medical Issues.* Columbus, Ohio: Ross Laboratories; 1991.

21. Tuttle KR, DeFronzo RA, Stein JH. Treatment of diabetic nephropathy: a rational approach based on its pathophysiology. *Semin Nephrol.* 1991;11:220–235.

22. Mitch WE. Dietary protein restriction in patients with chronic renal failure. *Kidney Int.* 1991;40:326–341.

23. Kaysen GA. Albumin metabolism in the nephrotic syndrome: the effect of dietary protein intake. *Am J Kidney Dis.* 1988;12:461–480.

24. Kaysen GA, Gambertoglio J, Jimenez I, Jones H, Hutchinson FN. Effect of dietary protein intake on albumin homeostasis in nephrotic patients. *Kidney Int.* 1986;29:572–577.

25. Ihle BU, Becker GJ, Whitworth JA, Charlwood RA, Kincaid-Smith PS. The effect of protein restriction on the progression of renal insufficiency. *N Engl J Med.* 1989;321:1773–1777.

26. Lucas PA, Meadows JH, Roberts DE, Coles GA. The risks and benefits of a low protein-essential amino acid keto acid diet. *Kidney Int.* 1986;29:995–1003.

27. Kopple JD, Berg R, Houser H, Steinman TI, Teschan P. Nutritional status of patients with dif-

ferent levels of chronic renal insufficiency. *Kidney Int.* 1989;36(suppl):S184–S194.

28. Fluckiger R, Harmon W, Meier W, Loo S, Gabbay KH. Hemoglobin carbamylation in uremia. *Med Intell.* 1981;304:823–827.

29. Eggers PW. Mortality rates among dialysis patients in Medicare's End-Stage Renal Disease Program. *Am J Kidney Dis.* 1990;5:414–421.

30. Collins AJ, Hanson G, Umen A, Kjellstrand C, Keshaviah P. Changing risk factor demographics in end-stage renal disease patients entering hemodialysis and the impact on long-term mortality. *Kidney Dis.* 1990;5:422–432.

31. Miller DG, Levine S, Bistrian B, D'Elia JA. Diagnosis of protein calorie malnutrition in diabetic patients on hemodialysis and peritoneal dialysis. *Nephron.* 1983;33:127–132.

32. Slomowitz A, Monteon RJ, Grosvenor M, Laidlaw SA, Kopple JD. Effect of energy intake on nutritional status in maintenance hemodialysis patients. *Kidney Int.* 1989;35:704–711.

33. Nompleggi D, Bell SJ, Blackburn GL, Bistrian BR. Overview of gastrointestinal disorders due to diabetes mellitus: emphasis on nutritional support. *J Parenter Enter Nutr.* 1990;13:84–91.

34. Jones R, Poston L, Hinestrosa H, Parsons V, Williams R. Weight gain between dialyses in diabetics: possible significance of raised intracellular sodium content. *Br Med J.* 1980;19:153.

35. Avram MM, Antignani A, Goldwasser P, et al. Lipids in diabetic and nondiabetic hemodialysis and CAPD patients. *Trans Am Soc Artif Intern Org.* 1988;34:314–316.

36. Passlick J, Grabensee B. CAPD and transplantation in diabetics. *Clin Nephrol.* 1988;30:S18–S23.

37. Gokal R, Friedman EA, Rottenbourg J, Tzamaloukas AH. Peritoneal dialysis in diabetic ESRD patients. *Dial Transplant.* 1991;20:59–66.

38. Rubin J, Walsh D, Bower JD. Diabetes, dialysate losses, and serum lipids during continuous ambulatory peritoneal dialysis. *Am J Kidney Dis.* 1987;8:104–108.

39. Blumenkrantz MJ, Gahl GM, Kopple JD, et al. Protein losses during peritoneal dialysis. *Kidney Int.* 1981;19:593–602.

40. Bannister DK, Acchiardo SR, Moore LW, Kraus AP. Nutritional effects of peritonitis in continuous ambulatory peritoneal dialysis (CAPD) patients. *J Am Diet Assoc.* 1987;87:53–56.

41. Arfeen S, Goodship THJ, Kirkwood A, Ward MK. The nutritional and hormonal effects of 8 weeks of CAPD with a 1% amino acid solution. *Clin Nephrol.* 1990;33:192–199.

42. Aplasca EC, Rammohan M. The effect of

prednisone on the levels of serum albumin of 20 patients with renal transplants. *J Am Diet Assoc.* 1986;86:1404–1405.

43. Seagraves A, Moore EE, Moore FA, Weil R. Net protein catabolic rate after kidney transplantation: impact of corticosteroid immunosuppression. *J Parenter Enter Nutr.* 1986;10:453–455.

44. Whittier FC, Evans DH, Dutton S, et al. Nutrition in renal transplantation. *Am J Kidney Dis.* 1985;6:405–411.

45. Gammarino M. Renal transplant diet: recommendations for the acute phase. *Dial Transplant.* 1987;16:497–502.

46. Najarian JS. Operating on uremic diabetics. In: Friedman EA, L'Esperance FA Jr, eds. *The Diabetic Renal-Retinal Syndrome: Prevention and Management.* New York, NY: Grune & Stratton; 1981.

47. Abouna GM, Al-Adnani MS, Kremer GD. Reversal of diabetic nephropathy in human cadaveric kidney after transplantation and into nondiabetic recipient. *Lancet.* 1983;2:1274–1276.

48. Levine SE. Determining changes in nutritional status following renal transplantation. *CRN Q.* 1987;11:15.

8. NUTRITION RECOMMENDATIONS FOR INFANTS, CHILDREN, AND ADOLESCENTS WITH END-STAGE RENAL DISEASE

The goal in nutrition management of the child with ESRD is to promote optimal growth and development while minimizing the physiologic and biochemical consequences of uremia. This chapter provides the dietitian with suggested guidelines to be implemented with the full understanding that individuality, flexibility, and resourcefulness are essential to ensure diet compliance and successful outcomes in the areas of growth and development.

When working with the child, the dietitian must establish a rapport with both the child and the primary caretakers to enhance compliance with the nutritional regimen. The patient's age determines who becomes the focus of the dietitian's attention. With an infant, the parents or primary caretaker are responsible for food intake and should be instructed accordingly. The adolescent usually eats independently and must therefore receive information directly. With a child in grade school, the parents and the child should be involved in dietary management.

Children sometimes demonstrate erratic appetites and manipulative behavior regarding food selection. The dietitian can help the parents by explaining priorities in the diet and making suggestions for appropriate limit-setting techniques.

Full compliance with all dietary restrictions is not always a realistic expectation. Priorities must be set on an individual basis, depending on the patient's physical status, emotional needs, and social situation. While the ideal goal is full compliance with a regimen, partial compliance often becomes acceptable. Compliance may be enhanced through rapport with the patient and family members, simplified regimens, concrete explanation, and ongoing evaluation of comprehension.[1]

Assessment of Nutritional Status

Nutrition assessment in pediatric patients should be performed on a frequent, ongoing basis because of growth and developmental needs. Diet histories, biochemical parameters, fluid balance, bowel habits, urine output, and medications are evaluated in a manner similar to that for adults. Additional clinical manifestations such as the condition of the tongue, teeth, breath, and hair should also be noted.

Growth parameters, obtained by using standardized techniques, should be measured regularly.[2,3] The importance of a wall-mounted stadiometer for height and a board for measuring the length of infants cannot be overstated. Measurements are most accurate when taken by only one observer using the same equipment. Height, weight, and head circumference (for children 36 months of age or less) are plotted by age and sex on standardized growth charts developed by the National Center for Health Statistics.[4] Midarm circumference, midarm muscle circumference, and triceps skinfold are compared with values for healthy children of the same age and sex in the absence of "normal" values for children with renal disease.[5]

The age of the child can be evaluated in three different ways. The chronological age is the actual age of the child in months or years. The height age is the age at which the actual height of the child crosses the 50th percentile for height on the growth chart for the appropriate sex. The bone age is based on the epiphyseal maturation demonstrated by radiography of the hands and wrists.

These measurements are often discrepant. The chronological and height ages are more commonly used, because the bone age is frequently not readily available. When chronological and height ages are widely discrepant, one should individualize treatment. Particularly in the area of caloric needs, the lower of the two values may be used as a starting point for goal setting and increased as necessary.

Formulation of the Dietary Prescription

A nutrition care plan containing the diet prescription and the goals and objectives for expected patient skills and behavior is developed for each child on the bases of assessment and psychosocial factors. Objectives are both short and long term. The plan is modified as necessary according to changes in the child's nutritional status, renal function, dialytic therapy, medication regimen, and psychosocial situation.

Tables 8.1 to *8.4* outline suggested levels of nutrients in the various modalities of the treatment of the child with ESRD. Levels should be based on a nonedematous weight. Restrictions in nutrients should be imposed when there is a clear indication rather than an anticipated prophylactic need. Possible exceptions are restriction of protein in a predialysis patient and sodium in a transplant patient. When a range of values is given (ie, 1 to 3 mEq/kg), the upper end of the range should be used initially and decreased if necessary. In general, the more restrictive a diet is, the less likely it is that the child will receive adequate calorie intake, because he or she may become less willing to eat.

Calculation of "ideal" energy intake may be based on one of three methods. One is the ideal calories for chronological age, based on RDA.[6] Second is the RDA for calories for the height age. A third way may be used when the height is not available, by using 100 kcal/kg for the first 10 kg, 50 kcal/kg for the next 10 kg, and 20 kcal/kg for each additional kilogram.[7] For example, a 22-kg child would ideally require 1000 kcal for the first 10 kg plus 500 for the next 10 kg and 20 × 2 for the remaining 2 kg, for a total of 1540 kcal (or 70 kcal/kg). Measurements of resting energy expenditure, obtained by using indirect calorimetry, may be useful in determining caloric needs.

Protein needs should be calculated on the basis of chronological age or height age, whichever value is lower. Other nutrient needs may be estimated on the basis of chronological age.

Table 8.1
Daily Nutrient and Fluid Recommendations for the Child With ESRD—Predialysis

	Age			
	Infant (0–1 y)	*Toddler (1–3 y)*	*Child (4–10 y)*	*Adolescent (11–18 y)*
Energy	0–0.5 y: ≥108 kcal/kg 0.5–1 y: ≥98 kcal/kg	102 kcal/kg	4–6 y: 90 kcal/kg 7–10 y: 70 kcal/kg	Girls 11–14 y: 47 kcal/kg Girls 15–18 y: 40 kcal/kg Boys 11–14 y: 55 kcal/kg Boys 15–18 y: 45 kcal/kg
Protein	0–0.5 y: 2.2 g/kg 0.5–1.0 y: 1.6 g/kg	1.2 g/kg	4–6 y: 1.2 g/kg 7–10 y: 1.0 g/kg	11–14 y: 1.0 g/kg 15–18 y: 0.9 g/kg
Sodium	Generally unrestricted; 1–3 mEq/kg if edema or HTN present	Generally unrestricted; 1–3 mEq/kg if edema or HTN present	Generally unrestricted; 1–3 mEq/kg if edema or HTN present	Generally unrestricted; 1–3 mEq/kg if edema or HTN present
Potassium	1–3 mEq/kg if needed (usually not until GFR is <10% normal)	1–3 mEq/kg if needed (usually not until GFR is <10% normal)	1–3 mEq/kg if needed (usually not until GFR is <10% normal)	1–3 mEq/kg if needed (usually not until GFR is <10% normal)
Calcium	0–0.5 y: 400 mg/d 0.5–1.0 y: 600 mg/d (provided hypercalcemia does not occur and calcium-phosphorus product does not exceed 70)	800 mg/d (provided hypercalcemia does not occur and calcium-phosphorus product does not exceed 70)	800 mg/d (provided hypercalcemia does not occur and calcium-phosphorus product does not exceed 70)	1200 mg/d (provided hypercalcemia does not occur and calcium-phosphorus product does not exceed 70)
Phosphorus	Use low-content formula if serum levels of phosphate are elevated; restrict high-content foods	Usually 600–800 mg/d when serum levels are elevated	Usually 600–800 mg/d when serum levels are elevated	600–800 mg/d when serum levels are elevated

(Continued)

Table 8.1—continued
Daily Nutrient and Fluid Recommendations for the Child With ESRD—Predialysis

	Age			
	Infant (0–1 y)	*Toddler (1–3 y)*	*Child (4–10 y)*	*Adolescent (11–18 y)*
Vitamins	1 mL multivitamin drops; vitamin D metabolite if needed, based on serum calcium, PTH, and alkaline phosphatase levels	Multivitamin if needed; vitamin D metabolite if needed, based on serum calcium, PTH, and alkaline phosphatase levels	Multivitamin if needed; vitamin D metabolite if needed, based on serum calcium, PTH, and alkaline phosphatase levels	Multivitamin or just B complex + C if needed; vitamin D metabolite if needed, based on serum calcium, PTH, and alkaline phosphatase levels
Trace minerals	Supplement zinc, iron, or copper if needed	Supplement zinc, iron, or copper if needed	Supplement zinc, iron, or copper if needed	Supplement zinc, iron, or copper if needed
Fluid	Unrestricted unless needed; then replace insensible + urinary output	Unrestricted unless needed; then replace insensible + urinary output	Unrestricted unless needed; then replace insensible + urinary output	Unrestricted unless needed; then replace insensible + urinary output

HTN, hypertension; GFR, glomerular filtration rate; PTH, parathyroid hormone.

Table 8.2
Daily Nutrient and Fluid Recommendations for the Child With ESRD—Hemodialysis

	Age			
	Infant (0–1 y)	*Toddler (1–3 y)*	*Child (4–10 y)*	*Adolescent (11–18 y)*
Energy	Same as for predialysis	Same as for predialysis	Same as for predialysis	Same as for predialysis
Protein	0–0.5 y: 3.3 g/kg 0.5–1.0 y: 2.4 g/kg	≥1.8 g/kg	4–6 y: ≥1.8 g/kg 7–10 y: ≥1.5 g/kg	≥1.3–1.5 g/kg
Sodium	1–3 mEq/kg if needed	Same as for predialysis	Same as for predialysis	Same as for predialysis

	Age			
	Infant (0–1 y)	*Toddler (1–3 y)*	*Child (4–10 y)*	*Adolescent (11–18 y)*
Potassium	1–3 mEq/kg if needed	Same as for predialysis	Same as for predialysis	Same as for predialysis
Calcium	Same as for predialysis	Same as for predialysis	Same as for predialysis	Same as for predialysis
Phosphorus	Same as for predialysis	600–800 mg/d	600–800 mg/d	600–800 mg/d
Vitamins	1 mL multivitamin drops, 1 mg folic acid, and vitamin D metabolite (in most cases)	Multivitamin, 1 mg folic acid, and vitamin D metabolite as needed	B-complex vitamin containing 1 mg folic acid, 10 mg pyridoxine, 60 mg ascorbic acid, 5 mg pantothenic acid, 1.0 mg thiamin, 1.2 mg riboflavin; 3 μg B_{12}, 300 μg biotin, 15 mg niacin; active form of vitamin D as needed	B-complex vitamin containing 1 mg folic acid, 10 mg pyridoxine, 60 mg ascorbic acid, 10 mg pantothenic acid, 1.5 mg thiamin, 1.7 mg riboflavin; 6 μg B_{12}, 300 μg biotin, 20 mg niacin; active form of vitamin D as needed
Trace minerals	Supplement zinc or copper if needed. Iron is usually needed with recombinant erythropoietin	Supplement zinc or copper if needed. Iron is usually needed with recombinant erythropoietin	Supplement zinc or copper if needed. Iron is usually needed with recombinant erythropoietin	Supplement zinc or copper if needed. Iron is usually needed with recombinant erythropoietin
Fluid	Provide insensible + urinary output + ultrafiltration capacity (if possible)	Provide insensible + urinary output	Provide insensible + urinary output	Provide insensible + urinary output

Table 8.3
Daily Nutrient and Fluid Recommendations for the Child With ESRD—Peritoneal Dialysis

	Age			
	Infant (0–1 y)	*Toddler (1–3 y)*	*Child (4–10 y)*	*Adolescent (11–18 y)*
Energy	Same as for predialysis	Same as for predialysis	Same as for predialysis	Same as for predialysis
Protein	2.5–4.0 g/kg	2.0–2.5 g/kg	2.0–2.5 g/kg	1.5 g/kg
Sodium	Same as for predialysis	Same as for predialysis	Same as for predialysis	Same as for predialysis
Potassium	Same as for predialysis	Same as for predialysis	Same as for predialysis	Same as for predialysis
Calcium	Same as for predialysis	Same as for predialysis	Same as for predialysis	Same as for predialysis
Phosphorus	Same as for predialysis	Same as for hemodialysis	Same as for hemodialysis	Same as for hemodialysis
Vitamins	Same as for hemodialysis	Same as for hemodialysis	Same as for hemodialysis	Same as for hemodialysis
Trace minerals	Same as for hemodialysis	Same as for hemodialysis	Same as for hemodialysis	Same as for hemodialysis
Fluid	Same as for hemodialysis	Unrestricted unless needed	Unrestricted unless needed	Unrestricted unless needed

Table 8.4
Daily Nutrient and Fluid Recommendations for the Child With ESRD—Transplantation

	Age			
	Infant (0–1 y)	*Toddler (1–3 y)*	*Child (4–10 y)*	*Adolescent (11–18 y)*
Energy	Same as for predialysis after ideal weight/ length is achieved	Same as for predialysis after ideal weight/ height is achieved	Same as for predialysis after ideal weight/ height is achieved	Same as for predialysis after ideal weight/ height is achieved

	Age			
	Infant (0–1 y)	*Toddler (1–3 y)*	*Child (4–10 y)*	*Adolescent (11–18 y)*
Protein	Usually 3 g/kg initially; RDA after approximately 3 mo	Usually 2–3 g/kg initially; RDA after approximately 3 mo	2–3 g/kg initially; RDA after approximately 3 mo	2 g/kg initially; RDA after approximately 3 mo
Sodium	1–3 mEq/kg initially	1–2 g/d initially; unrestricted when HTN and edema no longer present	Usually 2–3 g/d initially; unrestricted when HTN and edema no longer present	Usually 2–4 g/d initially; unrestricted when HTN and edema no longer present
Potassium	Unrestricted unless needed	Unrestricted unless needed	Unrestricted unless needed	Unrestricted unless needed
Calcium	Ad lib; supplement if necessary to RDA	Ad lib; supplement if necessary to RDA	Ad lib; supplement if necessary	Ad lib; supplement if necessary
Phosphorus	May need very high intakes; supplement as necessary	May need very high intakes; supplement as necessary	May need very high intakes; supplement as necessary	May need very high intakes; supplement as necessary
Vitamins	Usually not necessary unless severely malnourished before transplantation; vitamin D as needed	Usually not necessary; vitamin D as needed	Usually not necessary; vitamin D as needed	Usually not necessary; vitamin D as needed
Trace minerals	Generally unnecessary; supplement iron as needed	Generally unnecessary; supplement iron as needed	Generally unnecessary; supplement iron as needed	Generally unnecessary; supplement iron as needed
Fluid	Ad lib	Ad lib	Ad lib	Ad lib

HTN, hypertension.

Nutrition Management

Predialysis

ENERGY

Energy needs for the child with progressive renal disease are at least equal to the RDA for normal children of the same height age (40 to 108 kcal/kg/d).[8] Because of the poor nutritional status often prevalent in this population, however, energy needs may be greater to promote body weight gain and linear growth.

Research in infants not being treated with dialysis intervention has indicated that diets providing energy intakes between 9 and 12 kcal/cm/d and protein intake that does not exceed 0.15 g/cm/d result in the promotion of growth sufficient for eventual renal transplantation yet do not exceed the excretory and regulatory limits of renal function.[9] Infants with renal insufficiency may require greater caloric density of formula than standard dilutions of 20 kcal/oz if a poor appetite leads to inadequate consumption or if a fluid restriction is necessary. Concentrated formulas have a higher protein and mineral content than most uremic infants can tolerate biochemically in the predialysis period. Therefore, instead of making a formula more concentrated by adding less water to the powder base or concentrate, it should be supplemented in calories by adding carbohydrate and fat modules.

A glucose polymer such as Polycose* has a low osmolality and is generally the initial supplemental module added to infant formula to raise caloric density to 24 kcal/oz. Older infants (8 to 12 months) may tolerate corn syrup or sugar, which are easily available and less costly. To increase the caloric content of formula to 27 kcal/oz, corn oil is a commonly chosen fat module for most infants. Other unsaturated oils and commercial fat modules may be used as well. Medium chain triglyceride (MCT) oil is generally not necessary in the absence of malabsorption.

Both carbohydrate and fat modules are eventually increased to raise the formula to as much as 40 to 45 kcal/oz. To promote digestibility, efforts are made to keep the same proportion of total fat to carbohydrate calories as are contained in the base formula. If diarrhea or vomiting develops and persists, the feeding regimen needs to be altered. It is important to give the infant at least 24 hours at each 2- to 4-kcal/oz incremental increase in concentration.

When infants begin taking small amounts of strained foods (at approximately 6 months of age, if developmentally ready) modular components of carbohydrate and fat may be added to these products and the formula. Addition of Polycose to strained fruit is an example.

High-calorie carbohydrate supplements are not often well accepted by children beyond infancy. Thus it is often easier to encourage common foods with high energy but relatively low protein and mineral content. Beverages such as soft drinks, powdered fruit drinks, and frozen fruit-flavored desserts rather than water should be suggested as most of the daily fluid intake. Some children may eat foods containing sugar, such as candy, jelly, honey, and other concentrated sweets, but the altered taste acuity associated with uremia may prevent acceptance of these suggestions.

Because of this altered taste acuity, as well as the prevalence of hypertriglyceridemia in people with chronic renal disease, the use of unsaturated fats may be preferable to concentrated carbohydrate for increasing calorie intake. Children and adolescents should be encouraged to use margarine on popcorn, bread, vegetables, rice, and noodles for added calories. It must be noted, however, that when significant azotemia (rising BUN concentration)

*Ross Laboratories, Columbus, OH 43215.

is present, the protein-sparing effect of added fat calories may not be as good as with concentrated carbohydrate calories.

Low protein wheat starch products, if available and affordable, are additional low protein, low mineral caloric sources for children of all ages. Jelly and margarine may be added to these products for further caloric fortification.

Infants and children should be encouraged to consume formula and food by mouth. At times, nasogastric or gastrostomy feedings in addition to oral feedings may be necessary to obtain adequate calorie intake.

PROTEIN

The RDA for protein for healthy infants is encouraged as a standard for infants with renal disease during the predialysis period. Most infants with renal insufficiency voluntarily consume at least this amount of protein in the first few months of life and are encouraged to do so to maximize physical growth and development. Because no extensive evidence exists to suggest that protein needs are increased in children with uremia, it seems reasonable to prescribe at least the minimal amounts for healthy children during the predialysis stage.[10]

Ensuring adequate caloric intake for children whose diets require protein restriction is challenging. At least 60% to 75% of the protein allowance should be protein of high biological value. This need places a limitation on many products made with regular wheat or corn flour, which contain lower-quality proteins, such as cereals, breads, pasta, and snack foods. Although some products are manufactured with wheat starch to reduce protein content, they are expensive, difficult to obtain, and unpalatable to many children. When possible, diets should be planned with a daily dispersion of high- and low-quality protein foods in limited quantities. Under many circumstances, when increasing azotemia becomes evident, additional nonprotein calories should be encouraged.

The feasibility and effectiveness of keto and amino forms of essential amino acid supplementation for children beyond infancy during the predialysis interval is currently under investigation.[11]

In nephrotic syndrome, protein should be given at the level of the RDA for age. Protein should not be supplemented to replace urinary losses, since this has been shown to increase the losses.[12]

SODIUM

An estimate of the infant's sodium needs is based on the sodium content of a 12- to 24-hour urine collection.[13] Infants with salt-wasting syndromes may need a sodium chloride supplement to maintain adequate serum levels of sodium. Infants with chronic renal insufficiency rarely require a sodium restriction unless edema or hypertension is present. Regular infant formulas may be used in the absence of potassium or phosphorous elevations, and solid foods may be introduced in the usual manner. Strained baby foods are generally low in sodium.

When necessary, a restriction of 1 to 4 g/d (depending on the body size) may be implemented. Priority should be given to limiting (although not necessarily eliminating) quantities of preferred high sodium foods, so that excessive intake of these foods may be curtailed. For example, luncheon meats may be in the diet in specific quantities while other high-sodium foods such as table salt, salty chips, canned soups, and pickles are eliminated totally. The judicious use of diuretics in combination with a mild sodium restriction may make the diet more palatable and acceptable. Individualized management and regular follow-up is imperative to optimize compliance with a sodium restriction.

POTASSIUM

A potassium-restricted diet is usually not necessary during the predialytic period. As renal function decreases, the potassium excretion capacity of each nephron increases until the GFR reaches 10% of normal.[14] At this point, the quantity of potassium secreted into the bowel increases as well. Some diuretics that are prescribed before the need for dialysis (such as furosemide) increase urinary potassium excretion to the degree that potassium-rich foods may be required. Therefore, restrictions of this mineral may not be necessary until the GFR falls to less than 10% of normal or dialysis is initiated. A restriction should be started when the serum potassium level is consistently greater than 5.0 mEq/L (after correction of acidosis).

When restrictions for infants are warranted, low electrolyte formulas such as SMA* and Similac PM 60/40[†] are used. Low potassium strained foods are initiated in the usual manner. When serum potassium levels are persistently elevated, even with good compliance on a restricted potassium diet, an ion-exchange resin (Kayexalate) may be prescribed in addition to the low potassium formula and food intake.

When elevated serum potassium levels require restriction of dietary potassium intake for children and adolescents, the first step is to eliminate concentrated sources of potassium, such as citrus fruits and juices, dark green leafy vegetables, and dried fruits. Altering methods of food preparation, such as soaking vegetables before cooking, help decrease potassium content. Other foods such as those containing chocolate may need to be used in moderation, because they are widely accepted and are excellent sources of calories. If restricted potassium intake seriously jeopardizes overall food intake or if noncompliance with such a regimen exists, Kayexalate may be prescribed for this age group as well.

CALCIUM AND PHOSPHORUS

The maintenance of normal serum calcium and phosphorus levels in children with renal disease is extremely important in efforts to deter the development of bone disease and to promote growth. Serum levels of calcium, phosphorus, parathyroid hormone, and alkaline phosphatase are closely monitored to prevent renal osteodystrophy. Radiographic and/or bone biopsy studies are used to diagnose the presence of renal osteodystrophy.

Elevated serum phosphorus levels are treated with (1) a low phosphorus diet, limiting dairy products and other high sources of phosphorus, and (2) phosphate binders ingested immediately after meals. Calcium carbonate and calcium acetate are the most commonly used binders and have an additional advantage of contributing to the oral calcium intake. Calcium citrate is not recommended, because of its effect of potentiating aluminum absorption from the gut. Aluminum-containing binders are not recommended on a long-term basis because of the potential for aluminum toxicity.

Low serum calcium levels are treated with active vitamin D metabolites and partially by means of calcium-containing phosphate binders. When used as calcium supplements, these phosphate binders may need to be taken between meals as well as with meals to increase calcium absorption.

In infants (0 to 1 year), serum phosphorus levels are normally higher (4.2 to 9.0 mg/dL) because of the need for rapid mineralization of growing cartilage and bone in this age group.[7]

*Wyeth-Ayerst Laboratories, Philadelphia, PA 19101.
[†]Ross Laboratories.

If serum phosphorus levels are even higher, a low phosphorus infant formula such as Similac PM 60/40 may be required in combination with phosphate binders to achieve desired serum phosphorus levels.

Phosphorus restriction for children and adolescents is concomitantly achieved when protein intake is restricted, because dairy products, eggs, and meats are the richest sources of this mineral. If significant protein restriction is not yet warranted, limitation of milk intake to 60 to 240 mL/d (or the equivalent phosphorus content of other dairy products, nuts, dried beans, or chocolate) is generally advised as the initial restriction. Nondairy creamers and certain frozen nondairy desserts may be used in place of milk and ice cream.

VITAMINS AND OTHER MINERALS

Vitamin and iron supplementation for infants may be indicated during the predialysis period if the volume of formula intake is limited. The formulas mentioned previously, as well as most commercial infant formulas, are fortified with vitamins and iron. Infants and young children are given a daily multivitamin preparation if their estimated intake is considerably less than the RDA.

Vitamin D metabolites are often started early in the treatment of renal failure, on the basis of serum parathyroid and alkaline phosphatase elevations above normal levels for age. Iron supplementation is usually required for infants, children, and adolescents in the predialysis period when depletion of iron stores is documented by laboratory studies. Patients receiving erythropoietin generally require iron supplementation, based on regular checking of serum iron levels. Zinc supplementation is not routinely administered to children during the predialysis phase. Since foods rich in zinc are often limited in protein-restricted diets or are unpalatable to children (rich sources include oysters, crabs, organ meats, and other meats), supplementation by pharmacological means on the basis of RDA standards for height age may be recommended if there is reason to suspect zinc deficiency. Fluoride supplementation is provided only when the water supply contains less than 3 ppm.

FLUID

In the predialysis period, fluid requirements depend on the cause of renal disease and level of GFR. Increased urine output, as in the salt-wasting syndrome, dictate increased fluid intake. To avoid blood volume depletion secondary to third-spaced fluid, fluids are generally not restricted in patients with active nephrotic syndrome.

Maintenance fluid needs are estimated by the following formula: 100 mL for the first 10 kg of body weight; 50 mL for each additional kilogram between 11 and 20 kg; and 20 mL for each additional kilogram.[7] For example, a 23-kg child would require 1000 mL for the first 10 kg, plus 500 mL for kilograms 11 through 20, and 3×20 mL for the remaining 3 kg, for a total of 1560 mL per 24 hours.

If fluid limitations become necessary because of edema or hypertension, the prescribed amount is based on insensible fluid needs plus measured urine output. Insensible needs are estimated at 1500 mL/m^2/24 h.[7]

In the outpatient population, insensible fluid losses may be increased with physical activity, dictating increased fluid requirements. Liquids and foods liquid at room temperature (gelatin, ice, ice pops, ice cream) are considered in the total fluid intake.

Hemodialysis

ENERGY

Caloric needs for the infant, child, and adolescent undergoing hemodialysis are similar to those recommended during the predialysis period. More frequent dialysis treatments, especially for ultrafiltration, may be necessary to allow the infant optimal nutritional intake by increasing the volume of formula ingested.

In the child and adolescent, the potential for adequate caloric intake is aided by minimizing the number of restrictions in the diet and keying in on the child's favorite foods as the basis for intake. Foods commonly found in the home will most likely have better acceptance than caloric supplements. Calorie-containing beverages should replace water. Monthly 3-day food records provide an opportunity for evaluation of caloric adequacy of the diet, as well as assessment of dry weight changes.

When necessary, energy supplementation may be accomplished by using carbohydrate and/or fat modules alone or in combination with protein. Commercial products such as powdered breakfast drinks, Pediasure*, Ensure*, or Sustacal† are available for children and adolescents. The cost and lack of third-party reimbursement, however, may deter use of these products. When necessary, special formulas may be prepared at home by using readily available foodstuffs. The need for initiating, continuing, or discontinuing energy supplements should be frequently evaluated.

PROTEIN

Protein requirements for infants, children, and adolescents undergoing hemodialysis are usually at least those of the RDA for children of the same height age,[15] with the continued encouragement of adequate caloric intakes, to avoid excessive protein catabolism.

Predialysis BUN levels greater than 100 mg/dL can result from a variety of reasons. The technical aspects of hemodialysis, including type of dialyzer and blood flow rates, need to be examined to ensure that adequate dialysis is occurring. Recirculation of blood secondary to the condition of the vascular access might be considered. Also, catabolic processes such as infection must be ruled out as a cause for excessive azotemia. Finally, dietary aspects including the ratio of nonprotein to protein calorie ingestion and percentage of high biological value protein to total protein content need to be evaluated. Food diaries are helpful to assess overall dietary intakes.

Kinetic modeling, which involves the estimation of protein catabolic rate (PCR) by calculation of the urea generation rate, is an essential part of the assessment and maintenance of hemodialysis patients. In stable patients, the PCR equals the dietary protein intake.[16] In the unstable patient, measurement of the PCR is determined so that dietary strategies can be planned and their effects monitored. For the pediatric patient, this technique offers a greater degree of nutrition control.

Persistently low BUN levels (less than 50 mg/dL in a child with minimal residual GFR) may indicate overall inadequate protein and caloric intake rather than good nonprotein caloric intake. Kinetic modeling and food records are valuable assessment tools. Periodic arm anthropometric measurements can document prolonged inadequate protein and caloric intake as manifested by decreasing protein stores. Serum levels of protein and albumin may not be decreased in hemodialysis patients unless adequate food ingestion is curtailed for prolonged periods.

*Ross Laboratories.
†Mead Johnson, Evansville, IN 47721.

FATS

Fats are a crucial source of calories in the hemodialysis patient. Fats in the form of margarine and appropriate oils are recommended. Achievement of a specific ratio of unsaturated to saturated fats is difficult because of children's erratic eating habits.

SODIUM

Sodium intake for infants, children, and adolescents undergoing hemodialysis is similar to that prescribed for the predialysis period. Presence of hypertension, interdialytic weight gain, and residual urine output are the primary factors influencing the quantity of sodium prescribed.

Sodium need not be restricted if a patient is not hypertensive and does not have excessive interdialytic weight gain (more than 1 kg with short-interval treatments such as between Monday and Wednesday and 2 kg for long intervals such as between Friday and Monday).

POTASSIUM

Daily potassium allowances for all age groups are based on serum levels. When the potassium level is persistently elevated and other contributing factors are ruled out, dietary restriction is indicated (see *Table 8.2*). Dietary potassium intake should be distributed throughout the day, and this should be emphasized when patients are briefed regarding this restriction. High serum concentrations of potassium can develop in children when a large quantity of potassium is ingested at one time, regardless of total dietary content for 1 day. High potassium foods may be permitted on a limited basis; however, they should be avoided during the longest interdialytic interval. Dietary restrictions regarding this mineral may be taught by using a point system (using milliequivalents) or by placing a limit on all concentrated food sources.

When serum potassium levels are repeatedly elevated before dialysis and the overall dietary intake is jeopardized, Kayexalate administration is most effective in the evening, after all meals and snacks have been ingested. The sodium content of this medication must be taken into consideration for the patient with hypertension or edema.

CALCIUM AND PHOSPHORUS

The guidelines for calcium and phosphorus intake with regard to specific foods, supplements, and medications are the same for children undergoing hemodialysis as those outlined previously for predialysis patients. A phosphorus-restricted diet and phosphate binders are generally required with both meals and snacks to control serum phosphate levels.

VITAMINS AND OTHER MINERALS

Supplements of water-soluble vitamins are indicated for pediatric patients undergoing hemodialysis, because of their dialyzability and when dietary intake is inadequate secondary to diet restrictions or poor intake.

The daily recommendations for adults undergoing hemodialysis are the following[17]: 1.5 mg thiamin, 1.8 mg riboflavin, 6 μg B$_{12}$, 300 μg biotin, 20 mg niacin or niacinamide, 10 mg pantothenic acid, 800 to 1000 μg folic acid, 60 mg vitamin C, and 10 mg pyridoxine. No studies for pediatric patients are available at this time. It seems prudent to supplement by using the above recommendations for adolescents and the RDA values for the same nutrients in children 4 to 10 years of age. Vitamin A should not be supplemented; vitamin D is supplemented according to parameters outlined in the predialysis section on calcium and phosphorus.

Children younger than 4 years may have difficulty taking vitamin tablets. A multivitamin with iron may be given as a chewable tablet or in a liquid form for even younger children and infants. Serum vitamin A levels should be monitored regularly. Folic acid may be given at a level of 0.5 to 1.0 mg/d in children younger than 4 years. Vitamin D is supplemented as needed.

Children of all ages usually require iron supplementation if they are receiving erythropoietin therapy. Iron levels should be studied regularly. Iron supplements may be administered orally or intravenously.

FLUID

Principles of fluid management for all groups undergoing hemodialysis are the same as outlined in the predialysis period. Acceptable interdialytic weight gains are individualized on the basis of body size, ultrafiltration capacity, and psychosocial factors involving compliance. This goal can be achieved in some children through a reward system in which, for example, a child might choose a favorite sticker or seal to wear or place on a wall chart kept in the dialysis unit as a symbol of his or her accomplishment.

Peritoneal Dialysis

One of several forms of peritoneal dialysis (PD) may be chosen, including continuous ambulatory peritoneal dialysis (CAPD), which involves exchanges performed daily during waking hours; nocturnal or continuous cyclic PD (CCPD), which involves a cycler that automatically performs exchanges at night while the patient sleeps; tidal PD, a variation of CCPD; and intermittent PD (IPD), in which a patient receives 10 hours of treatment three times a week in a dialysis center rather than at home. IPD has few advantages over hemodialysis because of the length of treatment time and the frequent need to restrict potassium, sodium, and fluid. In the following discussion and recommendations, *PD* will be used to refer to CAPD, CCPD, and tidal PD.

ENERGY

Total calorie intake for children undergoing all forms of PD is usually less than the RDA. Patients undergoing CAPD may not eat as much as they would normally because of a feeling of fullness from the indwelling dialysate exerting pressure on the stomach. The reduced intake is also attributable to the glucose level of the dialysate solution, which may affect the brain's appetite control center, thereby decreasing the desire for food. This problem is somewhat reduced with CCPD, performed at night with a smaller daytime dwell.

Salusky and associates reported that in 15 patients being treated with CAPD, the total caloric intake was 68 kcal/kg/d, corresponding to 82% of the RDA. Of the 68 kcal/kg/d, glucose absorbed from the dialysate solution accounted for approximately 7.8 kcal/kg/d.[18]

The RDA for the patient's height age or actual age, whichever is lower, initially is used as the basis for caloric recommendations; however, the actual requirements for energy intake may be higher, as previously mentioned for predialysis patients. The very malnourished or very active child will require energy above the RDA. Obesity is infrequently seen in preadolescent children, but may occur in adolescents.

Energy supplementation with commercially available products is similar to that described for hemodialysis patients.

PROTEIN

Protein requirements for children undergoing PD are higher because of protein and amino acid losses in the dialysate. Actual requirements for children treated with PD, however, have not been established. Salusky and colleagues reported protein losses of total protein and albumin in the dialysate in children undergoing CAPD to be 4.0 and 2.7 g/d, respectively.[19] Higher losses were found in younger children, because of a proportionally greater peritoneal surface area. The use of amino acids as an osmotic agent in the dialysate of patients undergoing PD may help to compensate for protein and amino acid losses and improve nitrogen balance.

Current protein recommendations are adapted from those recommended for adults undergoing PD and are based on the RDA for the patient's height age plus additional quantities to replace peritoneal losses. Suggested intake values for all age groups undergoing continuous forms of PD are given in *Table 8.3*.

Kinetic modeling is available for PD,[20] and standards are being developed for pediatric patients. For stable PD patients, the urea nitrogen appearance (UNA) may also be useful when estimating dietary protein intake. Correlation between protein intake and UNA is good, and the accuracy of food records can be verified in this manner.[21] A 24-hour collection of the dialysate and urine output (if present) is required. The following formula is used: UNA (grams per day) = urinary nitrogen (grams per day) + dialysate urea nitrogen (grams per day). For CAPD patients, the BUN level is assumed to be stable.

Approximately 60% to 70% of the recommended protein should be high biological value. Protein of low biological value is allowed in the diet to increase palatability. Use of high protein foods with a lower saturated fat content, such as poultry and fish, is encouraged because of the propensity for elevated serum cholesterol and triglyceride levels in patients undergoing PD. Eggs are limited to one per day, and milk (because of its high phosphorus content) is limited to 240 mL/d.

Some children undergoing PD dislike meats, which curtails adequate protein ingestion. The reason for this aversion is not apparent. At times, increased quantities of milk, milk products, and eggs must be given to meet the protein requirements of the child. Modular protein products added to formula, strained foods, juices, cereals, or other foods may be required when protein intake is persistently poor.

FATS

Elevated serum levels of cholesterol and triglycerides are seen in patients undergoing PD, in part because of increased protein losses through the dialysate, as well as the constant infusion of glucose during PD.[22] The child undergoing PD is encouraged to increase complex carbohydrate intake in lieu of simple sugars and concentrated sweets and to use unsaturated fats such as oils and margarines from corn, safflower, and soy to control hyperlipidemia.

Caloric fortification of formula and food for infants undergoing PD is altered to compensate for glucose absorption from the dialysate and the potential for hypertriglyceridemia. When the fasting serum triglyceride level is markedly elevated, the source of calorie fortification is altered to achieve a proportionally higher unsaturated fat to carbohydrate ratio, which may lessen the severity of this lipid abnormality.

SODIUM

The level of sodium tolerated by infants and children undergoing CAPD or CCPD is usually greater than that tolerated by children undergoing hemodialysis or IPD. Tolerance for sodium depends in part on the size of the child, original kidney disease, and residual renal function. Restriction of sodium intake is instituted if edema or hypertension is present.

When sodium restriction is required for an older child or adolescent undergoing PD, it is often minimal, consisting of approximately 3 to 4 g (130 to 174 mEq) per day. A palatable diet containing less than 2 g of sodium per day is difficult to achieve for a child older than 12. When a sodium restriction is required, the mildest limitation that is effective should be set. Most children do not require a sodium restriction while undergoing PD; in contrast, patients undergoing IPD frequently require such a restriction.

POTASSIUM

Most patients being treated with PD do not require a potassium restriction. Restrictions of dietary potassium are indicated when the serum level persistently exceeds the upper limit of normal, assuming the carbon dioxide level is within normal limits. For many patients, decreasing the intake of high potassium foods is sufficient to lower serum levels to within normal limits. Calculated limitation of dietary potassium may be necessary, however, as stated in *Table 8.3*. Also, improved protein and calorie intake can alleviate potassium elevation caused by catabolism.

Fecal excretion of potassium plays an important role in maintaining normal serum levels. Therefore, routine questioning about bowel habits should be part of the nutrition assessment and follow-up. Recommendations include as high a fiber content in the diet as possible and adequate (but not excessive) fluid intake. Stool softeners are needed only if these two measures cannot prevent constipation.

CALCIUM AND PHOSPHORUS

The calcium content of the diets of patients undergoing PD is low because of the continued need to limit phosphorus intake. Because calcium and phosphorus commonly occur together in foods, supplements of vitamin D metabolites and calcium are used to treat or prevent hypocalcemia and bone disease.

The need for serum phosphorus control continues for children undergoing PD, but dietary intake must be slightly higher to permit ingestion of higher protein foods. When other high biological value protein foods are taken in adequate quantities, milk should be limited to 240 mL/d (or an equivalent quantity of phosphorus taken in the form of milk products) for most older children. Infants undergoing PD may ingest formulas with higher phosphate concentrations as well as cow's milk (in varying quantities, depending on biochemical status), especially if residual renal function is present.

VITAMINS AND OTHER MINERALS

Recommendations for vitamins and minerals are the same as those described for hemodialysis.

FLUID

PD patients should have little need for fluid limitation if ultrafiltration capacity is adequate. Patients undergoing IPD are more likely to require restrictions because the dialysis is not continuous. If hypertension or edema is persistent, a dialysis solution with a higher glucose concentration can be used to increase ultrafiltration, and the sodium content of the diet can be decreased. Instead of water, beverages containing calories (such as juices) can be given to the child with less than optimal energy intake.

Transplantation

A well-functioning allograft is the treatment goal for most pediatric patients with ESRD. The nutrient needs after transplantation are not well defined. The following recommendations are for a well-functioning graft. Patients whose grafts function suboptimally should be managed according to predialysis, hemodialysis, or PD recommendations as appropriate. Newer immunosuppressive drugs may cause nausea, vomiting, diarrhea, or anorexia, which should be treated symptomatically.

ENERGY

The goal is to achieve and maintain ideal weight for height. Corticosteroids (prednisone) stimulate the appetite, making weight control a challenge, especially in the first 6 months after transplantation, when doses are highest.[23] Control of total caloric intake, behavior modification techniques, and exercise should be emphasized. The RDA for age and sex is used as the starting point, with calories adjusted as necessary.

The effects of corticosteroids on carbohydrate metabolism include increased insulin secretion causing glucose uptake by fat cells, impaired glucose tolerance, glycosuria, and relative resistance to insulin.[24] Carbohydrate restriction has been suggested to minimize the cushingoid effects of corticosteroids[25]; Liddle and Johnson recommend 1 g carbohydrate per kilogram per day in adults to minimize the cushingoid effects of corticosteroids.[26] This is too restrictive to meet caloric needs in children, because of their smaller body size. Therefore, sugar and concentrated sweets are eliminated from the diet for 6 weeks after transplantation. Complex carbohydrates, fruit, and juices are permitted, with a goal of 40% to 50% of the caloric intake from carbohydrates. The limitation of concentrated sweets has a secondary benefit of limiting nonnutritious calories, which is helpful in weight management.

PROTEIN

Protein metabolism is altered by immunosuppressive drugs (including corticosteroids), increased protein metabolism, decreased anabolism through decreased uptake of amino acids in muscle tissue, and increased liver uptake of amino acids.[27] Azathioprine has been shown to inhibit DNA and RNA synthesis.[28] Protein intake is recommended at a level of 2 to 3 g/kg/d in the immediate posttransplantation period, tapering to the RDA after approximately 3 months.

FAT

Hypercholesterolemia and hyperlipidemia have been described after transplantation.[29] Part of the ongoing nutrition education includes recommendations for monounsaturated and polyunsaturated fats, overall fat intake of 30% to 35% of total calories, and use of lean meats.

SODIUM

Corticosteroids and cyclosporine can cause hypertension as a side effect, with enhanced sodium retention. Sodium is prophylactically restricted in the immediate posttransplantation period to 2 to 4 g/d. When hypertension is no longer present, the sodium intake may be liberalized.

POTASSIUM

Hyperkalemia may result from cyclosporine use, apparently from suppression of renin and aldosterone levels.[30] This primarily occurs when levels are excessively elevated. No routine potassium restriction is initiated.

CALCIUM AND PHOSPHORUS

Corticosteroids affect calcium metabolism through decreased absorption from the intestine and increased calcium resorption. If the serum levels decrease, supplements may be prescribed. Phosphorus supplements generally are required in addition to a liberal dietary intake of dairy products, because of impaired reabsorption in the renal tubules.[29]

VITAMINS AND MINERALS

Generally, supplements are not necessary, because of the increased appetite from immunosuppressive drugs. Vitamin D may need to be supplemented. A magnesium supplement is usually required by patients taking cyclosporine initially. Iron may be supplemented in patients who have low iron stores.

FLUIDS

Fluids are recommended ad libitum, with a minimum of 2 L/d encouraged, especially in older patients. Water rather than calorie-containing beverages is encouraged.

References

1. De Motte C. Renal nutrition and the non-compliant patient: some guidelines. *Nephrology News Issues.* 1990;3:14.

2. Nelson P, Stover J. Principles of nutritional assessment and management of the child with ESRD. In: Fine RN, Gruskin A, eds. *End-Stage Renal Disease in Children.* Philadelphia, Pa: WB Saunders; 1984:209.

3. Massie M, Niimi K, Yang W, et al. Nutritional assessment of children with chronic renal insufficiency. *J Renal Nutr.* 1992;2:2.

4. *National Center for Health Statistics Growth Curves for Children 0-18 years.* United States Vital and Health Statistics. Series II, no. 165. Washington, DC: Health Resources Administration, US Government Printing Office; 1977.

5. Frisancho RA. Triceps skinfolds and upper arm muscle size norms for assessment of nutritional status. *Am J Clin Nutr.* 1974;27:1052.

6. Food and Nutrition Board, National Academy of Sciences, National Research Council. *Recommended Dietary Allowances.* 10th ed. Washington, DC: National Academy Press; 1989.

7. Greene MD, ed. *The Harriet Lane Handbook.* 12th ed. St Louis, Mo: Mosby–Year Book; 1991:271.

8. Kurtin PS, Shapiro AC. Effect of defined caloric supplementation on growth of children with renal disease. *J Renal Nutr.* 1992;2:13.

9. Grupe WE, Spinozzi NS, Harmon WE. Nutritional management to postpone dialysis in infants. *Pediatr Res.* 1987;21:476.

10. Raymond NG, Dwyer JT, Nevins P, et al. An approach to protein restriction in children with renal insufficiency. *Pediatr Nephrol.* 1990;4:145.

11. Jureirdini KF, Hogg RJ, Van Renen MJ, et al. Evaluation of long term aggressive dietary management of chronic renal failure in children. *Pediatr Nephrol.* 1990;4:1.

12. Kaysen GA, Gambertoglio J, Jimenez I, et al. Effect of dietary protein intake on albumin homeostasis in nephrotic patients. *Kidney Int.* 1986;29:572.

13. Winters RW. Maintenance fluid therapy. In: Winters RW, ed. *The Body Fluids in Pediatrics.* Boston, Mass: Little, Brown, and Co; 1973:130.

14. Holliday MA, McHenry-Richardson K, Portale A, et al. Nutritional management of chronic renal disease. *Med Clin North Am.* 1979;63:945.

15. Grupe WE, Spinozzi NS, Harmon WE. Protein balance more dependent on protein intake than on energy intake in hemodialysed children. *Kidney Int.* 1983;23:149.

16. Levine J, Bernard DB. The role of urea kinetic modeling, TAC urea, and KT/V in achieving optimal dialysis: a critical reappraisal. *Am J Kidney*

Dis. 1990;15:285.

17. Makoff R. Water-soluble vitamin status in patients with renal disease treated with hemodialysis or peritoneal dialysis. *J Renal Nutr.* 1991;1:56.

18. Salusky IB, Lucullo L, Nelson PA, et al. Continuous ambulatory peritoneal dialysis in children. *Pediatr Clin North Am.* 1982;29:1005.

19. Salusky IB, Fine RN, Nelson PA, et al. Nutritional status of pediatric patients undergoing CAPD. *Kidney Int.* 1982;21:177.

20. Teehan BP, Brown JM, Schleifer CR. Kinetic modeling in peritoneal dialysis. In: Nissensen AR, Fine RN, Gentile DE, ed. *Clinical Dialysis.* Norwalk, Conn: Appleton and Lange; 1990.

21. Blumenkrantz MJ, Kopple JD, Moran JK, et al. Nitrogen and urea metabolism during continuous ambulatory peritoneal dialysis. *Kidney Int.* 1981;20:78.

22. Blumenkrantz MJ, Schmidt WR. Managing the nutritional concerns of the patient undergoing peritoneal dialysis. In: Nolph KD, ed. *Peritoneal Dialysis.* The Hague, The Netherlands: Martinus Nijhoff; 1981:295.

23. Ettenger RB, Rosenthal T, Marik J, et al. Cadaver renal transplantation in children: results with long-term cyclosporin immunosuppression. *Clin Transplant.* 1991;5:197.

24. Hill CM, Douglas JF, Kumar KV, et al. Glycosuria and hyperlipidemia after kidney transplantation. *Lancet.* 1974;2:490.

25. Whittier FC, Evans DH, Dutton S, et al. Nutrition in renal transplantation. *Am J Kidney Dis.* 1985;6:405.

26. Liddle VR, Johnson HK. Dietary therapy in renal transplantation. *Proc Dial Transplant Forum.* 1979;9:219.

27. Liddle VR, Walker PJ, Johnson HK, et al. Diet in transplantation. *Dial Transplant.* 1977;5:9.

28. Gradus D, Ettenger RB. Renal transplantation in children. *Pediatr Clin North Am.* 1982;29:1005.

29. Weil SE. Nutrition in the kidney transplant recipient. In: Danovitch GM, ed. *Handbook of Kidney Transplantation.* Boston, Mass: Little, Brown and Co; 1992:395.

30. Pagenkemper JL, Foulks CJ. Nutritional management of the adult renal transplant patient. *J Renal Nutr.* 1991;1:119.

9. Enteral Nutrition in End-Stage Renal Disease

The dietitian's ability to employ aggressive nutrition therapy strategies to offset malnutrition or to correct existing nutritional deficiencies may have a significant impact on the overall medical status of renal patients. Protein-energy malnutrition in renal disease is associated with delayed wound healing, increased incidence of infection, poor rehabilitation, and diminished overall quality of life.[1] Suboptimal dietary intake and the metabolic changes occurring in kidney failure lead to an increased incidence of nutritional wasting.[2] Periodic episodes of anorexia, common in this patient population, may be attributed to accumulation of uremic toxins, impaired taste acuity, psychological depression, and unpalatable diet. Despite these deterrents, adequate nutrition support can be achieved with the use of enteral feedings.

Dietary Supplementation

Nutrient requirements can be adequately supplied in many cases by voluntary food intake. Keeping the dietary restrictions as liberal as is medically possible can alleviate some of the boredom associated with the regimented renal diets. Providing small amounts of food at frequent intervals is of particular value in patients who experience the early satiety and gastric discomfort associated with gastroparesis, a condition common in patients with diabetes. Calorie-dense foods such as casseroles, custards, powdered breakfast beverage mixes, and puddings are often well tolerated by patients suffering from gastroparesis or nausea. Most of the aforementioned foods contain significant amounts of fluid and restricted nutrients (eg, potassium and phosphorus); however, since overall food intake is diminished, the total daily intake of nutrients will not exceed the dietary restrictions. When small frequent feedings of high phosphorus nourishments are given, the phosphate-binding medication dosage and administration may need to be modified.

There is an array of commercial formula feedings available that vary in nutrient content. The practitioner can take advantage of this assortment when planning individualized nutrition therapy. The majority of the formulas are convenient, requiring little or no preparation. Palatability, availability, and cost can directly influence patient acceptance. Patients may prefer consuming food items versus pharmaceutically prepared supplements.

Feeding modules *(Table 9.1)*, which are concentrated sources of one nutrient (eg, protein, carbohydrate, fat) are designed to be combined with food items or formula diets. Carbohydrate and/or fat modules are employed to increase the energy content of the diet and are of particular value for people who must follow protein-restricted diets. The electrolyte

Table 9.1
Feeding Modules

Formula	Kilocalories (per 100 g)	Carbohydrate (g) (per 100 g)	Protein (g) (per 100 g)	Nutrient Source	Supplier
Carbohydrates:					
Polycose powder	380	94		Glucose polymers	Ross Laboratories
Moducal	380	95		Maltodextrin	Mead Johnson
Sumacal powder	380	95		Maltodextrin	Sherwood Medical
Protein:					
Propac	395		75	Whey protein	Sherwood Medical
ProMod	318		75	Whey protein	Ross Laboratories
Casec	370		88	Casinate	Mead Johnson
ProMix	360		75	Whey protein	Corpac

	Volume to provide 1000 Kcal (cc)	Fat (g/cc)	Nutrient Source	Supplier
Fats:				
Microlipid	222	4.5	Safflower oil	Sherwood Medical
MCT Oil	130	7.7	Fractionated coconut oil	Mead Johnson

content of these formulas varies and is an important consideration in renal failure. Protein feeding modules may be of benefit to patients whose protein intake is impaired by poor appetite or meat aversions, or who have increased requirements for dietary protein (eg, peritonitis, wound healing).

Formula feedings vary in osmolality and nutrient composition. Patients may present with nonrelated medical conditions that cause malabsorption syndromes such as lactose intolerance. Feeding selection thus depends on the patient's ability to digest and absorb specific nutrients. Minimization of electrolyte ingestion may prove critical to the overall management of the medically unstable renal patient; thus, the electrolyte content of the formula may be the deciding factor in its use. Offering of supplements with a low mineral content has the additional benefit of allowing the patient to incorporate a higher percentage of electrolyte intake from actual foods. Commercially prepared supplements are generally available in liquid or pudding form. When fluid is restricted, the use of calorie-dense formulas providing 1.5 or 2.0 kcal/mL is beneficial.

Tube Feedings

Tube Feeding Sites

When appetite is depressed but the gastrointestinal tract is functional, the use of a feeding tube provides an alternate method of enteral support. Compared with parenteral nutrition, enteral feeding is easier to maintain, is less costly to use, and is associated with fewer serious complications.[3] Enteral access may be gained by nasogastric or nasointestinal passage, percutaneous endoscopic methods, or by surgical gastrostomy or jejunostomy.[4] Selection of the feeding site is dependent on the patient's medical condition and the estimated duration of feeding.

Nasoenteric tubes are most commonly used for short-term enteral feedings (less than 4 to 6 weeks).[4,5] These include nasogastric, nasoduodenal, and nasojejunal tubes. The nasopharynx, oropharynx, and esophagus must be patent for these tubes to be used.[5] Flexible silicone or polyurethane small-bore feeding tubes in diameters of 8 to 12 French are well tolerated by most patients. Careful placement of the tube is critical; the stylets and guidewires used for tube placement may contribute to perforation of the bronchus, esophagus, or stomach.[4] It is recommended that postplacement radiographs be obtained to evaluate tube placement before initiation of feedings. This will reduce complications of pneumothorax, hydrothorax, or tracheobronchial intubation.

Feeding directly into the stomach is contraindicated when there is gastric atony or gastric obstruction or when the patient lacks an intact gag reflex.[3] In these situations, transpyloric feedings via nasointestinal feeding tubes or jejunostomy are recommended. A nasointestinal feeding tube is generally longer than a nasogastric tube (43 in versus 36 in).[5]

Enterostomies are the preferred route for long-term enteral feeding, with gastrostomy or jejunostomy feeding tubes being the most common. An operative gastrostomy may be placed in patients who are not at risk for aspiration, by using local or general anesthesia, depending on the individual situation.[5] The simplest procedure is the Stamm gastrostomy, which involves suturing a catheter into the stomach.[3,4] The main disadvantage of this procedure is the fact that should the tube be accidentally removed, the tract will close within a few hours.[3] One possible complication associated with gastrostomies is external leakage around the site.[4] Jejunostomies are indicated in patients who have an incompetent gag reflex, gastric obstruction or bleeding, or who have a postsurgical ileus.[4,5]

Percutaneous endoscopic gastrostomy (PEG), developed in 1980, has the two advantages of requiring the use of local, rather than general, anesthesia and of taking only 10 to 15 minutes for placement.[6] Although complications of gastrocolic fistula formation, intraperitoneal leakage, and cutaneous stomal enlargement have been reported,[5] most practitioners find the PEG to be a relatively safe mode of feeding.[6] The PEG can be easily removed, and the stoma closes within 1 to 2 days.[3]

Formula Selection

It is usually the dietitian who recommends the formula for tube feeding (*Table 9.2*). Whenever it is appropriate, patients are encouraged to supplement intake by food consumption, particularly solids.

Fluid allowance is the key in deciding which formula to use in oliguric patients. Intravenous medications, dietary supplements, and any liquids required for administration of oral medications must be deducted from the daily allotment of fluid. For example, a daily fluid restriction of 1500 mL, with 210 mL required for water with medications and 90 mL required for tube flushing (15 mL every 4 hours), leaves a total volume of 1200 mL for the tube feeding. In this situation, a calorie-dense formula (1.5 to 2.0 kcal/mL) would facilitate the attainment of nutritional requisites. A variety of these formulas are on the market today; feeding modules also may be used to increase energy value (*Tables 9.1, 9.3*). Another strategy is the use of safflower or corn oil, which can be given in a 5- to 10-mL bolus directly into the feeding tube several times daily; this can substantially improve energy intake with negligible addition of electrolytes and provides essential fatty acids. The oil should not be directly mixed with the tube feeding because the addition of medium chain triglyceride oil and other oil preparations have caused clumping in some tube feeding preparations.[7]

The protein intolerance associated with renal failure may be exacerbated in situations in which dialysis is suboptimal or cannot be instituted. At these times, it is necessary to limit protein ingestion markedly. Some clinicians prefer to use an essential amino acid and histidine formula rather than a mixed essential and nonessential amino acid formulation when intake of protein is restricted,[8] although use of this product remains a controversial issue. The lack of scientific support regarding the appropriateness of an essential amino acid formulation and its high expense often preclude its clinical use. Similar debates exist regarding the beneficial effects of enteral formulas supplying a high concentration of branched-chain amino acids in improving nitrogen retention and visceral protein synthesis in stress.[9]

Daily ingestion of sodium, potassium, phosphorus, calcium, and magnesium must be scrutinized to prevent electrolyte imbalance. The mineral (phosphorus, calcium, and magnesium) and electrolyte (sodium, chlorine, and potassium) contents of commercial formula diets vary greatly.[10] Patients receiving nutrients from formula diets alone may ingest less than the prescribed levels of certain electrolytes. In these instances, the physician should be notified so that adjustment in the dialysate composition and/or supplementation of these nutrients can be initiated. During anabolism, renal patients may experience hypophosphatemia; thus, serum phosphorus levels should be closely monitored and adequate supplementation provided if low (approximately 1200 to 1500 mg/d). While most feedings provide the RDA levels for vitamins and minerals, some fortification of folate and other vitamins may be needed to achieve levels recommended in patients with uremia.[8] Liquid vitamin and mineral preparations designed for parenteral nutrition delivery can be added directly to the prepared feeding.

Table 9.2
Renal and Calorie–dense Formulas

Formula	kcal/mL	Protein (g/L)	Fat (g/L)	Carbohydrate (g/L)	mOsm/kg	Na (mg/L)	K (mg/L)	Volume to Meet RDA
Renal (Predialysis)								
Amin-Aid* Kendall McGaw	2.0	19	47.1	366	1095	345	234	No vitamins provided in formula
Travasorb Renal† Baxter-Travenol	1.35	23	18	271	590	0	0	2100 mL
Suplena‡ Ross Laboratories	2.0	30	95.6	255.2	615	783	1116	947 mL
Calorie-dense								
Nepro Ross Laboratories	2.0	70	96	215	635	830	1056	960 mL
Two Cal HN Ross Laboratories	2.0	83	90	216	740	1052	2316	950 mL
Ensure Plus HN Ross Laboratories	1.5	63	50	200	650	1184	1818	940 mL
Ensure Plus Ross Laboratories	1.5	55	53	200	600	1141	2325	1600 mL
Magnacal Sherwood Medical	2.0	70	80	250	590	1000	1250	1000 mL
Deliver 2.0 Mead Johnson	2.0	75	91	225	690	800	1400	1500 mL
Sustacal Plus Mead Johnson	1.5	61	58	190	650	840	1480	1200 mL
Isotein Sandoz	1.2	68.5	34	156	300	620	1070	1770 mL

(Continued)

Table 9.2—continued
Renal and Calorie–dense Formulas

	kcal/8 oz	Protein (g)	Fat (g)	Carbohydrate (g)	Na (mg)	K (mg)
Other						
(Per 8-oz serving)						
LoPro (Milk Substitute) Med Diet	87	2.35	3.7	11.2	96	260

*Amin-Aid: Crystalline essential amino acids, including histidine, provide a source of nitrogen; very low in electrolytes, lactose-free.
†Travasorb Renal: Low protein (60% essential amino acids and selected nonessential amino acids); product designed for patients requiring attention to fluid and electrolyte balance; water-soluble vitamins provided, but essentially electrolyte-free.
‡Suplena: Low protein (mixed essential and nonessential amino acids), calorically dense product for patients requiring protein, electrolyte, and fluid restrictions; provides at least 100% of recommended vitamins and minerals for patients with renal disease.

Table 9.3 Fortifying Commercial Feedings

Nutritional Goal: 1800 kcal, 70 g protein, 2 g Na+, 2 g K+, <1000 mg Phos, 1200 mL fluid

Item	Amount	Carbohydrate (g)	Protein (g)	Fat (g)	kcal	Na+ (mg)	K+ (mg)	Phosphate (mg)
Sample 1								
Isocal	1 L	132	34	44	1060	528	1319	528
Propac	47 g	0	36	4	180	108	241	145
Safflower oil	62 g	0	0	62	558	0	0	0
Total		132	70	110	1798	636	1560	673
Sample 2								
Magnacal	900 cc	225	63	72	1800	900	1125	900
Propac	10 g	0	7	0.8	35	22	50	30
Total		225	70	72.8	1835	922	1175	930
Sample 3								
Osmolite HN	1 L	141	44.4	36.8	1060	930	1564	757
Polycose (powder)	152 g	143	0	0	578	167	<45	<8
Propac	34 g	0	26	2.8	129	79	174	105
Total		284	70.4	39.6	1767	1176	1783	870

Administration of Tube Feedings

CONTINUOUS DRIP

In acute care situations, initiation of tube feeding by continuous drip is generally preferred. This method of delivery improves patient tolerance because the osmolality remains constant, and the incidence of gastric retention, aspiration, and vomiting are decreased.[10] This delivery technique is recommended for use in small bowel feedings and may prove beneficial in gastric feedings of the critically ill patient.

A feeding pump facilitates the delivery of the feeding at a constant rate of flow, and the feeding is usually infused continuously throughout the day.[3] By ensuring a constant flow when the feeding rate is slow (20 to 40 mL/min), this device may also diminish the incidence of clogging of the tube,[4] although proper flushing of the tube with water appears to have the greatest effect on tube patency. Because of the necessity of restricting fluid intake in renal disease, feedings should be started full strength, at initial rates of delivery of at least 20 to 30 mL/h. The rate of delivery is then increased as tolerated, by daily increments of 15 to 25 mL.

BOLUS METHOD

Bolus delivery of gastric feeding may be implemented in medically stable patients and is most often used in long-term care settings for patients stabilized on tube feeding regimens. Feedings are usually administered by using a syringe or bulb. The 300 to 400 mL of feeding is infused over a period of 10 minutes or less.[3] Tolerance to this feeding is dependent on gut function.

INTERMITTENT METHOD

Intermittent feeding involves the delivery of 300 to 400 mL of solution, usually administered by gravity drip over a period of 30 minutes, every 3 to 6 hours.[3] This method is not recommended for the critically ill, because it may be associated with gastric reflux and volume intolerance.

CYCLIC METHOD

The cyclic feeding method involves delivery of nutrients, usually over a period of 8 to 16 hours per day.[3] This method is typically employed for transitional feedings and practicality, with delivery rates controlled by use of a feeding pump. Patients are encouraged to eat during the day, and intake is supplemented by nocturnal tube feeding. Adequate nutritional intake can be ensured by use of calorie-dense formulas.

Monitoring Tube Feedings

The tube feeding should be closely monitored to reduce the risk of aspiration or gastric reflux. Hanging times vary; to prevent bacterial contamination, hanging of diluted feedings for no longer than 4 hours is recommended.[3] Full-strength feedings may be administered over 4 to 8 hours.

Protocols for monitoring tube feedings vary from institution to institution. Elevation of the head by 30 to 45 degrees during and for 1 to 2 hours after tube feeding reduces nausea, vomiting, and potential aspiration.[3] The gastric residuals are generally checked several times per day.[3,11] When patients are receiving bolus feedings or eating foods in conjunction with the tube feeding, residuals should be measured at least 1 hour following food or feeding ingestion. If the aspirate is greater than 150 mL, the tube is clamped for 1 hour, and the aspirate is checked again. If there is no change in volume, the physician is notified of the delayed gastric emptying.

Patients with symptomatic uremia or undergoing dialysis may experience delayed gastric emptying.[12] Medications that promote gastric motility may then be prescribed (eg, metaclopramide). The feeding will need to be stopped if vomiting, decreased gastric motility, or gastric obstruction develops.[3]

When blood pressure drops during hemodialysis, the tube-fed patient may be placed in the Trendelenburg position (legs elevated above the level of the head), thereby increasing the potential for aspiration. Bolus feedings should be terminated at least 1 hour before the hemodialysis treatment, and continuous drip feeding should be withheld during hemodialysis. Because of the extended length of time that patients undergo peritoneal dialysis (intermittent peritoneal dialysis is approximately 10 hours per treatment, and continuous ambulatory peritoneal dialysis is ongoing), it is impractical to discontinue tube feeding during therapy. Furthermore, severe shifts in blood pressure during peritoneal dialysis are uncommon; thus, patients are rarely placed in the Trendelenburg position.

Complications of Tube Feedings

Mechanical, gastrointestinal, and/or metabolic complications have been associated with enteral feeding therapy. Close monitoring of the feeding regimen may prevent these risks.

MECHANICAL COMPLICATIONS

Mechanical problems include irritation, erosion ulcers, obstruction of the tube lumen, aspiration, and tube displacement.[3] Tube displacement is the most common complication, typically resulting from the patient accidentally or intentionally removing the tube.[11,14] In a study involving 45 hospitalized patients, Barclay and Litchford[14] noted that 39% of the tubes were pulled out by the patients, with the majority removed within 1 to 5 days of placement. Only 10% of the tubes were removed because of occlusion. The tubes may also become displaced by "falling out" or "falling in" or simply by breaking.[4] Coughing or vomiting may also result in accidental tube removal.[3]

Given time, all feeding tubes ultimately clog.[4,7] An increased incidence of tube occlusion has been associated with the use of fiber-containing formulas or with the administration of crushed medications via the tube.[11,14,15] Liquid forms of medications should be used whenever possible.[16] If the medication solution is highly viscous, it should be diluted with 20 to 30 mL of water to facilitate delivery.[15] Medications should be administered separately, and the feeding tube should be flushed with water after administration to remove any particles of medication that may adhere to the tubing.

The protein source of the formula and the interactions of these feedings with the pH of the local environment have also been suggested to play a role in tube occlusion.[7,11] Cutie and associates noted that pharmaceutical syrups with a pH greater than 4 are likely to clump tube feeding formulas, whereas other acidic elixirs presented no compatibility problems when added slowly and with rapid stirring.[7] The best method to prevent clogging is to flush the tube with water routinely and to use a water rinse following administration of medication via the tube.[6,10,14]

GASTROINTESTINAL COMPLICATIONS

Inappropriate formula administration (eg, a too-rapid delivery rate) may result in diarrhea, cramping, distention, bloating, nausea, vomiting, and delayed gastric emptying.[3] Impaired gastric motility increases the risk of pulmonary aspiration.

Diarrhea occurs in as many as 60% of critically ill patients receiving liquid formula diets.[17] It has been defined as increased frequency of more than three stools daily or as increased stool weight above the 200-g normal fecal weight.[18] It is accompanied by urgency, perianal discomfort, or incontinence.

Diarrhea may be caused by antibiotics, cathartics, magnesium-containing antacids, and H-2 antagonists or by the delivery of hyperosmotic medications via the feeding tube.[10,14] Bacterial contamination of the feeding due to improper handling techniques or extended hanging times can also induce diarrhea. Patients with a lactase deficiency or a malabsorption disease (eg, Crohn disease, short bowel syndrome) often experience this symptom. Starvation hypoalbuminemia is believed to result in an increased frequency of diarrhea.[3] Patterson et al,[19] however, reported that there was no statistical difference to enteral feeding tolerance in patients with serum albumin levels less than 2.5 g/dL as compared with hospitalized patients with normal serum concentrations of this protein.

Gradual advancement of formula rate and concentration and the use of proper handling techniques may alleviate diarrhea caused by inappropriate formula administration. Patients with hypoalbuminemia or malabsorption diseases may benefit from an elemental or lactose-free formula. *Lactobacillus* granules or other antidiarrheal agents may be beneficial for patients with diarrhea due to antibiotic therapy. Promotional materials used to market fiber-containing formulas extol their benefits in reducing the incidence of diarrhea; still, it should be noted that there have been no controlled studies that support those claims.[18,20] While pectin has been shown to reduce diarrhea in tube-fed patients, none of the marketed fiber-containing feedings has pectin as the main source of fiber.[20]

Constipation in the enterally fed patient is associated with inadequate water intake, reduced gastric motility, inadequate bulk, or drug therapy.[3] At present, there are no definitive studies identifying fluid requirements as fiber intake increases; however, care should be taken to provide adequate amounts of water during administration of fiber-containing formulas.[20] In a fluid-restricted renal patient, provision of adequate water may prove difficult, and the risk of constipation or intestinal blockage may increase.

METABOLIC COMPLICATIONS

Vanlandingham and coworkers reported that 30% to 40% of 100 tube-fed patients studied experienced at least one metabolic complication, with hyperkalemia, hyponatremia, hypophosphatemia, and hyperglycemia being the most commonly observed.[21] Renal patients receiving enteral tube feedings with low electrolyte and mineral content have been reported to experience hypocalcemia, hypophosphatemia, and hyponatremia.[22] Most of the commercially prepared formulas contain a low electrolyte content; consequently, supplementation may be needed. Electrolyte solutions are extremely hyperosmolar (eg, potassium phosphate injection of 3 mmol of phosphorus per milliliter has an osmolality of 5450 mmol/kg), and their administration may trigger gastrointestinal symptoms.[18] The addition of electrolytes to the formula, rather than bolus administration, is therefore preferred.

Monitoring Progress in Enteral Feedings

Ongoing appraisal of patient response to nutrition intervention is essential to facilitate identification of any nutritional deficiencies and to plan appropriate nutrient supplementation. Decreased body weight and elevated serum sodium may be indicative of dehydration.

Hyperglycemia has been noted in renal failure.[18] In diabetic renal patients, serum blood glucose levels below 200 mg/dL may be a target goal. Persistent hyperglycemia may be managed by lowering the carbohydrate content of the feeding or by providing insulin or other hypoglycemic agents.[3,18]

Protein intake in early renal failure may be dependent on the degree of renal function, whereas in ESRD, it is related to the type of dialysis therapy given. While excessive protein intake can result in a gradual rise in blood urea nitrogen concentration, in extreme stress with endogenous protein catabolism, a sudden elevation of urea appearance of up to five times that caused by dietary protein has been reported.[23]

Most formula feedings provide the RDA for vitamins and minerals in volumes of 1 to 3 L/d.[18] Deficiencies of certain vitamins may develop when patients receive quantities less than this amount. Additional supplementation with folate (1 mg/d), ascorbic acid (to achieve a total intake of 60 to 100 mg/d), and vitamin B$_6$ (10 mg/d) may be prudent for the dialysis population.

Serum concentrations of phosphorus, potassium, sodium, and magnesium should be monitored several times during the first week of tube feeding in medically unstable patients. Supplementation of phosphorus is recommended when serum levels fall below 2 mg/dL, and additional magnesium may be needed when serum levels fall below 1 mEq/L.[18] Once a maintenance tube feeding regimen has been achieved, monitoring of these laboratory values on a weekly basis should prove sufficient.

Daily energy and protein intake should be recorded and patients monitored with evaluation of renal function and uremic status, fluid status, daily weight and blood pressure measurements, and a review of medical and/or surgical treatment plans. Anthropometric measurements (body weight, midarm muscle circumference, triceps skinfold thickness) and serum albumin concentrations should be recorded monthly to assess changes in body composition and in visceral protein stores. Serum transferrin levels may be monitored on a biweekly basis to assess visceral protein stores, but these may be variable due to fluctuations in iron status (see chapter 2, Nutrition Assessment in Chronic Renal Failure).

Modification of the formulation and/or delivery of the selected feeding program should be implemented as needed. Adjustments in the dialysis procedure to accommodate increased fluid or nutrient intake may be feasible in some cases. For instance, the frequency or length of treatment may be prolonged to facilitate greater removal of toxins and/or fluid. It may be possible to improve removal of potassium by lowering the potassium content of the dialysate in hemodialysis patients. Close collaboration with the nephrologist will ensure the delivery of optimal nutrition care.

References

1. Blumenkrantz MJ, Kopple JD, Gutman RA, et al. Methods for assessing nutritional status of patients with renal failure. *Am J Clin Nutr.* 1980;33:1567.

2. Feinstein EI. Nutritional hemodialysis. *Kidney Int.* 1987;32(suppl 22):S167.

3. Krey S, Porcelli K, Lockette G, et al. Enteral nutrition. In: Shronts E, ed. *Nutrition Support Dietetics Core Curriculum.* 1989. Silver Spring, Md: American Society for Parenteral and Enteral Nutrition; 1989.

4. Kirkland ML. Enteral and parenteral access. In: Skipper A, ed. *Dietitian's Handbook of Enteral and Parenteral Nutrition.* Rockville, Md: Aspen; 1989.

5. Monturo CA. Enteral access device selection. *Nutr Clin Pract.* 1990;5:207.

6. Gaziano JH. Percutaneous endoscopic gastrostomy: experience in a community hospital. *Nutr Support Serv.* 1987;7:23.

7. Cutie AJ, Altman E, Lenkel L. Compatibility of enteral products with commonly employed drug additives. *JPEN J Parenter Enter Nutr.* 1983;7:186.

8. Kopple JD. Nutritional therapy in kidney failure. *Nutr Rev.* 1981;39:139.

9. Shronts EP, Konstantinides NN, Teasley KM, et al. Modified amino acid support in metabolic stress: enteral vs parenteral. *Nutr Supp Serv.* 1987;7:12.

10. Fleming CR, Nelson J. Nutritional options. In: Kinney JM, Jeejeebhoy KN, Hill GL, Owen OE, eds. *Nutrition and Metabolism in Patient Care.* Philadelphia, Pa: WB Saunders; 1988.

11. Benson DW, Griggs BA, Hamilton F, et al. Clogging of feeding tubes: a randomized trial of a newly designed tube. *Nutr Clin Pract.* 1990;5:107.

12. Collins BJ. Gastric emptying in chronic renal failure. *Br Med J.* 1985;291:310.

13. Grodstein G, Harrison A, Roberts C, et al. Impaired gastric emptying in hemodialysis patients (abstr). *Proceedings of the American Society of Nephrology.* 1979.

14. Barclay BA, Litchford MD. Incidence of nasoduodenal tube occlusions and patient removal of tubes: a prospective study. *J Am Diet Assoc.* 1991;91:220.

15. Wright B, Robinson L. Enteral feeding tubes as drug delivery systems. *Nutr Supp Serv.* 1986;6:33.

16. Inquire Here. *Dietitians in Nutrition Support Newsletter.* 1990;12(4):12.

17. Palacio JC, Rombeau JL. Dietary fiber: a brief review and potential application to enteral nutrition. *Nutr Clin Pract.* 1990;5:107.

18. Skipper A. Monitoring complications of enteral feeding. In: Skipper A, ed. *Dietitian's Handbook of Enteral and Parenteral Nutrition.* Rockville, Md: Aspen; 1989.

19. Patterson ML, Dominguez JM, Lyman B, et al. Enteral feeding in the hypoalbuminemic patient. *JPEN J Parenter Enter Nutr.* 1990;14:364.

20. Slavin J. Commercially available enteral formulas with fiber and bowel function measures. *Nutr Clin Pract.* 1990;5:247.

21. Vanlandingham S, Simpson S, Daniel P, et al. Metabolic abnormalities in patients supported with enteral tube feeding. *JPEN J Parenter Enter Nutr.* 1981;5:322.

22. Rammohan M, Roxe DM. Recognition and management of sodium, calcium and phosphorus abnormalities with enteral tube feeding in renal failure patient. *Nutr Supp Serv.* 1986;6(2a):8.

23. Giordano C, DeSanto NG, Senatore R. The effect of catabolic stress in acute and chronic renal failure. *Am J Clin Nutr.* 1978;31:1561.

10. Parenteral Nutrition for the Patient With Renal Failure

When enteral nutrition support is not feasible or not tolerated, various forms of parenteral nutrition have been used for patients with renal failure. The following discussion is divided into four sections: total parenteral nutrition (TPN), peripheral parenteral nutrition (PPN), intradialytic parenteral nutrition (IDPN), and intraperitoneal parenteral nutrition (IPPN).

Total Parenteral Nutrition

Acute Renal Failure

Provision of parenteral nutrition for the patient with renal failure always presents a difficult challenge. The patient with acute renal failure presents further challenges complicated by postsurgical stress, trauma, and/or sepsis with resulting multiple organ failure. Such patients are often unable to ingest or absorb nutrients, are oliguric, and require TPN.

Despite treatment, mortality in this population is extremely high. This is due to the associated complications of underlying disease(s), infections, and poor wound healing rather than from renal failure itself.[1-3] Preexisting malnutrition may be present secondary to underlying disease or may occur rapidly in a catabolic patient who is unable to eat. This adversely affects healing of the renal injury.[4] Malnutrition is also associated with poor wound healing and reduced immunocompetence, increasing the risk of infection and sepsis.[5] Provision of nutrition therapy has a role in reducing catabolism and any underlying malnutrition, repairing cellular damage with perhaps an improved rate of recovery from acute renal failure, and improving immunocompetence, which may be important in improving prognosis.[6]

Careful management of nutrition therapy to avoid electrolyte abnormalities and fluid overload is essential. Usually, the one limiting factor in providing adequate nutrition support to patients with acute renal failure is the fluid allowance. Dialytic therapy is often necessary to allow provision of the volume of TPN needed to meet the protein and calorie needs of the patient, as well as to avoid uremic toxicity. Thus, the goals of nutrition management of patients with acute renal failure are to improve and maintain adequate nutritional status without inducing uremic toxicity or disturbing fluid or electrolyte balance, while facilitating healing of the injured kidney.[7]

The nutrition requirements of patients with acute renal failure vary widely with the clinical setting, degree of catabolism, degree of renal failure, and whether dialysis is used. Many patients with acute renal failure are very catabolic.[6,8] Amino acid losses during dialysis also add to the protein requirement. For the stressed patient, the rate of protein breakdown may be as great as 150 to 200 g/d, necessitating as much as 2 to 2.5 g of protein per kilogram per day.[9,10] The protein requirement for a nonstressed patient is comparable to that in a patient with chronic renal failure (CRF) in the predialysis phase (0.6 to 0.8 g/kg/d), or undergoing either hemodialysis (1.1 to 1.4 g/kg/d) or peritoneal dialysis (1.2 to 1.5 g/kg/d).[11,12] Because of the wide variation in protein needs, use of an objective measurement such as calculation of the protein catabolic rate may be helpful for individualizing protein requirements.[13]

Historically, only essential amino acids rather than mixed solutions of both essential and nonessential amino acids were infused in patients with acute renal failure. This practice was based on the theory that nitrogen from urea could be used to synthesize nonessential amino acids. Studies have shown, however, that insignificant amounts of urea nitrogen are recycled.[10,13–15] An amino acid solution containing both essential and nonessential amino acids is therefore currently recommended.[11]

The resting energy expenditure for patients with acute renal failure associated with multiple trauma, sepsis, and postsurgical complications may be 20% to 50% greater than normal, with an average increase of 26%.[11,16] Acute renal failure per se, however, is not likely to cause any increase in energy expenditure. Therefore, although energy requirements are markedly different for individual patients, they rarely exceed 35 kcal/kg/d.[5] Hirschberg and Kopple make recommendations based on the Harris-Benedict equation with an adjustment factor based on the underlying disease.[11] Ideally, measurements of caloric expenditure by using indirect calorimetry would provide objective data to more closely estimate actual needs.

Energy requirements should be provided with infusions of both glucose and fat. Hypertonic dextrose (70%) and 20% lipid solutions may be useful in providing a concentrated source of calories in the least amount of fluid volume. It is known, however, that glucose metabolism is impaired in patients with multiple trauma, sepsis, or uremia. These disturbances may be exacerbated by diabetes mellitus, pancreatic insufficiency, and glucocorticoid administration. Also, patients undergoing peritoneal dialysis can absorb large amounts of glucose transperitoneally.[17]

Efforts to avoid hyperglycemia and promote cellular uptake of glucose may require the use of exogenous insulin in about half of all patients with acute renal failure receiving TPN. Insulin added directly to the parenteral nutrition solution has the benefit of maintaining a constant glucose-insulin infusion. Some severely glucose-intolerant patients, however, may require a continuous insulin drip to maintain adequate control. In any case, maximum glucose infusion should not exceed 5 mg/kg/min.[18]

Reduction of the glucose infused by increasing the proportion of lipids provided may also be helpful for patients who are very glucose intolerant. A maximum of 60% of the calories can be provided by lipids if they are well tolerated. Because the rate of fat utilization is slower than normal in both acute and chronic renal failure, triglyceride clearance must be monitored.[19] One gram per kilogram of body weight or 30% to 40% of total calories has been found to be a safe amount.[20]

Alterations in serum sodium for patients with renal failure usually represent changes in body water. Hyponatremia rarely represents an absolute deficit of sodium, but rather a dilutional effect with oliguria. Hyponatremia can also be seen with extraordinary fluid losses at surgery, such as with nasogastric suction and fistula drainage. Hypernatremia, on the other hand, may occur with high urine output as a result of depressed antidiuretic hormone secretion, as in nephrogenic diabetes insipidus, which frequently occurs in the recovery phase of acute renal failure.

When hyponatremia exists, the sodium content of the TPN solution may need to be increased, while the total fluid volume given the patient is limited. To correct hypernatremia, the sodium content of the TPN would be decreased and total free water given increased. A general recommendation for the sodium content of TPN solutions provided to patients with renal failure is 40 to 50 mmol/L, given as sodium chloride, sodium acetate, or sodium phosphate (when phosphate is needed).[11]

Increased serum potassium levels may be seen as a result of decreased renal excretion, metabolic acidosis, and/or catabolism. High levels may produce electrocardiographic changes and thus need to be medically treated in conjunction with an alteration in the TPN potassium content. It is important to use potassium-free TPN solutions for patients demonstrating gradually increasing potassium levels or with oliguric renal failure and sudden renal shutdown.

Hypokalemia may occur as the patient is nutritionally replenished or as urine output increases and renal function improves. In general, potassium does not need to be added to TPN solutions until the patient's serum potassium is less than 3 mEq/L.

Oliguric renal failure usually necessitates some decrease in the magnesium content of the TPN because of decreased excretion; however, this would be tempered by gastrointestinal or fistula losses. Estimated TPN requirements are 4 mmol/d, given as magnesium sulfate.[11]

Metabolic acidosis, which is typical of renal failure and more severe in sepsis and hypercatabolic states, can be reduced by adding acetate to the TPN solution. Thirty or more milliequivalents per liter, given usually as sodium acetate, may be initially provided to reduce the acidotic state worsened by concentrated amino acid infusions. Addition of acetate to the TPN solution also reduces the need for an additional bicarbonate drip, which may be important in consolidating fluid volume delivery.

Abnormalities of calcium and phosphorus metabolism occur in both acute and chronic renal failure. Severe hypocalcemia secondary to a reduction in plasma ionized calcium in part due to elevated plasma calcitonin may develop in patients with sepsis and acute renal failure.[11] Standard amounts of calcium may be given in TPN solution (approximately 5 mmol/d) and adjusted upward cautiously after hyperphosphatemia has been corrected. This is necessary to avoid a high calcium-phosphorus product, which could cause precipitation of calcium phosphate from the serum, promoting soft-tissue calcification. Initial TPN solutions must have phosphorus limited or removed when hyperphosphatemia is present. This hyperphosphatemia is worsened by the presence of decreased renal excretion, metabolic acidosis, increased catabolism, and tissue breakdown.

During nutritional repletion with refeeding, phosphorus supplementation may be needed by the fifth to eighth day of TPN therapy, to avoid hypophosphatemia. Maintenance of a TPN solution with phosphorus concentration of 8 mmol/d, given as sodium or potassium phosphate in a patient who is not hyperphosphatemic, may help avoid the frequently inevitable drop in phosphorus to dangerously low levels.

Vitamin requirements are altered in patients with CRF, but those for patients with complicated acute renal failure are poorly defined and based on limited scientific data.[11] Generally, TPN recommendations are based on requirements for patients with CRF and undergoing maintenance dialysis. The need for water-soluble vitamins, especially pyridoxine and folic acid, is increased with renal failure. Dialytic therapy generally increases the need for all water-soluble vitamins except vitamin B_{12} because of losses through the dialysate.

The need for fat-soluble vitamins is still undetermined.[3,13] It is known, however, that serum levels of vitamin A increase in patients with renal failure, and toxicosis has been observed in a few cases where patients were receiving TPN containing vitamin A.[21] It is suggested that patients treated with TPN are more susceptible to this when their protein status is poor (as in malnutrition and stress) and retinol-binding capabilities are exceeded.[22] In practice, vitamin A toxicosis is rarely seen, perhaps because TPN is infrequently given to these patients long enough to produce symptoms. Also, actual stability and availability of vitamin A in TPN solutions may be limited.[22] In any case, it is not generally recommended that vitamin A be added to TPN solutions. When vitamin A is given for practical reasons, however, malnourished patients should be monitored for signs and symptoms of toxicosis.

Vitamin D in the form found in TPN additives cannot be used by the nonfunctioning kidney. Small amounts of active vitamin D_3 (1,25-dihydroxycholecalciferol) can be given intravenously during hemodialysis for severely hypocalcemic patients.[11] The suggested dosage is 0.25 μg/d or 0.5 to 1.0 μg given during dialysis treatments three times per week.[11] This vitamin is not added directly to the TPN solutions.

Vitamin K is not routinely added to the TPN solution because of instability beyond a 24-hour period, but its need can be determined by monitoring prothrombin times.[23] It can be added to the TPN solution in the amount of 1.0 mg/d. Hirschberg and Kopple suggest 7.5 mg of vitamin K per week for patients with renal failure.[11]

Zinc, manganese, copper, and chromium may be deficient in both chronic and acute renal failure.[24,25] Thus, although data are still limited, standard amounts of trace elements should probably be added daily to the TPN solution.

The use of iron in patients with renal failure must be closely monitored. Frequent transfusions combined with decreased erythropoiesis in renal failure can lead to hemosiderosis. The advent of recombinant human erythropoietin therapy has created the need for more iron as more red blood cells are produced. Percentage iron saturation levels may indicate that iron needs to be given (up to 100 mg in five to ten doses) in addition to the 1 to 2 mg/d often given in TPN solutions.[11] See appendix C for more information.

Chronic Renal Failure

Patients with CRF may need to receive parenteral nutrition if comorbid conditions such as severe pancreatitis, short bowel syndrome, inflammatory bowel disease, radiation enteritis, or ischemic gut develop. As in acute renal failure, the needs may vary, depending on the degree of stress from the concurrent illness as well as from any preexisting malnutrition. Generally, the protein requirements for patients with CRF who are nonstressed are the same as for nonstressed patients with acute renal failure. Again, whether dialysis is being used and its specific modality must be taken into consideration.

Caloric needs are generally not less than 35 kcal/kg/d for a patient with CRF who is receiving TPN. A patient with a relative body weight of more than 120% may require fewer calories, and one who is stressed may require more. The amount of sodium, potassium, phosphorus, magnesium, and calcium in these solutions needs to be individualized, as discussed for patients with acute renal failure. Water-soluble vitamins and trace elements should also be added to the TPN solution, and vitamin K should be given as previously discussed.

Table 10.1 presents suggested composition of TPN solutions for patients with acute or chronic renal failure and *Table 10.2* lists monitoring parameters for patients receiving TPN.

Table 10.1
Suggested Composition of TPN Solution for Adults With Acute or Chronic Renal Failure*

Component	Recommendations
Amino acids (essential and nonessential free crystalline amino acids)	Stressed patient (undergoing dialysis): 1.5–2.5 g/kg/d Nonstressed patients 　No dialysis: 0.6–0.8 g/kg/d 　Hemodialysis: 1.1–1.4 g/kg/d 　Peritoneal dialysis: 1.2–1.5 g/kg/d
Calories	Energy sources include dextrose monohydrate (3.4 kcal/g) 70% dextrose solutions may be used to minimize fluid volume Maximum glucose infusion should be 5 mg/kg/min 20% lipid emulsions (2 kcal/mL) may be used to minimize fluid volume Up to 60% of total kilocalories may be from fat, 1 g/kg/d or 30%–40% of total kilocalories is ideal Generally, 35 kcal/kg/d is provided to nonstressed patients undergoing hemodialysis, peritoneal dialysis, or no dialysis (include glucose absorbed from dialysate solutions); 20%–50% additional kilocalories per day may be needed for the stressed patient.
Minerals	
Sodium	40–50 mmol/L
Chloride	25–35 mmol/L
Potassium	about 35 mmol/d
Phosphorus	8 mmol/d
Calcium	5 mmol/d
Magnesium	4 mmol/d
Iron	2 mg/d
Vitamins	
D	See text
K	7.5 mg/wk (may be doubled during antibiotic therapy)
E	10 IU/d
Niacin	20 mg/d
Thiamin HCl	2 mg/d
Riboflavin	2 mg/d
Pyridoxine HCl	10 mg/d
Pantothenic acid	10 mg/d
Ascorbic acid	60 mg/d
Biotin	200 μg/d
Folic acid	1 mg/d
Vitamin B_{12}	3 μg/d

*Please refer to the body of the text for discussion of TPN additives because specific minerals may periodically need to be omitted from solutions.

Adapted with permission from Hirschberg R, Kopple J. Nutritional therapy in patients with renal failure. In: Levine D, ed. *Care of the Renal Patient.* Philadelphia, Pa: WB Saunders; 1991:169–180.

Table 10.2
Monitoring Parameters for Patients Treated With TPN

Serum Values	Initially	Daily	Weekly	Three Times per Week
Glucose	x	x		
Creatinine	x	x		
Cholesterol	x			
Triglycerides	x		x	
Liver enzymes	x		x	
Bilirubin	x		x	
Total protein	x		x	
Albumin	x		x	
Calcium	x			x
Phosphorus	x			x
BUN	x	x		
Magnesium	x		x	
Electrolytes	x	x		
Transferrin	x		x	
CBC with differential	x			x
Ferritin	x			
Iron	x			
Total iron-binding capacity	x			
Prothrombin time	x			x
Weight	x	x		
Intake/output	x	x		

Peripheral Parenteral Nutrition

Peripheral parenteral nutrition can be used as a temporary feeding route for the hospitalized patient who is moderately depleted and unable to consume adequate oral nutrition or who is not currently eligible for central access placement. Generally, 10 days is the maximum duration for PPN, but it has been used for longer periods without ill effects for the non-renal patient. The advantages of PPN include easy access by nonsurgical personnel and minimal risk of serious complications.[8] However, for the patient with renal failure, PPN generally has limited applicability because of the need for fluid constraints in this population and also because of the frequent problem with poor or limited peripheral vein access sites, which are more readily subject to thrombosis.

PPN solutions are hypertonic, and vein thrombosis is a risk even for patients with good peripheral veins. For this reason, the osmolality of PPN solutions must not exceed 900 mOsm/L, necessitating low concentrations of dextrose and amino acids. Solutions containing 10% dextrose with up to 8.5% amino acids or 20% dextrose with no more than 5.5% amino acids may be used. The use of lipid emulsions in conjunction with dextrose and amino acids is important in PPN solutions for two major reasons. First, they provide the main source of calories in these solutions, and second, they offer some degree of protection for the peripheral vein when provided along with dextrose and amino acids. Because lipid emulsions are isotonic, the osmolality of the total infusion is lowered. In any case, because of the need to limit total volume of fluid given to patients with renal failure, PPN can rarely provide sufficient caloric support to warrant its use for more than a few days.

Intradialytic Parenteral Nutrition

Malnutrition is common in the hemodialysis population and frequently independent of other medical conditions.[26-28] When usual means of nutrition and medical therapy such as provision of frequent small feedings, calorically dense foods, oral supplements, and antiemetics have been used without improved nutritional response, IDPN may be considered. IDPN is a method of providing protein and calories intravenously in conjunction with the patient's dialysis treatment. It may be used in the outpatient setting and has the advantage of not requiring placement of a central line for delivery to the patient. IDPN solution is infused directly into the venous drip chamber of the hemodialysis machine.

Anecdotal and small-sample studies have reported nutritional benefits from IDPN,[29-33] but large controlled studies have not been conducted, nor has the ideal maximum solution been identified.[34] For these reasons and because the high cost of IDPN is borne by third-party reimbursement (Medicare Part B), the criteria for using IDPN are very specific.[35] These criteria include a documented primary diagnosis of gastrointestinal abnormality that precludes absorption of adequate protein and calories to maintain weight, such as uremic malabsorption, chronic malabsorption syndrome, gastroparesis secondary to diabetes or uremia, chronic pancreatitis, liver disease, gastrointestinal obstruction, radiation enteritis, inflammatory bowel disease, or short bowel syndrome. Also, the gastrointestinal abnormality must be chronic and anticipated to require intravenous hyperalimentation for at least 3 months.

Unfortunately, the hemodialysis patient who has the "dialysis dwindles syndrome" and may be the best candidate for IDPN is often excluded for lack of a primary diagnosis.[26] Thus, the dietitian's role in documenting various nutrition parameters indicating poor or deteriorating nutritional status is critical.[26,29] Various authors[27,28,36] have suggested specific nutrition assessment indices for identifying IDPN candidates and monitoring patients receiving IDPN therapy. A list of these indices follows.

Subjective data
- History of nausea, vomiting, diarrhea, anorexia, intolerance to oral nutrition

Objective data
- Weight loss: 10% to 15% over 6 months
- Ideal body weight: <90%
- Triceps skinfold values: <6 mm (males) and <12 mm (females)
- Protein catabolic rate: < 0.8 g/kg/d
- Albumin: < 3.5 g/dL (A recent study suggests that a serum albumin level <4.0 g/dL is predictive of greatly increased mortality risk.[37])

Once the IDPN candidate has been identified, there are several considerations for determining the appropriate formula for individual patients. These considerations include:
1. Mixed amino acid solutions containing essential and nonessential amino acids are used, generally providing 50 to 60 g of protein. It has been shown that approximately 90% of

the amino acids given by way of IDPN are retained, thus offsetting amino acid losses during each hemodialysis treatment.[38]

2. Glucose infusions of 3 to 5 mg/kg/min avoid exceeding the maximal oxidative rate; excess is converted to fat.[18]

3. The caloric contribution of lipids should be maximized, but should not exceed 2.5 g/kg/d.[36] To avoid fat overload, lipids should not provide more than 60% of the total calories, and triglyceride levels should be monitored.

4. Vitamins and minerals are not usually added because of loss in the dialysate, although specific minerals may be added if this loss is considerable and the patient requires such replacement.

5. Initial solutions are suggested to be half of the goal volume, to allow monitoring of the patient's insulin response. Serum glucose should be monitored before treatment, 1 hour into the treatment, at midtreatment, and after treatment. If glucose levels are elevated 1 hour into the treatment or at midtreatment (300 mg/dL or higher), insulin may be added to the IDPN solution, taking into consideration the amount of remaining solution. Five units of regular insulin can be added per 1000 mL of IDPN solution as an initial dose, with increments of 2 units for each treatment until satisfactory glucose levels are consistently achieved.[28] If the patient's serum glucose level is less than 200 mg/dL after treatment, a snack such as juice and crackers is suggested. The patient should be monitored for 1 hour after the first IDPN infusion for signs of reactive hypoglycemia. The dialysis unit protocol should indicate appropriate therapy for both hyperglycemia and hypoglycemia.

6. Initial IDPN solutions usually do not contain lipids, in efforts to establish overall tolerance to the infusion separately from the possibility (3%) of an anaphylactic lipid reaction.[33,34] Allergic reactions to lipids include nausea, vomiting, headache, fever, flushes, sleepiness, pain in the chest and back, slight pressure over the eye, dizziness, and irritation at the site of the infusion.

7. Parameters to monitor in a patient receiving IDPN include predialysis electrolytes and phosphorus until the patient is stable. Serum triglyceride levels should also be evaluated before the first infusion of lipids and at least before the second infusion, to assess clearance of serum triglycerides. Ongoing evaluation of these parameters in conjunction with monthly evaluation of biochemical values is then suggested.

Table 10.3 lists sample IDPN solutions that meet the criteria discussed in this section.

Intraperitoneal Parenteral Nutrition

Maintaining good nutritional status can be especially difficult for patients undergoing peritoneal dialysis. Protein losses in the dialysate have been reported to vary between 5 and 15 g/d and to increase by 50% to 100% during episodes of peritonitis.[39] Poor appetite can result in inadequate protein intake and a further decline in protein status.

Some recent studies, as described below, have shown that the infusion of amino acid solutions in place of dextrose may improve nutritional status in patients undergoing peritoneal dialysis. Amino acid solutions might also be beneficial by reducing the glucose load delivered during peritoneal dialysis. This could be especially helpful for patients with insulin-dependent diabetes or hypertriglyceridemia. For the patient undergoing peritoneal dialysis and unable to tolerate adequate enteral feedings, amino acids infused through the dialysis exchange can be used in place of parenteral amino acids.

Table 10.3 Composition of Commonly Used IDPN Solutions

Prescription	Rate (mL/h)	Protein (g)	Carbohy- drate (g)	Fat (g)	Kilo- calories	Percentage of Total Kilocalories
Initial						
250 mL (11.4% amino acids)	125	28.5			114	21
250 mL (50% dextrose)			125		425	79
With Lipids						
500 mL (11.4% amino acids)	250	57			228	19.8
250 mL (50% dextrose)			125		425	37
250 mL (20% lipid)				50	500	43.2
Lipid-free						
500 mL (11.4% amino acids)	250	57			228	21
500 mL (50% dextrose)			250		850	79

When providing 42 g of protein via the peritoneal cavity along with intravenous lipids, Giordano et al were able to maintain positive nitrogen balance and body weight and prevent protein catabolism in patients undergoing peritoneal dialysis.[40]

In several studies, 2 L of 1% amino acids have been successfully substituted in place of dextrose in one or two exchanges per day.[41–44] Ultrafiltration was between that of a 1.5% and 2.5% dextrose solution. Patients on an ad lib diet showed an improvement in nutritional status (increased transferrin and albumin levels and/or improved amino acid profile) with the amino acid dialysate.

After 6 hours, the absorption of a 1% amino acid solution was 87%, and after 8 hours, absorption was 92%.[42] A 2% amino acid solution has also been shown to be well tolerated, with 80% to 90% of the amino acids being absorbed after 6 hours.[45]

While the use of IPPN is increasing, there are several concerns that must be addressed before initiation of this therapy. They are as follows:

1. The patient and/or caregiver must be thoroughly instructed as to appropriate hygenic procedures, as for home parenteral nutrition administration.

2. An experienced supplier must be identified. Currently, IPPN can be supplied through the peritoneal dialysate contractor or a home care company (typically the IDPN supplier).

3. It is not yet determined if third party reimbursement to the supplier will be available through private insurance or Medicare for IPPN therapy.

With the above concerns kept in mind, IPPN may present an option for the many older and sicker patients with diabetes for whom peritoneal dialysis is the chosen modality of treatment.

References

1. Blumenkrantz M, Kopple J, Koffler A, et al. Total parenteral nutrition in the management of acute renal failure. *Am J Clin Nutr.* 1978;31:1831–1839.

2. Knochel J. Complications of total parenteral nutrition. *Kidney Int.* 1985;27:489–496.

3. Mirtallo J, Kudsk K, Ebbert M. Nutritional support of patients with renal disease. *Clin Pharm.* 1984;3:253–263.

4. Toback FG, Havener LJ, Dodd C, et al. Phospholipid metabolism during renal regeneration after acute tubular necrosis. *Am J Physiol.* 1977;232:216–222.

5. Alvestrand A, Bergstrom J. Renal diseases. In: Kinney J, Jeejeebhoy KN, Hill G, Owen O, eds. *Nutrition and Metabolism in Patient Care.* Philadelphia, Pa: WB Saunders; 1988;531–557.

6. Feinstein E. Nutrition in acute renal failure. In: Rombeau J, Caldwell MD, eds. *Clinical Nutrition.* Philadelphia, Pa: WB Saunders; 1984;595–601.

7. Kopple J, Cianiciaruso B. Nutritional management of acute renal failure. In: Fischer JE, ed. *Surgical Nutrition.* Boston, Mass: Little, Brown and Co; 1983;567.

8. Steffe W. Nutrition support in renal failure. *Surg Clin North Am.* 1981;61:661-670.

9. Feinstein EI, Blumenkrantz MJ, Healy M, et al. Clinical and metabolic responses to parenteral nutrition in acute renal failure. *Medicine.* 1981;60:124–137.

10. Feinstein EI. Total parenteral nutritional support of patients with acute renal failure. *Nutr Clin Pract.* 1988;3:3–9.

11. Hirschberg R, Kopple J. Nutritional therapy in patients with renal failure. In: Levine D, ed. *Care of the Renal Patient.* Philadelphia, Pa: WB Saunders; 1991;169–180.

12. Alvestrand A. Nutritional requirements of hemodialysis patients. In: Mitch WE, Klahr S, eds. *Nutrition and the Kidney.* Boston, Mass: Little, Brown and Co; 1988;192.

13. Davis M. Use of PCR to monitor nutrition in patients with renal dysfunction. *Support Line (DNS Newsletter).* 1991;13(2):4–5.

14. Mitch W, Walser M. Effects of oral neomycin and kanamycin in chronic uremic patients. 2. Nitrogen balance. *Kidney Int.* 1977;11:116–122.

15. Walser M. Nutritional support in renal failure: future directions. *Lancet.* 1983;1:340–341.

16. Mault JR, Bartlett RH, Dechert RE, et al. Starvation: a major contribution to mortality in acute renal failure. *Trans Am Soc Artif Org.* 1983;29:390–395.

17. Abel R. Nutritional support in the patient with acute renal failure. *J Am Coll Nutr.* 1983;2:33–44.

18. Reilly J, Gerhardt A. Modern surgical nutrition. *Curr Probl Surg.* 1985;22:1–81.

19. Druml W, Laggner A, Widhalm K, et al. Lipid metabolism in acute renal failure. *Kidney Int.* 1983;24:S139–S142.

20. Druml W, Widhalm K, Laggner A, et al. Fat elimination in acute renal failure. *Clin Nutr.* 1982;1:109–115.

21. Gleghorn E, Eisenberg L, Hack S, et al. Observations of vitamin A toxicity in 3 patients with renal failure receiving parenteral alimentation. *Am J Clin Nutr.* 1986;44:107–112.

22. Muth I. Implications of hypervitaminosis A in chronic renal failure. *J Renal Nutr.* 1991;1(1):2–8.

23. Louie N, Niemiec P. Parenteral nutrition solutions. In: Rombeau J, Caldwell M, eds. *Clinical Nutrition.* Philadelphia, Pa: WB Saunders; 1986;272–305.

24. Burge J, Schemmel R, Park H, et al. Taste acuity and zinc status in chronic renal disease. *J Am Diet Assoc.* 1984;84:1203–1209.

25. Sanstead H. Trace elements in uremia and hemodialysis. *Am J Clin Nutr.* 1980;33:1501–1508.

26. Bilbrey QL, Cohen TL. Identification and treatment of protein-calorie malnutrition in chronic hemodialysis patients. *Dial Transplant.* 1989; 18:669–678.

27. Foulkes CJ. Nutrition evaluation and management of patients on maintenance hemodialysis treatments. *CRN Q.* 1989;13:10–13.

28. Goldstein JD, Strom JA. Intradialytic parenteral nutrition: evolutions and current concepts. *J Renal Nutr.* 1991;1:9–22.

29. Cano N, Labastie-Coeyrebourg J, Lacombe P, et al. Predialytic parenteral nutrition with lipids and amino acids in hemodialysis patients. *Am J Clin Nutr.* 1990;52:726.

30. Heidland A, Kult J. Long term effects of essential amino acid supplementation in patients on regular dialysis treatments. *Clin Nephrol.* 1975;3:234–239.

31. Olshan A, Bruce J, Schwartz A. Intradialytic parenteral nutrition administration dur-

ing outpatient hemodialysis. *Dial Transplant.* 1987;16:495–496.

32. Piraino A, Firpo J, Powers D. Prolonged hyperalimentation in catabolic chronic dialysis treatment patients. *JPEN J Parenter Enter Nutr.* 1981;5:463–477.

33. Moore L, Acchiardo S. Aggressive nutrition supplementation in chronic hemodialysis patients. *CRN Q.* 1987;11:13.

34. Heyman MB. General and specialized parenteral amino acid formulations for nutrition support. *J Am Diet Assoc.* 1990;90:491–411.

35. *PEN Suppliers Guide to Medicare.* Columbia, SC: Medicare; January 1989.

36. Holmes J. Intradialytic parenteral nutrition: concerns and issues. *Contemp Dial Nephrol.* 1990;11:50–54.

37. Lowrie E, Lew NL. Death risk in hemodialysis patients: the predictive value of commonly measured variables and an evaluation of death rate differences between facilities. *Am J Kidney Dis.* 1990;15:458–482.

38. Wolfson M, Jones MR, Kopple JD. Amino acid losses during hemodialysis with infusion of amino acids and glucose. *Kidney Int.* 1982;21:500–506.

39. Lindholm B, Bergstrom J. Protein and amino acid metabolism in patients undergoing continuous ambulatory peritoneal dialysis (CAPD). *Clin Nephrol.* 1988;30:S59–S63.

40. Giordano C, Capodicosa G, DeSanto N. Artificial jut for total parenteral nutrition through the peritoneal cavity. *Int J Artif Org.* 1980;3:325–330.

41. Bruno M, Bagnis C, Maranzella M, et al. CAPD with an amino acid dialysis solution: a long term cross–over study. *Kidney Int.* 1989;35: 1189–1194.

42. Arfeen S, Goodship THJ, Kirkwood A. The nutritional/metabolic and hormonal effects of 8 weeks of continuous ambulatory peritoneal dialysis with a 1% amino acid solution. *Clin Nephrol.* 1990;33:192–199.

43. Oren A, Wu G, Anderson G, et al. Effective use of amino acid dialysate over four weeks in CAPD patients. *Perit Dial Bull.* 1983;3:66–73.

44. Young GA, Dibble JB, Hobson SM, et al. The use of an amino acid based CAPD fluid over 12 weeks. *Nephrol Dial Transplant.* 1989;4:285–292.

45. Williams P, Anderson G, et al. Amino acid following intra-peritoneal administration on CAPD patients. *Perit Dial Bull.* 1982;2:124–130.

11. Medications Commonly Prescribed in Chronic Renal Failure

The purpose of this chapter is to give an overview of selected drugs commonly prescribed during the course of renal failure and how they may affect nutritional status. (See Appendix K for a listing of manufacturer information.)

Table 11.1
Overview of Selected Drugs

Indications and Uses	Drugs	Possible Gastrointestinal Effects	Nutritional Implications and Other Side Effects	Dietary and Medical Management
Aluminum chelating agent				
Used in treatment of: (1) aluminum overload in patients with CRF (usually on dialysis); (2) aluminum-related bone disease, encephalopathy, and microcytic anemia; (3) iron intoxication by binding iron and other trace metals	Deferoxamine (Desferal)	Nausea, vomiting, diarrhea, abdominal discomfort	Mobilizes aluminum from bone and other tissues Long-term use may cause ocular abnormalities Hypotension may occur during hemodialysis Decreased serum calcium may occur due to facilitation of calcium entry into bone after removal of aluminum	Patients should be hemodynamically stable before initiating therapy with this drug Patients receiving this drug should have routine opthalmologic examinations Monitor serum aluminum, iron, ferritin, and calcium levels

(Continued)

Table 11.1—continued
Overview of Selected Drugs

Indications and Uses	Drugs	Possible Gastrointestinal Effects	Nutritional Implications and Other Side Effects	Dietary and Medical Management
Aluminum chelating agent (continued)			Iron deficiency microcytic anemia may develop in patients with marginal iron stores Recently associated with a serious fungal infection (mucormycosis)	
Anabolic-androgenic hormones				
Used to treat anemia due to damaged bone marrow, ineffective erythropoiesis, hemolytic anemia, or neutropenia; currently used infrequently to treat anemia resulting from inadequate erythropoietin production, due to the success of recombinant human erythropoietin	Danazol (Danocrine) Nandrolone decanoate (Deca-Durabolin) Nandrolone phenpropionate (Durabolin)	All of these drugs may cause increased appetite, or nausea, vomiting, diarrhea, and/or mild to moderate liver damage with abnormal values of liver function testing	All of these drugs may cause: dry weight gain commonly seen within 3 mo (due to increased muscle mass); elevated creatinine and triglyceride levels; retention of fluid, sodium, potassium, nitrogen, and phosphorus; and excretion of calcium	A diet adequate in calories, protein, vitamins, and minerals should be provided Monitor serum levels of BUN, creatinine, electrolytes, calcium, and phosphorus, as well as fluid status

Indications and Uses	Drugs	Possible Gastrointestinal Effects	Nutritional Implications and Other Side Effects	Dietary and Medical Management
Anticonvulsant drugs				
Used to control seizures	Phenobarbital Phenytoin (Dilantin) Primidone (Mysoline)	Constipation, gastric irritation, vomiting, nausea, diarrhea, dry mouth, glossitis, stomatitis, decreased taste acuity	Possible decreased serum levels of folate, pyridoxine, vitamins B_{12} and B_6, and calcium Phenytoin has caused increased triglyceride, VLDL cholesterol, glucose, and alkaline phosphatase levels	May need to monitor folate, calcium, or 25-(OH) D_3 levels of patients taking phenytoin; supplements of these vitamins and minerals may be needed
			Phenobarbital and phenytoin cause increased turnover of vitamin D Tube feedings may decrease the bioavailability of phenytoin The sedating effects of ETOH are potentiated by all of these drugs	To minimize gastric irritation, these drugs should be taken with food If constipation develops, prescribe a high fiber diet or supplement Monitor blood levels of phenytoin closely if patient is also receiving tube feedings; may need to give this drug during a break in the feeding regimen
Antihypertensive drugs				
Used to control blood pressure	Atenelol (Tenormin)	Diarrhea, nausea	This beta blocker may mask signs of hypoglycemia in diabetic patients and cause dry mouth, dizziness, drowsiness, and mental confusion (especially in the elderly)	May take with food Monitor serum glucose, potassium, and triglycerides

(Continued)

Table 11.1—continued
Overview of Selected Drugs

Indications and Uses	Drugs	Possible Gastrointestinal Effects	Nutritional Implications and Other Side Effects	Dietary and Medical Management
Antihypertensive drugs (continued)			May cause elevated serum BUN, triglycerides, and potassium	
	Captopril (Capoten)	None noted	This angiotensin-converting enzyme inhibitor may cause hyperkalemia	Take captopril 1 hour before meals on an empty stomach
	Clonidine (Catapres)	Abdominal pain, nausea, constipation, anorexia, vomiting, dry mouth	May cause fluid retention and rebound hypotension when discontinued	Gastrointestinal distress may be less if these drugs are given after meals (all except captopril)
	Enalapril (Vasotec)	May cause diarrhea, nausea, vomiting, abdominal pain	This angiotensin-converting enzyme inhibitor may cause hyperkalemia, increased BUN and creatinine, altered taste, and hyperglycemia (if patient is diabetic)	A low sodium, low potassium diet may be needed (captopril and enalapril) Monitor fluid status due to sodium retention with many of these drugs
	Hydralazine (Apresoline)	Anorexia, nausea, vomiting, diarrhea, constipation	May deplete pyridoxine levels, cause sodium retention, congestive heart failure, and/or anemia	May need to supplement pyridoxine and monitor fluid status and other serum parameters for anemia

Indications and Uses	Drugs	Possible Gastrointestinal Effects	Nutritional Implications and Other Side Effects	Dietary and Medical Management
Antihypertensive drugs (continued)				
	Methyldopa (Aldomet)	May cause flatus, nausea, vomiting, constipation, diarrhea, distention, and/or weight gain	May cause sodium retention, edema, and/or anemia May cause sore mouth	
	Metoprolol (Lopressor) Pindolol (Visken)	Diarrhea, abdominal pain, flatulence, constipation, heartburn	These beta blockers may mask signs of hypoglycemia (diabetic patients) and cause confusion, fatigue, dizziness, or dry mouth	Take with food (enhances absorption) Monitor glucose
	Minoxidil (Loniten)	Nausea and vomiting	May cause marked fluid and sodium retention, which can potentiate congestive heart failure unless given in combination with a beta blocker and a diuretic or dialysis therapy; also causes hirsutism and increased BUN and creatinine	A low sodium diet may be indicated Fluid status should be monitored
	Nitroprusside (Nipride)	Nausea, substernal distress	Decreased vitamin B_{12} levels	May need to supplement vitamin B_{12}
	Prazosin (Minipress)	Abdominal pain, vomiting, constipation, diarrhea, nausea, dry mouth, mild gastrointestinal upset, anorexia	Increased creatinine levels	

(Continued)

Table 11.1—continued
Overview of Selected Drugs

Indications and Uses	Drugs	Possible Gastrointestinal Effects	Nutritional Implications and Other Side Effects	Dietary and Medical Management
Antihypertensive drugs (continued)				
	Propranolol (Inderal)	Constipation, gastrotintestinal distress, nausea	This beta blocker may cause hypoglycemia, elevated potassium and triglyceride levels, and increased liver function test values	Monitor glucose, potassium, and triglyceride levels and liver function
Calcium replacements				
Used to treat hypocalcemia due to secondary hyperparathyroidism and renal osteodystrophy; also used as phosphate binder of choice, rather than aluminum-containing binders; may also be used to neutralize gastric acidity	Calcium acetate Calcium carbonate Calcium citrate Calcium glubionate Calcium gluconate Calcium lactate (Brand names of these drugs are listed in *Tables 11.4* and *11.6*)	Constipation, anorexia, nausea, belching, flatulence	For optimal calcium absorption, active vitamin D is required Hypercalcemia may develop	Acceptable serum calcium levels are 10.5–11.0 mg/dL Recommended doses of elemental calcium are often initiated at approximately 1000 mg/d, but the serum calcium level needs regular monitoring, especially when active vitamin D is being given Low calcium–containing dialysate may be required to continue calcium supplements used for phosphate binding

Indications and Uses	Drugs	Possible Gastrointestinal Effects	Nutritional Implications and Other Side Effects	Dietary and Medical Management
Calcium replacements (continued)				Calcium supplements are frequently avoided until the calcium-phosphorus product is ≤70
			Calcium absorption is impaired by the presence of ferrous salts, corticosteroids, and food sources of oxalic acid and phytic acid	Corticosteroids (if possible) and ferrous salts should not be given at the same time as calcium supplements
				To increase serum calcium only, these drugs should be taken 1 to 1.5 h after meals
				To reduce serum phosphate, these drugs should be taken with or immediately after meals
				All of these drugs should be prescribed according to the amount of phosphorus ingested to prevent hypercalcemia
				Precipitated calcium carbonate tablets should be chewed for gastrointestinal absorption

(Continued)

Table 11.1—continued
Overview of Selected Drugs

Indications and Uses	Drugs	Possible Gastrointestinal Effects	Nutritional Implications and Other Side Effects	Dietary and Medical Management
Calcium replacements (continued)				A high fiber diet or fiber supplement may be prescribed for constipation
			Calcium citrate increases aluminum absorption from other medications or sources	Calcium citrate should not be given if aluminum-containing phosphate binders are prescribed
Cardiac drugs—antianginals Used to control anginal symptoms	Nifedipine (Procardia) Verapamil (Calan); also used as an anti-arrhythmic Diltiazem (Cardizem)	Nausea, diarrhea, constipation, cramps, flatulence	These calcium channel blockers may cause weakness, headache, dizziness, altered taste, hyperglycemia, or increased liver function values	Take with food or milk allowance and monitor glucose (for diabetic patients)
	Nitroglycerin (Nitro-Bid, Nitro-Dur-Patch)	Nausea, vomiting, abdominal pain	May cause headache, dizziness, dry mouth, blurred vision, or flushing	Avoid alcohol and foods containing nitrates

Indications and Uses	Drugs	Possible Gastrointestinal Effects	Nutritional Implications and Other Side Effects	Dietary and Medical Management
Cardiac drugs—antiarrhythmics				
Used to control cardiac arrhythmias	Quinidine (Duraquin, Quinaglute) Amiodarone (Cordarone)	Constipation or diarrhea, abdominal pain, anorexia, nausea and vomiting	Bitter taste, dizziness, visual problems, headache, toxicosis (fast heart rate, loss of consciousness) May cause vitamin K deficiency when taken with anticoagulants	Ideally taken on an empty stomach; take with food or milk allowance if gastrointestinal distress is experienced
Cardiac drugs—glycosides				
Used to strengthen heart muscle contractions and control congestive heart failure	Digoxin (Lanoxin, Lanoxicaps, Digoxin) Digitoxin (Crystodigin)	Anorexia, gastrointestinal irritation, nausea, vomiting (especially with toxic high levels of this drug)	Hypokalemia and magnesium deficiency may increase toxicity Hypercalcemia may increase drug effects and result in arrhythmia High fiber meals or supplements may decrease absorption	Appetite will return with dose adjustment if anorexia occurs Monitor serum magnesium and potassium; may not want to use a low or zero potassium dialysate if this drug is prescribed Monitor serum calcium levels Take this drug 0.5 h before or 2 h after high fiber or high calcium foods or medication

(Continued)

Table 11.1—continued
Overview of Selected Drugs

Indications and Uses	Drugs	Possible Gastrointestinal Effects	Nutritional Implications and Other Side Effects	Dietary and Medical Management
Corticosteroids Used as anti-inflammatory agents in collagen vascular diseases (such as systemic lupus erythmatosus) and immunosuppressive agents in organ transplantation and chemotherapy	Hydrocortisone (Hydrocortone) Methylprednisolone (Medrol) Prednisolone Prednisone (Deltasone, Prednisone)	Gastrointestinal distress, increased appetite, nausea, vomiting, diarrhea, gastric ulcer	Increased serum levels of glucose, cholesterol, and triglycerides may occur Sodium and fluid retention Obesity due to increased appetite and intakes High doses of prednisone over time may cause cushingoid appearance, muscle wasting, and aseptic necrosis of the bones Negative nitrogen balance may occur due to increased protein catabolism Decreased absorption of calcium and phosphorus Vitamin D metabolism is accelerated Excessive loss of potassium may occur	Low carbohydrate, low sodium, low fat diets may minimize some effects for those treated with long-term corticosteroid therapy; monitor fluid status, weight, serum glucose, cholesterol, and triglyceride levels Insulin may be necessary for those who become glucose intolerant (insulin-dependent diabetic patients may need higher insulin doses) Encourage adequate protein, potassium, calcium and phosphorus intake; may take oral preparations with food These drugs should not be discontinued suddenly; gradually taper over several months

Indications and Uses	Drugs	Possible Gastrointestinal Effects	Nutritional Implications and Other Side Effects	Dietary and Medical Management
Diuretics				
To promote sodium and water excretion	Bumetanide (Bumex)	Abdominal pain, cramps, nausea, vomiting, diarrhea	Increases sodium, potassium, and magnesium excretion and may cause glucose intolerance, headache, dry mouth and dizziness	Monitor serum potassium, magnesium, and glucose; may need to increase dietary potassium or provide supplements
	Ethacrynic acid (Edecrin)			
	Furosemide (Lasix)			
	Metolazone (Zaroxolyn)	Diarrhea, abdominal cramps, anorexia		
	Spironolactone (Aldactone)		Potassium retention, altered taste, thirst	Monitor serum potassium levels
Gastrointestinal stimulant				
Used to stimulate gastric emptying; frequently used for diabetic gastroparesis	Metaclopramide (Reglan)	Nausea or diarrhea may occur	Given to prevent the nausea, vomiting, and/or early satiety due to diabetic gastroparesis and/or uremia	Take 0.5 h before meals and at bedtime
			May also cause drowsiness, dizziness, headache, sedation, dry mouth, or lactation	Consider this drug when mental status changes occur in a patient for whom it is prescribed
			May alter insulin requirements for diabetic patients	Monitor glucose levels for diabetic patients

(Continued)

Table 11.1—continued
Overview of Selected Drugs

Indications and Uses	Drugs	Possible Gastrointestinal Effects	Nutritional Implications and Other Side Effects	Dietary and Medical Management
Iron preparations				
Used to treat iron deficiency anemia caused by hemolysis, blood loss, lack of erythropoietin production, and inadequate iron intake; necessary to support erythropoeisis (see section on recombinant human erythropoietin)	Ferrous fumarate Ferrous gluconate Ferrous sulfate	Constipation, diarrhea, nausea, vomiting, altered taste, abdominal cramps, gastrointestinal irritation, dark stools	Iron absorption is impaired by calcium carbonate, magnesium hydroxide, fiber, phytates, tannates, certain sulfur-containing compounds, and cholesterol-lowering drugs Geophagia (the practice of eating clay) also interferes with iron absorption	Iron supplements should be taken before or between meals to minimize the interference that certain substances may exert on iron (may need to be taken with some food if stomach upset occurs)
			Iron absorption may be enhanced by ascorbic acid, fructose, sorbitol, vitamin E, and certain organic acids, including succinic, lactic, pyruvic, and citric acids	Some iron supplements also contain vitamin C and other B-complex vitamins, which should be noted when considering vitamin recommendations for the renal population (see *Table 11.5*) Iron supplements should not be taken within 1 h of taking all antacids and phosphate binders Slow-release iron preparations are not absorbed as well and should be avoided

Indications and Uses	Drugs	Possible Gastrointestinal Effects	Nutritional Implications and Other Side Effects	Dietary and Medical Management
Iron preparations (continued)				
	Polysaccharide iron complex	Polysaccharide iron formulations may produce less gastrointestinal intolerance than others	Polysaccharide formulations are more concentrated in elemental iron, thus requiring a smaller dosage	Monitor serum iron, hematocrit, and ferritin
To provide adequate iron stores when iron deficiency is present and oral iron supplements are not effective	Iron dextran injections		Iron dextran injections may cause falsely decreased serum calcium values	If oral iron is not feasible or effective, injectable iron is advised
	(Refer to *Tables 11.5* and *11.6* for lists of drugs by brand name)			Iron dextran injections are given intravenously for patients prior to initiation of dialysis and for those treated with peritoneal dialysis, or during hemodialysis
Phosphate binders				
Used to control hyperphosphatemia by binding the phosphorus from ingested food in the gastrointestinal tract	Oral calcium preparations (refer to section on calcium replacements)	Constipation, anorexia, nausea, vomiting	Calcium preparations are the preferred phosphate binders due to the potential for aluminum toxicosis	Acceptable serum levels of phosphorus are generally 4.5–6.0 mg/dL
	Aluminum hydroxide		Aluminum toxicosis can result in encephalopathy, osteomalacia, proximal myopathy, and anemia	These drugs should be taken at least 1 h before or after taking iron supplements
	Aluminum carbonate			
	(Refer to *Tables 11.4* and *11.6* for lists of drugs by brand name)		All of these drugs interfere with iron as well as phosphate absorption	Dietary phosphorus should be restricted in conjunction with these drugs

(Continued)

Table 11.1—continued
Overview of Selected Drugs

Indications and Uses	Drugs	Possible Gastrointestinal Effects	Nutritional Implications and Other Side Effects	Dietary and Medical Management
Phosphate binders (continued)				The appropriate dose should be based on phosphorus content of meals and snacks Monitor aluminum levels for patients taking aluminum binders; try to decrease or stop these drugs as soon as serum phosphorus normalizes
Potassium exchange resin				
Used to treat hyperkalemia	Sodium polystyrene sulfonate (Kayexalate)	Constipation, fecal impaction, anorexia, gastric irritation, nausea, vomiting, and diarrhea	This drug binds magnesium and aluminum, as well as potassium, by exchanging sodium for them in the gastrointestinal tract and eliminating them from the body through the stool This drug is ineffective if given without a laxative due to its constipating effect May cause decreased calcium absorption and sodium retention	This drug should not be given with fruit juices because the potassium in the juice, rather than in the gastrointestinal tract, will bind it Give this drug with sorbitol Monitor serum potassium, magnesium, calcium, and volume status

Indications and Uses	Drugs	Possible Gastrointestinal Effects	Nutritional Implications and Other Side Effects	Dietary and Medical Management
Recombinant human erythropoietin				
To replace erythropoietin for patients with CRF who do not produce this hormone in adequate amounts; it is used to treat the anemia of CRF	Epoetin alfa (Epogen, Procrit)	Gastrointestinal distress	Increased appetite, blood pressure, serum creatinine, urea, potassium, and phosphorus levels may occur May promote iron deficiency and low folate and vitamin B_{12} stores Polycythemia may occur if the hematocrit is not carefully monitored	All hematologic parameters, as well as iron status, should be monitored regularly Iron supplementation frequently required in conjunction with this therapy Vitamins containing folate and vitamin B_{12} should be provided Blood pressure, BUN, creatinine, potassium, phosphorus, and uric acid should be monitored regularly This drug may be contraindicated for patients with uncontrolled hypertension

(Continued)

Table 11.1—continued
Overview of Selected Drugs

Indications and Uses	Drugs	Possible Gastrointestinal Effects	Nutritional Implications and Other Side Effects	Dietary and Medical Management
Vitamins Used to treat or prevent vitamin deficiencies caused by removal of water-soluble vitamins by dialysis, decreased absorption from the gastrointestinal tract, inadequate intake, and/or "leaching" by cooking techniques	(See *Table 11.3* for various vitamins available and used in the renal population); when using vitamins containing large amounts of vitamin C (>100 mg), the potential for oxalate retention in the renal population must be considered	Gastrointestinal irritation, nausea, vomiting	Patients with CRF may require vitamin supplementation before undergoing dialysis if they have inadequate nutrient intakes due to poor appetite or dietary restrictions, hyperemesis, malabsorption diarrhea, drug-alcohol abuse, and/or other medical complications The status of vitamin C, pyridoxine, and folate is affected by uremia, especially if intakes are inadequate Patients with CRF do not need vitamin A supplements; the potential for vitamin A toxicosis exists Vitamin supplements may be given after renal transplantation if nutrition is inadequate	See individual sections for vitamin recommendations during various phases of renal failure

Indications and Uses	*Drugs*	*Possible Gastrointestinal Effects*	*Nutritional Implications and Other Side Effects*	*Dietary and Medical Management*
Vitamin D preparations				
Used to provide the active form of vitamin D, which is not adequately produced in CRF; often necessary to treat secondary hyperparathyroidism and resulting renal osteodystrophy	Calcitriol (Rocaltrol) Calcitriol injection (Calcijex)	Nausea, vomiting, and constipation	Active vitamin D is necessary for absorption of calcium from the gut These drugs should not be given if hypercalcemia or vitamin D toxicosis is evident Prolonged therapy with these drugs may cause elevated BUN, albuminuria, elevated cholesterol, or hypervitaminosis D Mineral oil and cholestyramine impair intestinal absorption of vitamin D preparations	Monitor serum calcium, phosphorus, and parathyroid hormone levels These drugs should generally not be given until the serum phosphorus level is within normal range (4.5–6.0 mg/dL) Acceptable serum calcium levels are generally 10.5–11.0 mg/dL Maintain the calcium-phosphorus product at ≤70 to prevent metastatic calcification

Table 11.2
Effects of Selected Drugs on Biochemical Indices

Biochemical Index	Increased	Decreased
Potassium	Triamterene Spironolactone Amiloride Penicillin G potassium Phosphorus replacements (Fleet Phospho-Soda, K-Phos Neutral, Neutra- Phos, Neutra-Phos K) Anabolic androgenic hormones Potassium supplements Atenelol Captopril Enalapril Propranolol	Penicillin G sodium Laxatives Corticosteroids Furosemide Ethacrynic acid IV sodium bicarbonate Hypertonic glucose and insulin IV Hydrochlorothiazide Kayexalate Bumetanide Metolazone
Calcium	Aluminum hydroxide gel Aluminum carbonate gel Vitamin D preparations Calcium replacements Triamterene Spironolactone Amiloride Hydrochlorothiazide Anabolic androgenic hormones	Tetracycline Corticosteroids Furosemide Ethacrynic acid Anticonvulsants Phosphorus replacements Kayexalate Deferoxamine
Phosphorus	Phosphorus replacements Vitamin D preparations Anabolic androgenic hormones Epoetin alfa	Aluminum hydroxide gel Aluminum carbonate gel Magnesium hydroxide Dilantin Calcium replacements Glucose Sucralfate Vitamin D Corticosteroids
Creatinine	Anabolic androgenic hormones Diazoxide Enalapril Epoetin alfa Minoxidil Na nitroprusside Prazosin	

Biochemical Index	*Increased*	*Decreased*
Urea/nitrogen	Allopurinol Coricosteroids Furosemide Ethacrynic acid Vitamin D preparations Anabolic androgenic hormones Tetracycline Beta blockers Diazoxide Guanethidine Minoxidil Enalapril	Glucose
Iron	Iron preparations Ascorbic acid Sorbitol Vitamin E Amino acids (especially cysteine) Epoetin alfa Oral contraceptives	Cimetidine Clofibrate Aluminum hydroxide gel Aluminum carbonate gel Phosphorus replacements Calcium carbonate Sodium bicarbonate Magnesium hydroxide Tetracycline Deferoxamine Allopurinol Cortisone
Glucose	Corticosteroids Furosemide Hydrochlorothiazide Diazoxide Dilantin	Insulin Oral hypoglycemic drugs Bisacodyl Clofibrate Propranolol
Lipids	Allopurinol Anabolic androgenic hormones Corticosteroids Dilantin Vitamin D preparations Beta blockers Atenelol Propranolol	Clofibrate Cholestyramine Colestipol hydrochloride Gemfibrozil Probucol Niacin Lovastatin Heparin Antidiabetic drugs
Albumin	Heparin (in large doses)	Aspirin Heroin Niacin Oral contraceptives Penicillin

Table 11.3
Nutrient Content of Selected Vitamins

Available Vitamin Supplements	Vitamin C (mg)	Thiamin/B₁ (mg)	Riboflavin/B₂ (mg)	Niacin (mg)
Albee With C*	300	15	10.2	50
Albee With C Alternative†	300	15	10	50
Berocca‡	500	15	15	100
Biotin Forte§	200	10	10	40
Biotin Forte Extra Strength§	100	10	10	40
Dialyvite‖	100	1.5	1.7	20
Iberet¶	150	6	6	30
Iberet 500¶	500	6	6	30
Iberet Folic 500¶	500	6	6	30
Lifeline#	600	15	15	100
Longs Balanced B Complex**	100	10	10	10
Longs Balanced B 100**	100	100	100	100
Nature Made Stress††	600	15	15	100
Nature Made Super B Complex††	150	100	20	25
Nature Made B Complex & C††	300	15	10.2	50
Nephrocaps‡‡§§	100	1.5	1.7	20
Nephro-Vites‖ ‖	60	1.5	1.7	20
Nephro-Vite RX‡‡ ‖ ‖	60	1.5	1.7	20
Safeway High Potency¶¶	500	15	10	100
StressCap##	300	10	10	100
Stress Formula With Biotin and Folic Acid†	600	15	15	100
Stress Tab High Potency##	500	15	10	100
Stress Tab With Iron##	600	15	10	100
Surbex Alternative†	500	15	10	100
Surbex With C¶	250	6	6	30
Tabron Filmseal***	500	6	6	30
Theragran Stress†††	600	15	15	100
Z-Bec Alternative†	600	15	10.2	—

When using vitamins containing large amounts of vitamin C (>100 mg), the potential for oxalate retention in patients with renal failure must be considered.

*A.H. Robins Co., Richmond, Va.

†AARP Pharmacy Service, Alexandria, Va (members only).

‡Roche Laboratories, Nutley, NJ.

§Vitaline Formulas, Incline Village, Nev.

‖Hillestad, San Jose, Calif.

¶Abbott Pharmaceuticals, North Chicago, Ill.

#Lifeline Nutritional Products, Hayward, Calif.

Pyridoxine/B_6 (mg)	Cyanocobelamin /B_{12} (µg)	Folate (µg)	Pantothenic Acid (mg)	Biotin (µg)	Vitamin E (IU)	Iron—Elemental (mg)	Zinc (mg)
5	—	—	10	—	—	—	—
5	—	—	10	—	—	—	—
4	5	500	18	—	—	—	—
25	10	800	10	3000	—	—	30
25	10	800	10	5000	—	—	—
10	6	1000	10	300	—	—	—
5	25	—	10	—	—	105	—
5	25	—	10	—	—	105	—
5	25	800	10	—	—	105	—
5	12	400	20	45	30	—	—
10	—	100	50	10	15	—	—
100	100	400	100	100	—	—	—
5	12	—	20	45	30	—	—
2	15	—	5.5	—	—	—	—
5	—	—	10	—	—	—	—
10	10	1000	10	300	—	—	—
10	6	800	10	300	—	—	—
10	6	1000	10	300	—	—	—
5	12	400	20	45	30	—	—
2	6	—	20	—	—	—	—
5	12	400	20	45	30	—	—
5	12	400	20	45	30	—	—
5	12	400	20	45	30	27	—
5	10	—	20	—	—	—	—
2.5	5	—	10	—	—	—	—
5	25	1000	10	—	30	100	—
25	12	400	20	45	30	27	—
10	6	—	25	—	45	—	—

**Longs Drugs, Walnut Creek, Calif.
††Nature Made Nutritional Products, Los Angeles, Calif.
‡‡Denotes prescription required.
§§Fleming and Co., Fenton, Mo.
‖ ‖R and D Laboratories, Marina del Rey, Calif.
¶¶Safeway Stores, Inc, Los Angeles, Calif.
##Lederle, Pearl River, NY.
***Parke-Davis, Morris Plains, NY.
†††E.R. Squibb and Sons, Princeton, NJ.
Reprinted with permission from McCann L. Selecting an appropriate vitamin supplement. *J Renal Nutr.* 1991;1:95.

Table 11.4
Mineral Content of Selected Drugs

Drug	Dose	K^+ (mg)	Na^+ (mg)	Elemental Ca^{++} (mg)	PO_4 (mg)	Al (mg)	$Mg(OH)_2$ (mg)
Aluminum hydroxide or carbonate							
Alterna gel	5 mL		< 2.5			204	
Alu-Cap or Alu-Tab	1 cap 1 tab		< 2.0			162	
Amphojel							
0.3 g	1 tab		1.8			102	
0.6 g	1 tab		3.0			204	
Susp	5 mL		2.3			109	
Basaljel							
Tablet	1 tab		2.1			140	
Capsule	1 cap		2.8			140	
Reg susp	5 mL		3.0			92	
Extra-strength susp	5 mL		23.0			230	
Dialume	1 cap		1.2			170	
Calcium acetate							
Phos-Lo 667	1 tab			169			
Calcium carbonate							
Alka-Mints	1 tab		< 0.5	340			
Calcium Carbonate 650	1 tab			260			
Calci-Chew	1 tab			500			
Calci-Mix	1 cap			500			
Caltrate 600	1 tab			600			
Dicarbosil	1 tab			200			
Equilet	1 tab		0.3	200			
Nephro-Calci	1 tab			600			
Oscal 500	1 tab			500			
Titralac							
Tablet	1 tab		0.3	168			
Liquid	5 mL		11.0	400			
Calcium carbonate (precipitated)							
Tums							
Regular	1 tab		≤ 2.0	200	3.5		
Extra-strength	1 tab		≤ 2.0	300	5.3		
Liquid	5 mL		≤ 5.0	400	2.6		Trace
Calcium citrate							
Citracal 950	1 tab			200			

Drug	Dose	K^+ (mg)	Na^+ (mg)	Elemental Ca^{++} (mg)	PO_4 (mg)	Al (mg)	$Mg(OH)_2$ (mg)
Calcium glubionate							
Neo-Calglucon	5 mL			115			
Calcium gluconate							
1000 mg	1 tab			93			
485 mg	1 tab			47			
Calcium lactate							
325 mg	1 tab			42			
648 mg	1 tab			84			
Magnesium oxide or hydroxide							
Gelusil							
Tablet	1 tab		1.6			68	200
Liquid	5 mL		0.69			68	200
Maalox							
Tablet	1 tab					68	200
Liquid	5 mL					68	200
Mylanta							
Tablet	1 tab					68	200
Liquid	5 mL					68	200
Phillips Milk							
of Magnesia	5 mL		0.6				405
Miscellaneous							
Alka-Seltzer							
Regular	1 tab		311				
Extra-Strength	1 tab		588				
Kayexalate	1 tsp		345				
K-Phos Neutral	1 tab	45	298		250		
Metamucil							
Effervescent							
powder	1 pkt	290–310	2.0				
Regular powder	1 dose	31	10				
Neutra-Phos	1 cap	278	164		250		
Neutra-Phos K	1 cap	556			250		
Rolaids							
Regular	1 tab		50				15–20
Sodium-free							
and calcium-							
rich	1 tab			130–220			64
Sodium-free,							
extra-strength	1 tab			400			
Sodium bicarbonate	1 tab		177				

Table 11.5
Iron and Vitamin Content of Selected Iron Preparations

Drug	Dose	Elemental Iron(mg)	Vitamin C (mg)	Vitamin B
Ferrous fumarate				
Chromagen	1 cap	66	250	10 μg B$_{12}$
Ferro-Sequels	1 tab	50		
Hemocyte	1 tab	106		
Nephro-Fer	1 tab	115		
Trinsicon	1 cap	110		
Hemaspan	1 tab	110	75	15 μg B$_{12}$
Ferro-Gradumet	1 tab	105	500	
Ferrous gluconate				
Ferrous Gluconate (5 g)	1 tab	39		
Fergon Plus	1 cap	58	75	
Ferrous sulfate				
Feosol				
Tablet	1 tab	65		
Capsule	1 cap	50		
Irospan				
Tablet or capsule	1 tab or cap	60	100	
Slow Fe	1 tab	50		
Polysaccharide iron complex				
Niferex	1 cap	150		
Niferex150 Forte	1 cap	150		25 μg B$_{12}$/1 mg folic acid
Niferex with				
Vitamin C	1 tab	50	100–150	
Nu-Iron				
Capsule	1 cap	150		
Elixir	5 mL	100		

Table 11.6
Percentage of Iron, Calcium, and Aluminum of Selected Drugs

Percentage of Aluminum	*Percentage of Elemental Calcium*	*Percentage of Elemental Iron*

Aluminum hydroxide 34%
  Alternagel
  AluCap
  AluTab
  Amphojel
  Dialume
	Calcium carbonate 40%
	  Calci-Chew
	  Calci-Mix
	  Caltrate
	  Equilet
	  Nephro-Calci
	  Oscal
		Ferrous fumarate 33%
		  Chromagen
		  Feostat
		  Ferro-Sequels
		  Fumerin
		  Hemaspan
		  Hemocyte
		  Nephro-Fer

Aluminum carbonate 23% Basaljel	Titralac Tums	Tabron Trinsicon

Aluminum phosphate 22%
  Phosphajel
	Calcium chloride 27%
	
	Calcium citrate 24%
	  Citracal
		Ferrous gluconate 12%
		  Fergon
		  Ferralet
		  Simron

Sucralfate 20%
  Carafate
	Calcium glubionate 6.5%
	  Neo-Calglucon
	
	Calcium gluconate 9.0%
	
	Calcium lactate 13%
	
	Calcium acetate 25%
	  Phos-Lo
	
	Dibasic calcium
	  phosphate 23%
	
	Tribasic calcium phosphate
	  38%
	  Posture
		Ferrous sulfate 20%–30%
		  Feosol
		  Feratab
		  Ferro-Gradumet
		  Irospan
		  Mol-Iron
		  Slow Fe
		
		Iron dextran 100%
		  In FeD
		
		Polysaccharide
		  Iron-complex 100%
		  Niferex
		  Niferex-150 Forte
		  Niferex with Vitamin C
		  Nu-Iron

Figure 11.1
Sample Patient Information Drug Card

Name of drug: <u>Calcium carbonate (Oscal, Titralac, Tums)</u>

Your Dose:_____

Take _____ tablets/capsules_____ times per day.

The Purpose of Taking This Medicine:

This drug is being used to prevent or treat hypocalcemia (not enough calcium in your blood). You will get the calcium that your body needs from taking this medicine.

This drug may also be used as a phosphate binder and as an antacid to relieve heartburn, sour stomach, or acid indigestion.

Calcium is a mineral that is needed by the body to build and maintain bones and teeth.

In kidney disease, too much phosphorus may accumulate in the blood, causing loss of calcium from the bones. As a result, the bones become brittle or fragile and break very easily.

Possible Side Effects:

Belching, chalky taste, swelling of stomach or gas, constipation (mild).

Check with your physician if any of the following side effects occur: loss of appetite, mood or mental changes, nervousness or restlessness, unusual tiredness or weakness. If you notice any other side effects not listed, please also discuss them with your physician.

Other Information to Know About This Medicine:

As a calcium supplement, it is best that this drug be taken 1 to 1-1/2 hours after meals unless otherwise directed by your physician.

As a phosphate binder, this medicine should be taken with or immediately after your meals.

If you are taking the chewable form of this medicine, chew the tablets well before swallowing. This is to allow the medicine to work faster and be more effective.

Prepared by Peggy Wright Harris, RD, Shreveport Regional Dialysis Center, Shreveport, La. Used by permission.

References

Abreo K. Use of deferoxamine in the treatment of aluminum overload in dialysis patients. *Semin Dial.* 1988;1:55–61.

Allen AM. *Food/Medication Interactions.* 7th ed. Phoenix, Ariz: Food Medication Interactions; 1991.

Boelaert JR, Fenves AZ, Coburn JW. Deferoxamine therapy and mucormycosis in dialysis patients: report of an international registry. *Am J Kidney Dis.* 1991;8: 660–667.

Consumer Reports Books: Drug Information for the Consumer. Mount Vernon, NY: Consumers Union; 1992.

Food and Nutrition Board, National Academy of Sciences, National Research Council. *Recommended Dietary Allowances.* 10th ed. Washington, DC: National Academy Press; 1989.

Grant A, DeHoog S. Drug and nutrient interactions. In: Grant A, DeHoog S, eds. *Nutritional Assessment and Support.* Seattle, Wash: Grant and DeHoog; 1991:153–180.

Makoff R. Water-soluble vitamin status in patients with renal disease treated with hemodialysis or peritoneal dialysis. *J Renal Nutr.* 1991;1:56–73.
McCann L. Selecting an appropriate vitamin supplement. *J Renal Nutr.* 1991;1:94–95.

Physicians' Desk Reference. 46th ed. Oradell, NJ: Medical Economics; 1993.

Shangraw RE. Factors affecting dissolution and absorption of calcium supplements. *Fl Pharm J.* 1987;10–11.

Schmitt J. Selection of an appropriate iron supplement. *J Renal Nutr.* 1992;2:126–128.

Slatapolsky E, Martin K: *Management of Hypocalcemia and Secondary Hyperparathyroidism in Patients with Chronic Renal Disease.* St. Louis, Mo: Renal Division, Department of Internal Medicine, Washington University School of Medicine; 1987.

12. RENAL OSTEODYSTROPHY

Renal osteodystrophy is a generic term that encompasses the bone lesions associated with renal failure. The kidneys' role in mineral homeostasis is so crucial, it is not surprising that metabolic bone diseases develop in patients with chronic renal disease. The kidneys maintain external balance for calcium, phosphorus, and magnesium; produce calcitriol; and degrade parathyroid hormone (PTH). Renal bone disease develops in the early stages of renal insufficiency. When the glomerular filtration rate (GFR) falls to 50% of normal, more than 50% of patients exhibit bone abnormalities at histologic evaluation. When ESRD occurs, nearly all patients have bone abnormalities.[1]

It has been suggested that distribution of the different types of renal osteodystrophy in peritoneal dialysis (PD) patients is similar to that found in hemodialysis patients[2]; however, a recent study of 445 patients showed PD patients to have more adynamic bone disease.[3] The treatment of secondary hyperparathyroidism is the same as for patients undergoing long-term hemodialysis.

Renal bone disease can be divided into four groups. These groups are not completely separate entities, and bone can transform from one form to another. The four types of bone disease are osteitis fibrosa, osteomalacia, mixed lesions, and adynamic bone disease.

Types of Bone Disease

Osteitis Fibrosa

Osteitis fibrosa is seen in approximately 5% to 30% of dialyzed patients.[1] This bone disease is associated with secondary hyperparathyroidism; high levels of PTH lead to the development of osteitis fibrosis. Histologic findings at evaluation of bone include increased numbers of osteoclasts and osteoblasts, excess amounts of woven osteoid, fibrosis, and increased bone turnover.[4] Normally, 80% to 90% of bone matrix is mineralized, and 10% is made of collagen strands soon to be mineralized osteoid. In excessive bone turnover, however, the normal arrangement of collagen fibrils is lost; instead, fibrils are deposited in a random fashion, creating woven bone. Because mineralization of the bone is deficient and haphazard, the bone is prone to fracture.

Hypocalcemia is a powerful stimulant of PTH secretion, but hypocalcemia does not seem to be the sole cause of hyperparathyroidism.[5] Factors that play a role in hypocalcemia and secondary hyperparathyroidism in CRF are phosphate retention, altered vitamin D metabolism, skeletal resistance to the biological effect of PTH, altered "set point" for calcium-regulated PTH secretion, and decreased rates of PTH degradation.

PHOSPHORUS RETENTION

As renal function deteriorates, excretion of phosphorus per unit of glomerular filtration increases in response to increased secretion of PTH. Therefore, phosphorus levels usually remain normal until the GFR decreases to approximately 0.5 mL/s (30 mL/min).[6] Studies of animals have shown that long-term feeding of a high phosphorus diet can lead to hyperplasia of the parathyroid gland, increased intact PTH (i-PTH), and a mild reduction in serum calcium levels.[7,8]

Further studies, in azotemic dogs, have illustrated that decreasing dietary phosphate in proportion to the decrease in GFR can prevent development of secondary hyperparathyroidism over short and long periods.[9,10] Similar results have been found in humans with mild renal failure.[11] In advanced renal failure, however, while reduced phosphate intake resulted in a substantial drop in i-PTH, levels remained elevated.[12] Studies of dialysis patients have correlated serum i-PTH levels with the degree of hyperphosphatemia.[13]

In a study of a group of dogs with advanced renal failure fed a progressively lower phosphorus and calcium diet, ionized calcium decreased, as did serum phosphorus. Serum levels of $1,25\text{-}(OH)_2D_3$ (calcitriol) remained low, but i-PTH gradually decreased. This study suggests that a reduction in dietary phosphorus in advanced renal disease may improve secondary hyperparathyroidism by a mechanism that is independent of serum ionized calcium or the level of $1,25\text{-}(OH)_2D_3$.[5] Thus, hyperphosphatemia plays a role in causing parathyroid hypersecretion, particularly in advanced renal failure.

ALTERED VITAMIN D METABOLISM

The kidneys are the major site for the production of the active form of vitamin D, $1,25\text{-}(OH)_2D_3$. There is controversy, however, regarding the level of kidney function at which vitamin D metabolism becomes abnormal. Slatopolsky and associates found levels of $1,25\text{-}(OH)_2D_3$ to be normal with creatinine clearances greater than 0.67 mL/s (40 mL/min) and low in those with more advanced disease.[14] Others found low circulating levels of $1,25\text{-}(OH)_2D_3$ in patients with moderate renal failure (creatinine clearance of 0.7 to 0.8 mL/s or 40 to 50 mL/min).[15] Patients with a mild degree of renal insufficiency (serum creatinine level less than 221 µmol/L, or 2.5 mg/dL) do not have calcium malabsorption.[16] There is little evidence for low serum values of calcitriol in most patients with early renal insufficiency.

SKELETAL RESISTANCE

An important cause of hypocalcemia in patients with renal insufficiency may be skeletal resistance to the calcemic action of PTH. This means higher circulatory levels of PTH, and parathyroid hyperplasia may be needed for the maintenance of normal serum calcium levels in patients with renal failure. This is based on studies showing a delayed recovery from induced hypocalcemia in patients with mild renal insufficiency compared with results in healthy subjects.[17] Studies in dogs suggest that low levels of circulating $1,25(OH)_2D_3$ are not directly responsible for the skeletal resistance to PTH in CRF. They further suggest that desensitization to high levels of endogenous PTH in uremia prevents a normal calcemic response to the administration of exogenous PTH.[18]

ALTERED SET POINT FOR CALCIUM

One cause of increased PTH levels in CRF may be a shift in the "set point" for calcium.[19] The set point is defined as the ionized calcium concentration required to suppress the secretion of PTH by 50%. It has been shown that the calcium level required to suppress PTH production is higher in patients with renal failure than in healthy persons. Therefore, the normal concentration of serum calcium may not be sufficient to suppress hyperplastic glands, and serum calcium levels may have to be increased to the upper limits of normal to control the release of PTH in patients with secondary hyperparathyroidism.

REDUCED DEGRADATION OF PTH

The major factor responsible for the high plasma levels of i-PTH in patients with renal insufficiency is the increased secretion of PTH. A contributing factor could be decreased catabolism, because the kidneys play an important role in the degradation of PTH. Because the kidneys are the only organs responsible for the removal of carboxy-terminal fragments, there is a marked accumulation of these fragments in renal failure patients. Therefore, high levels of i-PTH result partially from increased secretion, as well as from decreased catabolism secondary to the decreased number of nephrons.[20]

Osteomalacia

Osteomalacia is characterized by a reduction in the number of bone-forming and bone-resorbing cells in association with an accumulation of lamellar osteoid or unmineralized bone collagen. To make the diagnosis of osteomalacia, an abnormal mineralization front must be present. The turnover rate of bone is low in patients with osteomalacia. There is no evidence of secondary hyperparathyroidism in hemodialysis patients with pure osteomalacia. Aluminum toxicosis (in which stainable aluminum deposits are seen at the bone osteoid surface) currently accounts for most of the cases of osteomalacia.

Mixed Lesions

Approximately 45% to 85% of patients undergoing dialysis and most patients with ESRD show evidence of both osteitis fibrosa and osteomalacia at bone biopsy. This is called *"mixed lesions" renal osteodystrophy*.[21] These patients show biochemical findings that are characteristic of high PTH, in addition to features that are associated with signs of vitamin D deficiency, that is, impaired bone formation and mineralization. Mixed lesions are seen in patients with osteitis fibrosa and in whom aluminum-related bone disease is developing.

Bone biopsy is a technique that allows accurate determination of the severity of hyperparathyroidism, the amount of aluminum stored in the bone, the presence of osteomalacia and mixed bone diseases, as well as the state of iron stores. Indications for biopsy include[22]:
1. To assess the severity and consequences of aluminum accumulation.
2. To determine the cause of hypercalcemia.
3. To evaluate bone status prior to parathyroidectomy.
4. To assess bone pain and discomfort.

Adynamic Bone Disease

Adynamic bone disease refers to bone histologic findings that show normal amounts of osteoid, no fibrosis, decreased numbers of osteoblasts and osteoclasts, and low rates of bone formation. PTH levels tend to be low. The development of adynamic bone disease is poorly understood; thus, specific elements of treatment remain largely undefined.

Treatment and Prevention

Much work has been done in determining means to prevent and treat renal osteodystrophy. Control of phosphorus and calcium, use of vitamin D sterols, avoidance of aluminum, and parathyroidectomy have all been extensively studied. Each patient must be considered individually when determining the options available for treatment of renal osteodystrophy.

Control of Phosphorus

The control of phosphorus is accomplished through multiple means. These include a low phosphorus diet, use of phosphate binding medications, and removal of phosphorus by means of dialysis. Ultimately, attention must be given to all of these aspects in each patient to achieve ideal control of phosphorus. Phosphorus levels should be in the range of 1.45 to 1.78 mmol/L (4.5 to 5.5 mg/dL) before dialysis for hemodialysis patients and 1.3 to 1.6 mmol/L (4 to 5 mg/dL) for PD patients. Low levels of phosphorus below 1.1 mmol/L (3.5 mg/dL) should be avoided because of possible development of osteomalacia.

LOW PHOSPHORUS DIET

Approximately 32 to 85 mmol (1000 to 1800 mg) of phosphorus is eaten per day in an average western diet. From this, about 60% to 70% is absorbed, primarily in the jejunum and duodenum.

All foods that are high in protein, such as meat, fish, eggs, poultry, milk, and dried beans and peas, are high in phosphorus. Therefore, the intake of phosphorus is largely related to the protein content of the diet. Phosphorus can be further lowered in the diet by excluding from each food group the foods that contribute the greatest amount of phosphorus yet can be eliminated without affecting the nutritional content of the diet. Examples include avoidance of milk and milk products while relying on meat, fish, and poultry to provide high biological protein, and replacement of whole-grain bread with white bread. Liquid nondairy creamers and other nondairy milk substitutes that contain low levels of phosphorus can be used in place of milk. High phosphorus foods that are not a necessary part of the diet should be automatically eliminated. Examples are liver, peanut butter, canned salmon, beer, colas, dried beans and peas, whole-grain and bran cereals and breads, chocolate, and nuts. *Table 12.1* provides phosphorus content information for several high phosphorus foods.

For hemodialysis patients who require 1 g protein per kilogram of ideal body weight, the dietitian can provide a diet that contains approximately 25.8 to 29 mmol (800 to 900 mg) of phosphorus per day. This applies to diets that contain up to approximately 70 g of protein. Beyond this level it is difficult to keep phosphorus intake under 29 mmol/d (900 mg). A diet with 1.2 to 1.5 g protein per kilogram of ideal body weight has been recommended for PD patients. In spite of elimination of food sources with a high phosphorus content, this leads to an obligate ingestion of more than 32.3 mmol (1000 mg) of phosphorus per day. Diets that are very low in protein (0.6 g/kg) are often used for patients who have renal insufficiency but are not yet being treated with dialysis. These diets may provide only 16.1 to 22.6 mmol (500 to 700 mg) of phosphorus, depending on the meal plan.[23] Because protein nutrition remains a higher priority than dietary phosphorus control, it is important for the dietitian to provide patients with a diet containing the least possible amount of phosphorus while achieving protein needs. It is equally important that patients become knowledgeable regarding phosphorus content of food. A commonly overlooked fact is that consumption of several low phos-

Table 12.1
High Phosphorus Foods

Foods (Ready to Eat)	Portion Size	Phosphorus Content (mg)
Dairy		
Cheese, all types	1 oz	110–220
Half and half	1/2 cup	103
Cream pies or desserts	1/8	100
Custard	1/2 cup	155
Frozen custard	1/2 cup	100
Ice cream	1/2 cup	77
Ice milk	1/2 cup	80
Milk, all kinds	1/2 cup	123
Pudding	1/2 cup	123
Yogurt	1/2 cup	110–160
Protein foods		
Braunschweiger	1 oz	70
Eggs	1 large	103
Liver	1 oz	152
Peanut butter	2 tbsp	122
Salmon	1 oz	70–80
Sardines	1 oz	70–141
Tuna	1 oz	55–70
Vegetables		
Baked beans and pork and beans	1/2 cup	132
Dried beans	1/2 cup	130
Dried peas	1/2 cup	89
Lentils	1/2 cup	90
Mixed vegetables	1/2 cup	58
Soybeans	1/2 cup	161
Bread and cereals		
Barley	1/2 cup	189
Bran	1/2 cup	350
Cornbread (from mix)	2 1/2 x 2 1/2 x 1 3/8-in	209
Waffles (from mix)	7-in diameter	257
Whole-grain breads	1 slice	60
Miscellaneous		
Chocolate	1 oz	65
Nuts	1 oz	102
Beverages		
Beer	12 oz	50
Colas	12 oz	54

Data from *Agriculture Handbook No. 456.* Washington, DC: US Department of Agriculture, US Government Printing Office; 1975.

Pennington JAT. *Bowes and Church's Food Values of Portions Commonly Used.* 15th ed. Philadelphia, Pa: JB Lippincott; 1989.

phorus foods can contribute as much phosphorus to the daily total as one or more servings of high phosphorus foods. Thus, a patient who consumes low phosphorus foods in excess of his regular diet plan will exceed the total phosphorus allowance for the day. It is often not enough simply to avoid high phosphorus foods.

PHOSPHORUS REMOVAL

A study by Hou and colleagues[24] evaluated phosphorus removal in patients undergoing conventional dialysis with a blood flow of 300 mL/min and dialysate flow of 500 mL/min. Predialysis phosphorus levels averaged 2.1 mmol/L (6.7 mg/dL). There was a high rate of phosphorus removal early in dialysis that progressively declined during the 4-hour treatment. The decrease was attributed to the lowering of serum phosphorus levels and the slow movement of phosphorus from the intracellular space and/or bone to extracellular space. Overall, 32.5 mmol (1006 mg) were removed with each treatment. Further studies failed to find an effect of dialyzer membrane type[25] or differences between hemodialysis, hemodiafiltration, and hemofiltration on net phosphorus removal.[26] Corrected anemia through the use of erythropoietin has been shown to decrease the removal of phosphorus by 13% in hemodialysis patients.[27] There does not seem to be an effect of dialysate calcium concentration[24] or buffer[28] on phosphorus removal.

In continuous ambulatory PD (CAPD) patients, the clearance of phosphorus is approximately 4.7 mL/min in a 4-hour exchange.[29] In patients with a mean phosphorus level of 1.7 mmol/L (5.26 mg/dL), 2.1 mmol (65 mg) was removed with each 1.5% dextrose exchange and 3.6 mmol (111.5 mg) with each 4.25% dextrose exchange for a daily phosphorus removal rate of 9.9 mmol (306.6 mg). Therefore, on a weekly basis, CAPD removes no more and possibly less phosphorus than does hemodialysis.

PHOSPHATE BINDERS

Because dialysis cannot remove the amount of phosphorus that is absorbed from the ingestion of currently recommended diets, compounds that bind phosphorus in the bowel, thus preventing absorption, are necessary to control serum phosphorus levels. Bound phosphorus becomes part of the fecal material and is eliminated as such. Various preparations have been used to bind phosphorus, including binders containing aluminum, calcium, and magnesium.

ALUMINUM-CONTAINING BINDERS

Historically, phosphate binding medications were those that contain aluminum. They were considered to be very effective in binding phosphorus[30] and contributed no toxic side effects. Patients, however, complained of constipation, which was often a factor affecting compliance. In spite of adequate water purification following reported epidemics of encephalopathy, osteomalacia, and myopathy when dialysate was contaminated with aluminum, sporadic cases of aluminum toxicosis continued to be reported. Subsequently, it was discovered that aluminum was being absorbed from aluminum binders.[31] Patients who faithfully took the aluminum binders had lower phosphorus and PTH levels and less severe changes of osteitis fibrosa. Unfortunately, these same patients showed clear evidence of aluminum overload.[32] Children and young adults with renal failure who ingest aluminum binders also show evidence of aluminum accumulation at bone biopsy.[33]

Severe aluminum overload leads to osteomalacia, encephalopathy, proximal myopathy, and microcytic anemia. For this reason it is better, when possible, to avoid the use of aluminum binders altogether. These binders are primarily useful for lowering phosphorus in the severely hyperphosphatemic patient. Once phosphorus levels decrease, the patient should be gradually switched to calcium-containing phosphate binders. For dialysis patients who already have been exposed to aluminum and may exhibit evidence of aluminum accumulation, the avoidance of further use will allow for gradual reduction in aluminum levels.[34,35]

Avoidance may be superior to the use of deferoxamine (DFO), a chelating agent, for the removal of aluminum. Although DFO removes substantial aluminum after several months of treatment and results in improved symptoms, several serious side effects have been documented. These include cataract formation, retinitis, neurotoxicity, thrombocytopenia, sepsis, and fatal rhizopus infections.[35]

In spite of inducing side effects when used in larger amounts to remove aluminum, DFO is also a useful diagnostic tool. When it is given in the dose of 20 to 30 mg/kg, an increase in the levels of serum aluminum is produced, because aluminum is released from the bone and other tissues. This test is a nonspecific, noninvasive tool in the diagnosis of aluminum accumulation in bone. Bone biopsy with aluminum staining is required for the most accurate diagnosis of aluminum-induced osteomalacia.

If it is determined that aluminum-containing binders are necessary for a given patient, the dose should remain very small. There is no good evidence that aluminum-containing binders taken together with calcium-containing binders interfere with each other's actions.

CALCIUM-CONTAINING BINDERS

Calcium carbonate has been a known phosphate binder for many years.[36] When problems associated with aluminum-containing binders became evident, a major increase occurred in the use of calcium carbonate as a sole drug to treat hyperphosphatemia and hypocalcemia. Since that time, many studies have illustrated the effectiveness of its use.[37-41]

In a study by Slatopolsky and colleagues, calcium carbonate was used with 20 patients.[42] Calcium content of the dialysate was maintained at 1.625 mmol/L (3.25 mEq/L). Good control of phosphorus and calcium was achieved during the study period of 2 months. The amount of calcium carbonate needed to attain predialysis phosphorus levels of 1.29 and 1.77 mmol/L (4.0 to 5.5 mg/dL) was variable, ranging from 62 to 424 mmol/d (2.5 to 17 g/d). Unfortunately, although the quantity of aluminum used to bind phosphorus was reduced by 80%, about one third of the patients continued to require aluminum binders to achieve target phosphorus levels. Additional aluminum binders were required because further increases of calcium carbonate in these patients induced hypercalcemia.

In further studies, the same investigators studied the long-term effects of a lower dialysate calcium level (1.25 mmol/L or 2.5 mEq/L) along with oral calcium carbonate as the phosphate binder in 21 patients.[43] Calcium and phosphorus were well controlled in these patients without use of additional aluminum binders. The average dose of calcium carbonate was 260.4 mmol/d (10.5 g/d). The calcium carbonate dose correlated well with dietary phosphorus intake, indicating that larger phosphorus loads in the diet required larger doses of binder to achieve acceptable phosphorus levels. Although not significant, PTH levels decreased by 20%. These studies and others point out the usefulness of a lower calcium dialysate in allowing for larger doses of calcium carbonate to lower phosphorus levels.

PD patients are usually maintained on standard dialysate containing 1.75 mmol/L (3.5 mEq/L) of calcium. When serum ionized calcium levels are maintained at the upper limits of normal, a patient absorbs about 0.25 mmol (10 mg) calcium with each 2-L 1.5% dextrose exchange, and 0.5 mmol (20 mg) of calcium are removed with a 4.25% dextrose exchange.[29]

The difference is explained by the increased ultrafiltration volume and solvent drag incurred with the solution of higher osmolality. This indicates that a PD patient would be at risk for development of a positive calcium balance if large amounts of calcium carbonate are used for phosphate binding while a standard dialysis regimen is used. It may be expected that a negative calcium flux of 2.5 to 5.0 mmol/d (100 to 200 mg/d) into dialysis occurs with the use of a 1.25 mmol/L (2.5 mEq/L) calcium dialysate.[44] Such a dialysate is commercially available. As with hemodialysis, this regimen of using a lower calcium dialysate may allow for larger amounts of calcium carbonate to be used for phosphate binding. Dialysate calcium should be lowered mainly to treat hypercalcemia. Hemodialysis patients at highest risk for hypercalcemia are those with low rates of bone turnover, as assessed by low PTH and osteo-calcin levels.[45]

Low calcium dialysate should not be used in all patients. Negative calcium balance and worsening of secondary hyperparathyroidism may develop in patients who do not take adequate oral calcium. The use of a lower calcium dialysate to minimize hypercalcemia in patients relying on large doses of calcium carbonate should be limited to patients who are compliant with the prescribed doses of calcium carbonate.

Long-term use of calcium carbonate to bind phosphorus in dialysis patients is of concern because of possible development of vascular and periarticular calcification. Studies evaluating these effects are limited. However, in a study of 32 hemodialysis patients treated for at least 24 months with calcium carbonate (approximately 80 mmol/d or 3.2 g/d elemental calcium), no difference in the incidence or extent of progressive extraskeletal calcification was found when results were compared retrospectively with those in a group of patients treated with vitamin D and aluminum-containing binders.[46] Additional long-term studies are necessary to confirm that calcium carbonate is safe in dialysis patients.

Another effective substance for phosphate binding is calcium acetate. In studies performed in healthy subjects and patients treated with long-term hemodialysis, calcium acetate appeared to bind approximately twice the amount of phosphorus per amount of calcium absorbed.[47,48] Few studies to evaluate the long-term effects of use of calcium acetate as a phosphate binder and calcium supplement have been performed.

In a study of 91 hemodialysis patients maintained with 1.625 mmol/L (3.25 mEq/L) calcium dialysate, the dose of elemental calcium necessary for phosphorus control was 10 to 15 mmol per meal (400 to 600 mg per meal). Transient hypercalcemia was seen in 17% of the patients.[49] Similar results have been found.[50]

A study comparing the efficacy of calcium acetate with carbonate showed the average daily dose of elemental calcium to be 25.4 ± 8.2 mmol (1018 ± 329 mg) with calcium acetate and 46.9 ± 23.9 mmol (1880 ± 960 mg) with calcium carbonate.[51] The incidence of hypercalcemia was not statistically different between the two. Results were similar in patients treated with oral calcitriol. Further studies using half the amount of elemental calcium in the form of calcium acetate showed control of calcium, phosphorus, and PTH levels comparable to those with calcium carbonate.[52] The incidence of hypercalcemia was the same.

Thus, it appears that calcium acetate is probably more efficient than calcium carbonate as a binder of phosphorus, but calcium acetate has not been shown superior to calcium carbonate in controlling calcium and phosphorus without resulting in hypercalcemia. Additional long-term comparative studies are necessary to evaluate further similarities or differences in the application of these substances.

Calcium citrate has been shown to have phosphate binding and calcium absorption properties similar to those of calcium carbonate. When compared with aluminum-containing binders, calcium citrate resulted in lower levels of serum phosphorus and lower calcium-phosphorus products.[53] Although calcium citrate appears to be effective in controlling calcium and phosphorus in hemodialysis patients, citrate enhances absorption of aluminum.[54]

Avoidance of aluminum-containing phosphate binders while taking calcium citrate may not be adequate to prevent aluminum absorption by citrate, since many other medicines contain substantial amounts of aluminum. Additional substances found in food and nutritional supplements may also enhance aluminum absorption.[55] When this is considered, it may be best to avoid the use of calcium citrate altogether. *Tables 12.2* and *12.3* illustrate the aluminum content of various medications and selected substances that enhance aluminum absorption.

Studies have shown a marked influence of calcium on iron absorption.[56,57] Calcium supplements inhibit the absorption of iron supplements and iron from food when taken with meals. Whereas calcium-containing binders are usually taken with meals, iron supplements should be taken between meals.

Table 12.2
Selected Aluminum-Containing Medications

Type	*Brand Names*
Antacids	Alternagel, Amphojel, Basaljel, Dialume, Gaviscon, Gelusil, Maalox, Mylanta, Riopan
Antidiarrheals	Donnagel, Kaopectate, Kaoline
Antiulceratives	Carafate
Buffered aspirins	Bufferin, Arthritis Strength Bufferin, Arthritis Pain Formula, Ascriptin
Douches	Massengil

From Lione A. Aluminum toxicology. *Pharm Ther.* 1985; 29:255–285.

Table 12.3
Selected Substances That May Enhance Aluminum Absorption

Substance	*Source*
Ascorbic acid	Citrus fruits, food additive, vitamin supplement
Citrate	Shohl's solution, Alka Seltzer, K-Lyte, Citracal
Citric acid	Citrus fruits, food additive

GUIDELINES FOR ADMINISTERING CALCIUM-CONTAINING PHOSPHORUS BINDERS

1. Lower phosphorus levels with diet control.
2. Use aluminum-containing phosphate binding agents, if necessary, to achieve serum phosphorus values in the range of 1.6 to 2.26 mmol/L (5 to 7 mg/dL).
3. Evaluate the phosphorus content of the diet and its distribution among meals and snacks.
4. Begin with approximately 12.5 to 25 mmol/d (500 to 1000 mg/d) elemental calcium from calcium carbonate or 7.5 to 17.5 mmol/d (300 to 700 mg/d) elemental calcium from calcium acetate at each meal.
5. Depending on the amount of phosphorus ingested each day and the distribution among meals and snacks, gradually increase the amount of calcium binder to correct the serum phosphorus level to normal. Add calcium binder to meals and snacks that are heaviest in phosphorus.
6. Once the phosphorus level has been corrected, aluminum binders can be tapered or stopped.
7. Serum total calcium may not be a reliable indication of the actual calcium status, since it underestimates the risk of hypercalcemia. Serum ionized calcium is the most accurate measure. If ionized calcium levels are not available, the second best alternative is a corrected calcium level, which adjusts for serum albumin. As a correcting factor, the following equation should be used: corrected calcium = total calcium in milligrams per deciliter + [0.8 × (4.5 − serum albumin in grams per deciliter)], although some practitioners prefer to use 4.0 − serum albumin in the corrected calcium formula (see chapter 2, Nutritional Assessment in Chronic Renal Failure).
8. If total or corrected serum calcium reaches 2.75 mmol/L (11 mg/dL) or ionized calcium exceeds 1.3 mmol/L (5.2 mg/dL), evaluate use of a lower-calcium dialysate. This allows for more oral calcium intake for phosphate control, yet avoids the use of aluminum-containing binders.
9. The goal of phosphorus control is to reach 1.45 to 1.78 mmol/L (4.5 to 5.5 mg/dL) before dialysis for hemodialysis and about 1.29 to 1.6 mmol/L (4 to 5 mg/dL) for peritoneal dialysis.
10. Phosphorus should not be allowed to drop below 1.13 mmol/L (3.5 mg/dL). Phosphate binders should be decreased in the presence of hypophosphatemia.
11. Additional calcium binders should be added for hyperphosphatemia.
12. When phosphorus levels are under good control but the calcium level is lower than recommended, calcium binders can be added away from meals, such as at bedtime. Vitamin D might be indicated to improve calcium absorption. Patients taking vitamin D may absorb additional phosphorus.
13. If hyperphosphatemia persists in the face of hypercalcemia, the patient should also receive a small dose of phosphate binders containing aluminum or a magnesium-containing binder along with a reduced magnesium dialysate.
14. Patients should be seen frequently by a dietitian and should be educated about all the complications of hyperphosphatemia.

MAGNESIUM-CONTAINING BINDERS

Various magnesium-containing supplements have been evaluated for their phosphate-binding properties. In healthy subjects using magnesium acetate, 28% of ingested phosphorus was absorbed with the maximum dose of 38 mmol (77.2 mEq).[58] In a study of 28 hemodialysis patients who were switched from dialysate containing 0.85 mmol/L (1.7 mEq/L) magnesium to dialysate containing none, magnesium carbonate in doses of 21 to 63 mmol/d (0.5 to 1.5 g/d) successfully controlled phosphorus for up to 2 years. The magnesium carbonate was well tolerated.[59] A similar study was performed in CAPD patients using a magnesium-free dialysate.[60]

Magnesium toxicosis results in muscle weakness, hypotension, electrocardiographic changes, sedation, and confusion.[59] However, when used with a zero magnesium dialysate, magnesium-containing phosphate binders may be useful in controlling the absorption of phosphorus. Unfortunately, magnesium given in high doses may cause severe diarrhea. Magnesium-containing phosphate binders may be most effective when used along with maximal doses of calcium carbonate to achieve phosphorus control while avoiding hypercalcemia. This strategy was reported to be successful when used with a reduction in dialysate magnesium.[46] Further work in this area is also required.

Why Hyperphosphatemia May Persist

COMPLIANCE

Poor compliance with diet and medications is a common problem in dialysis patients. It appears that compliance can be improved with aggressive education and encouragement. Frequent visits and positive reinforcement by the dietitian and others may be of benefit. Unfortunately, attempts to achieve adequate protein intake may interfere with dietary control of phosphorus. Patients on very limited budgets may be forced to rely on such high phosphorus foods as dried beans and peas or peanut butter. Staff awareness of these problems can prevent unnecessary chastisement of the patient. There may be no easy solution to this situation.

PRESCRIPTION ERRORS

A patient may not have been prescribed adequate binders to cover the phosphorus load of the diet. More important, since eating patterns are so variable from person to person or from day to day, it is critical that the binders be titrated to fit the phosphorus load at each meal or snack.

Schiller et al [61] found that the dosing schedule of calcium acetate had a marked effect on phosphorus and calcium absorption. When 25 mmol (1000 mg) of calcium from calcium acetate was given with a standard meal, the percentage of phosphorus absorbed decreased from a baseline of 78% to 31%. When calcium was given 2 hours after a meal or with the patient fasting, however, the percentage of phosphorus absorbed increased to approximately 42%. Calcium absorption averaged 21% when the binder was given with the meal compared with 40% when given in the fasting state. This information translates to some practical applications. For example, if a patient eats a large breakfast, skips lunch, and eats a medium-sized supper, he or she may ingest 45% of the phosphorus for breakfast and 55% at supper. It would not be wise to give this patient an equal number of calcium-containing binders three times a day. The first and last dose may be insufficient to bind the phosphorus ingested, and the middle dose may cause excess calcium absorption, resulting in unnecessary hypercalcemia. Rather, the proper regimen may be to give nearly equal doses at breakfast and supper and none in between. Patients' eating habits should be reviewed frequently and the dosing schedule adjusting accordingly.

PROBLEMS WITH DISSOLUTION

Not all calcium carbonate tablets are equal. Efficacy of different brands of calcium carbonate is varied. Because calcium carbonate is not a drug, according to the US Food and Drug Administration (FDA), it is not subjected to the same rigorous standards the FDA applies to drugs. At this writing, the only calcium-containing phosphate binder that has FDA approval for use is the PhosLo brand. All others are classified as supplements. The outer coating of some calcium carbonate supplements has been observed never to dissolve; other supplements appear to be overcompressed and do not disassociate or break apart. Some manufacturers, in an attempt to promote a starch-free product, have had the substance removed from their ingredients. Starch is a principal disintegrating ingredient.

An interesting report by Kobrin and colleagues[62] describes two dialysis patients with poor control of calcium and phosphorus despite ingestion of large amounts of calcium carbonate. Abdominal radiography showed undisintegrated tablets, and tablets were also recovered from fecal material. To solve the problem, these patients were switched to a brand of calcium carbonate with good dissolution rates. The authors suggest testing of calcium carbonate tablets that have an unknown dissolution rate. A tablet of calcium carbonate placed in 6 oz of vinegar at room temperature and stirred frequently should disintegrate within 30 minutes. This technique may be useful when allowing patients for whom finances are a major problem to use less expensive brands of calcium carbonate.

SEVERE BONE DISEASE

Some patients who have severe hyperparathyroidism and seem to be compliant with phosphate binders and dietary phosphorus persistently have hyperphosphatemia. In these patients the phosphorus may be emanating from the bone as a result of enhanced bone resorption.[63] Bone resorption might be achieved by suppressing PTH with calcitriol. This can be very difficult because calcitriol enhances the absorption of calcium and phosphorus, resulting in high calcium levels along with high phosphorus levels, which causes calcifications. Hyperplasia of the parathyroid glands is the major problem with suppression of PTH in patients with advanced hyperparathyroidism. The large amount of parathyroid tissue may prevent the attainment of significant suppression by calcitriol, requiring a subtotal parathyroidectomy in these patients.

Control of Calcium

Many factors are responsible for the regulation and secretion of PTH, although the most important cause of development of secondary hyperparathyroidism is a reduced level of ionized calcium.

CALCIUM SUPPLEMENTS

Patients with a GFR lower than 0.5 mL/s (30 mL/min) have a significant degree of calcium malabsorption. Restriction of dairy products due to phosphorus content can reduce dietary calcium to only 10 to 12.5 mmol (400 to 500 mg) of calcium per day. Therefore, patients with advanced renal insufficiency or those maintained with hemodialysis can be in constant negative calcium balance unless diets are supplemented. Positive or neutral calcium balance can be achieved in uremic patients when they receive supplemental calcium that results in a total calcium intake above 37.4 mmol/d (1.5 g/d).[64]

Indications for calcium supplementation differ with the stage of renal failure and the sex and age of the patient. Early in renal failure, calcium supplementation should be used primarily as a preventive measure against secondary hyperparathyroidism. Because calcium balance declines and gradually becomes negative at age 35 to 40 years, and women accelerate toward negative calcium balance because of the loss of estrogen in the postmenopausal years, calcium supplements would be indicated for females and older patients even without mild to moderate renal insufficiency. Therefore, older patients, especially women, have an additional need for calcium supplementation.

Hruska suggested the schedule shown in *Table 12.4* for supplementing calcium.[65] Age and sex may be factored in by using the upper ranges when necessary.

Table 12.4
Calcium Supplementation According to Stage of CRF

Stage of CRF	*Calcium Supplementation (mg)*
Early	500–1000
Moderate	1000–1200*
Advanced	1200–1500*
Dialysis	1200–1800*

*These values are for calcium taken apart from that used for phosphate binding. Calcium supplements should be taken when the stomach is empty.

Calcium should be supplemented with caution, however. Patients with marked hyperphosphatemia should not be given calcium supplements because of the risk of increasing the calcium-phosphorus product. A calcium-phosphorus product greater than 70 probably predisposes a patient to extraskeletal calcification.[66] Serum phosphorus levels should be under control before oral calcium supplements are given.

Calcium carbonate and calcium acetate are generally the choice as a source of supplemental calcium. While both forms are relatively well tolerated, calcium carbonate is tasteless, and generic brands are much less expensive. Calcium carbonate contains 40% elemental calcium, and calcium acetate contains 25% elemental calcium. Even though calcium levels appear to be controlled equally by calcium acetate, the number of pills required is often greater. Calcium acetate tablets currently contain less than half the elemental calcium (4.2 mmol or 167 mg) found in standard calcium carbonate tablets (12.5 mmol or 500 mg).

The serum calcium level should be maintained at the upper limits of normal (2.62 to 2.74 mmol/L or 10.5 to 11 mg/dL) because hyperplastic glands require a higher concentration of calcium to suppress the release of PTH than do normal glands. Calcium has a rapid suppressive effect (2 to 3 minutes) on PTH secretion. Also, an inverse correlation between messenger RNA levels and serum calcium concentrations has been demonstrated in rats.[67] Therefore, calcium may affect the steady-state levels of PTH messenger RNA following prolonged periods of hypercalcemia and hypocalcemia. The mechanism by which calcium decreases the syntheses of PTH is not completely understood.

Hypercalcemia can occur during the use of oral supplementation.[68] Most uremic patients with mild hypercalcemia (2.74 to 2.99 mmol/L or 11 to 12 mg/dL) are asymptomatic, but pruritus develops in some patients.[69] The common symptoms of hypercalcemia—nausea, vomiting, anorexia, mental confusion, and lethargy—can develop in other patients. If hypercalcemia occurs, calcium supplements should be discontinued temporarily until the serum calcium level returns to the normal range. Calcium supplementation can be restarted at a lower dose.

VITAMIN D

In healthy people, vitamin D is produced as 7-dehydrocholesterol, converted to previtamin D_3 in the skin, and converted to vitamin D_3 (cholecalciferol). Vitamin D_3 is then hydroxylated in the liver to form 25-hydroxycholecalciferol (25[OH]D_3). The conversion of 25(OH)D_3 to 1,25(OH)$_2$D$_3$ occurs in the renal proximal tubular mitochondria.[70]

Knowledge of the kidneys' role in producing 1,25(OH)$_2$D$_3$ and an understanding of the therapeutic use of vitamin D sterols has led to improved treatment of patients with renal osteodystrophy. In the past years, treatment focused on the use of such sterols at D_2 dihydrotachysterol, 25-hydroxyvitamin D_3 (calcifidiol) and 1 α-hydroxyvitamin (alphacalcidiol). Currently, 1,25-dihydroxyvitamin D_3 (calcitriol) has been the center of investigation and therapy. Calcitriol plays a key role in the day-to-day maintenance of calcium balance. It is the drug of choice in patients with severe hypocalcemia because it is extremely effective in stimulating intestinal absorption of calcium.

Many investigators have studied the benefits of using 1,25(OH)$_2$D$_3$ in treating patients with symptomatic renal osetodystrophy. Reported positive changes include decrease in bone pain, improvement in muscle strength, and lowering of plasma, immunoreactive PTH, and alkaline phosphatase levels. Studies on bone have revealed a prominent decrease in marrow fibrosis and other features of secondary hyperparathyroidism.[71,72]

Intravenous administration of calcitriol has been shown to reduce the serum levels of PTH markedly in hemodialysis patients.[73] PTH suppression with intravenous calcitriol was much greater in comparison with PTH levels achieved after raising calcium levels with oral calcium carbonate. Because the suppression of PTH secretion by calcitriol is dose-dependent, the presumed reason for the suppressive effect is the higher serum concentrations of calcitriol with intravenous administration over that with oral calcitriol. Early during the administration of calcitriol, before a significant increase in ionized calcium levels occurs, there is already a decrease in the concentration of i-PTH, suggesting a direct effect of calcitriol on PTH production.

Several studies have illustrated the direct effects of calcitriol on the synthesis and secretion of PTH.[74] The main effect appears to be related to inhibition of PTH gene transcription and synthesis of pre-pro-PTH messenger RNA. Calcitriol administration also appears to change the set point for PTH suppression by calcium by making the parathyroid gland more sensitive to lower calcium levels.[75] This indicates that, independent of the direct suppressive effects of calcitriol on PTH synthesis, calcitriol lowers the point at which calcium directly suppresses PTH production.

A receptor protein in the parathyroid cells is thought to mediate the control of gene transcription by calcitriol. Parathyroid glands from CRF patients contain fewer receptors. Although it has not been proved that the calcitriol receptor is involved in suppressing PTH synthesis and determining the set point for calcium, it is possible that the reduced number of receptors in parathyroid glands of uremic patients leave the glands less responsive to the inhibiting action of calcitriol. It is not yet known if the serum calcitriol level determines the number of receptors in parathyroid glands, although there is evidence for this in the intestine.[76]

Intravenous calcitriol should be given three times a week at the end of each dialysis. The dose should be started at 0.5 μg per dialysis and gradually increased every 2 weeks until the calcium level is maintained in the upper limits of normal. Initially, the dose necessary may be as high as 2 to 3 μg per treatment; however, over time, the patient may require only 1 to 2 μg. The goal is to give the highest dose possible, while avoiding hypercalcemia. Careful monitoring of serum phosphorus and calcium levels should be done weekly or every other week. Phosphorus levels tend to rise during calcitriol administration because of increased phosphorus absorption in the gut, and additional phosphate binders may be required. Hypercalcemia may occur after several weeks or months of treatment in patients who experience a favorable response to calcitriol. This may be preceded by a decrease or normalization in the plasma alkaline phosphatase level. Hypercalcemia may appear sooner in patients with aluminum-related bone disease or in those with severe secondary hyperparathyroidism who have calcium levels that are slightly above normal before treatment. These patients usually have very large parathyroid glands and often require subtotal parathyroidectomy.

Oral calcitriol has been used for many years to increase serum calcium levels and suppress PTH through suppressive effects of calcium on the gland. Low doses averaging 0.5 μg daily have been used for this purpose. Recent studies have shown that intermittent therapy with oral calcitriol (pulse therapy) is effective in suppressing PTH in hemodialysis patients.[77–79] With doses averaging 4 μg twice weekly, reductions in PTH levels were similar to reductions seen with intravenous therapy. Hypercalcemia was noted; thus, the calcium concentration of dialysate should be reduced to 1.25 mmol/L (2.5 mEq/L). Presumably the drug can be administered in the dialysis facility at the time of dialysis therapy, eliminating the problem of noncompliance. Further long-term studies are needed to confirm the efficacy and safety of this therapy.

Hypercalcemia may prevent the administration of large doses of calcitriol in renal disease patients. The recent development of vitamin D analogs that retain the properties of calcitriol with less calcemic activity may be useful in the treatment of secondary hyperparathyroidism and renal osteodystrophy. One of the compounds, 22-oxacalcitriol (OCT), which differs from calcitriol by the substitution of an oxygen atom for the methylene group at carbon 22, has been found to suppress PTH synthesis and secretion in animal models.[80,81] Studies in normal rats demonstrated that OCT has a significant suppressive effect on the pre-pro-PTH messenger RNA. Studies in dogs with CRF demonstrated that OCT decreases the levels of circulating PTH with no change in levels of serum ionized calcium. Thus, OCT, with similar properties of PTH synthesis and release as calcitriol without a calcemic effect, may prove to be a unique therapeutic tool in the treatment of secondary hyperparathyroidism in patients with CRF. To date, no clinical trials with patients have been performed.

Parathyroidectomy

Phosphorus and calcium control along with the use of vitamin D may not be successful in all patients. Reversal of the symptoms of bone disease and suppression of parathyroid hormone secretion may fail for a number of reasons, including noncompliance. When there is ample evidence of the presence of secondary hyperparathyroidism, parathyroidectomy may be indicated. Parathyroidectomy should be considered the treatment of last resort, and the presence of aluminum-related bone disease should be excluded before surgery. Indications for parathyroid surgery include (1) persistent hypercalcemia, particularly when symptomatic, (2) intractable pruritus that does not respond to dialysis or other medical treatment, (3) progressive extraskeletal calcification that occurs with a calcium-phosphorus product consistently greater than 75 to 80, (4) fractures, and (5) the appearance of ischemic soft-tissue and skin lesions and vascular calcification.[64] Bone biopsy for histologic verification is recommended.

Three types of parathyroidectomy are used. They include subtotal and total parathyroidectomy and total parathyroidectomy with autotransplantation (a small portion of the gland is implanted into the forearm, where it revascularizes and continues to function as normal tissue). Without good control of calcium and phosphorus, recurrent hyperplasia can occur in the remaining gland.

After parathyroidectomy, careful monitoring is required to ensure adequate serum calcium levels because calcium is rapidly taken up by bone. Oral or intravenous calcium supplementation is always needed to correct hypocalcemia. In cases of marked bone disease, hypocalcemia may persist for months following parathyroidectomy, despite use of large amounts of oral calcium and oral calcitriol. An abrupt decrease in serum phosphorus also immediately follows parathyroidectomy, perhaps because of reduced mobilization of phosphate from bone or its increase in bone. Hypophosphatemia may last as long as 1 year after the parathyroidectomy. By the third week after parathyroidectomy, the serum alkaline phosphatase level decreases steadily.[82] Hypocalcemia appears to be less pronounced in patients receiving intravenous calcitriol than in those treated with oral calcitriol, and the serum calcium levels in the former patients remain higher. Additionally, these patients have less pronounced hypophosphatemia, and PTH levels remain lower. Therefore, intravenous calcitriol may be particularly useful in parathyroidectomy patients.[83]

Measurement of PTH

Parathyroid hormone is an 84 amino polypeptide hormone. All of the structural information required for full biological activity is held in the 34 amino acids at the amino terminal portion. Studies of the middle region and C-terminal portions of the molecules have shown them to have no PTH activity. PTH assays are divided into categories on the basis of amino acid region of the PTH molecule they recognize. Examples include: carboxy (C)-terminal, amino (N) terminal, mid-region, and intact PTH.

Carboxy-terminal assays measure mainly biologically inactive fragments; however, because most hemodialysis patients have no residual glomerular filtration, the degradation of the mid- and carboxy-terminal fragments is constant. Therefore, changes in PTH levels are a result of changes in the rate of secretion from the gland. Acute changes in calcium levels do not change levels of PTH measured with the mid- and carboxy-terminal assay because of the prolonged half-life of these fragments in renal failure.

The amino-terminal measurement of PTH is sensitive to acute changes in PTH secretion because there is little detection of the large amounts of background fragments. Mid- and carboxy-terminal assays may be preferable for long-term assessment of parathyroid status in the dialysis population. The amino-terminal assay is better for assessing acute changes in PTH secretion.[84] The assay to detect intact molecules may be the gold standard, but cost is currently a factor in the selection of this assay.

There are different normal values for each individual PTH assay; thus, it is not practical to list them here. All clinicians are advised to become familiar with the normal range for the assay used in their facilities. Levels of ten times normal are generally associated with severe bone disease.

References

1. Malluche HH, Faugere MC. Effects of 1,25(OH)$_2$D$_3$ administration on bone in patients with renal failure. *Kidney Int*. 1990;29(suppl):S48–S53.

2. Malluche HH. Renal bone disease. *Nephrol Exchange*. 1991;1:7–18.

3. Pei Y, Hercz G, Greenwood C, et al. Non-invasive prediction of aluminum bone disease in hemo- and peritoneal dialysis patients. *Kidney Int*. 1992;4:1374–1382.

4. Coburn JW, Slatopolsky E. Vitamin D, parathyroid hormone, and renal osteodystrophy. In: Brenner, Rector, eds. *The Kidney*. 3rd ed. Philadelphia, Pa: WB Saunders; 1986:1657–1729.

5. Lopez-Hilker S, Dusso AS, Rapp NS, et al. Phosphorus restriction reverses hyperparathyroidism in uremia independent of changes in calcium and calcitriol. *Am J Physiol*. 1990;259:F432–F437.

6. Slatopolsky E, Bricker NS. The role of phosphate restriction in the prevention of secondary hyperparathyroidism in chronic renal disease. *Kidney Int*. 1973;4:141.

7. LaFlame GH, Jowsey J. Bone and soft tissue changes with oral phosphate supplements. *J Clin Invest*. 1972;51:2834–2839.

8. Jowsey J, Reiss E, Canterbury JM. Long-term effects of high phosphate intake on parathyroid hormone levels and bone metabolism. *Acta Orthop Scand*. 1974;45:801–806.

9. Slatopolsky E, Caglar S, Gradowska L, et al. On the prevention of secondary hyperparathyroidism in experimental chronic renal disease using "proportional reduction" of dietary phosphorus intake. *Kidney Int*. 1972;2:147–151.

10. Rutherford WE, Bordier P, Marie P, et al. Phosphate control and 25-hydroxycholecalciferol administration in preventing experimental renal osteodystrophy in the dog. *J Clin Invest*. 1977;60:332–341.

11. Llach F, Massry SG, Koffler A, et al. Secondary hyperparathyroidism in early renal failure: role of phosphate retention. *Kidney Int*. 1977;12:459–463.

12. Fotino S. Phosphate excretion in chronic renal failure: evidence for a mechanism other than circulating parathyroid hormone. *Clin Nephrol*. 1977;8:499–503.

13. Foumier AE, Armand CD, Johnson WJ, et al. Etiology of hyperparathyroidism and bone diseases during chronic hemodialysis. II. Factors affecting serum immunoreactive parathyroid hormone. *J Clin Invest*. 1971;50:599–605.

14. Slatopolsky E, Gray R, Adams ND, et al. The pathogenesis of secondary hyperparathyroidism in early renal failure. In: Norman A, ed. *Fourth International Workshop in Vitamin D*. Berlin, Germany: DeGruyer; 1979:1209–1213.

15. Juttman JR, Burman JC, Dekam E, et al. Serum concentrations of metabolites of vitamin D in patients with renal failure. *Clin Endocrinol*. 1981;14:225–232.

16. Coburn JW, Koppel MH, Brickman AS, et al. Study of intestinal absorption of calcium in patients with renal failure. *Kidney Int*. 1973;3:264–272.

17. Llach F, Massry SG, Singer FR, et al. Skeletal resistance of endogenous parathyroid hormone in patients with early renal failure: a possible cause for secondary hyperparathyroidism. *J Clin Endocrinol Metab*. 1975;41:339–345.

18. Galceran T, Martin KJ, Morrissey J, et al. Role of 1,25-dihydroxyvitamin D on the skeletal resistance to parathyroid hormone. *Kidney Int*. 1987;32:801–807.

19. Brown EM. Set point for calcium: its role in normal and abnormal parathyroid secretion. In: Cohn DV, Talmage RV, Mathews JL, eds. *Hormonal Control of Calcium Metabolism*. Amsterdam, The Netherlands: Excerpta Medica; 1981:35–43.

20. Freitag J, Martin KJ, Hruska KA, et al. Impaired parathyroid hormone metabolism in chronic renal failure. *N Engl J Med*. 1978;298:29–31.

21. Sherrard DJ, Baylink DJ, Wergedal JE, et al. Quantitative histological studies on the pathogenesis of uremic bone disease. *J Clin Endocrinol Metab*. 1974;39:119–135.

22. Kaye M. What are the most common errors in the management of renal osteodystrophy? *Semin Dial*. 1989;2:146–148.

23. Norwood K. An expanded role for the dietitian in the treatment of renal osteodystrophy and secondary hyperparathyroidism. *Cont Dial Nephrol*. 1987;8:16–20.

24. Hou SH, Zhao J, Ellman CF, et al. Calcium and phosphorus fluxes during hemodialysis with low calcium dialysate. *Am J Kidney Dis*. 1991;18:217–224.

25. Fleming LW, Hudson SW, Stewart WK. Improved phosphate clearances with polycarbonate membranes. *Clin Exp Dial Apheresis*. 1982; 6:211–222.

26. Man NK, Kuno CT, Poignet JL, et al. Phosphate removal during hemodialysis, hemodiafiltration, and hemofiltration: a reappraisal. *ASAIO Trans*. 1991;37:M463–M465.

27. Lim VS, Flanigan MJ, Fangman J. Effect of hematocrit on solute removal during high effi-

ciency hemodialysis. *Kidney Int.* 1990;37:1557–1562.

28. Miller JH, Gardner PW, Heinecken F, et al. Studies of inorganic phosphate removal during acetate and bicarbonate dialysis (abstr). *Proc Am Soc Artif Org.* 1983;12:57.

29. Delmez JA, Slatopolsky E, Martin KJ, et al. Minerals, vitamin D and parathyroid hormone in continuous ambulatory peritoneal dialysis. *Kidney Int.* 1982;21:862–867.

30. Clarkson EM, Luck VA, Hynson WV, et al. The effect of aluminum hydroxide on calcium, phosphorus and aluminum balances, the serum parathyroid hormone concentrations and the aluminum content of bone in patients with chronic renal failure. *Clin Sci.* 1972;43:519–531.

31. Alfrey AC. Aluminum metabolism. *Kidney Int.* 1986;18(suppl):S8–S11.

32. Delmez JA, Fallon MD, Harter HR, et al. Does strict phosphorus control potentiate renal osteomalacia? *J Clin Endocrinol Metab.* 1986;62:747–752.

33. Salusky IB, Foley J, Nelson P, et al. Aluminum accumulation during treatment with aluminum hydroxide and dialysis in children and young adults with chronic renal disease. *N Engl J Med.* 1991;324:527–531.

34. Finch JL, Bergfeld M, Martin KJ, et al. The effects of discontinuation of aluminum exposure on aluminum-induced osteomalacia. *Kidney Int.* 1986;30:318–324.

35. Delmez JA, Weerts C, Finch JL, et al. Accelerated removal of deferoxamine mesylate-chelated aluminum by charcoal hemoperfusion in hemodialysis patients. *Am J Kidney Dis.* 1989;13:308–311.

36. Clarkson EM, McDonald SJ, DeWardener HE. The effect of a high intake of calcium carbonate in normal subjects and patients with chronic renal failure. *Clin Sci.* 1966;30:425–438.

37. Alon U, Davidai G, Bentur L, et al. Oral calcium carbonate as phosphate-binder in infants and children with chronic renal failure. *Min Electrolyte Metab.* 1986;12:320–325.

38. Hercz G, Jeffrey AK, Andress DA, et al. Use of calcium carbonate as a phosphate binder in dialysis patients. *Min Electrolyte Metab.* 1986;12:314–319.

39. Salusky IB, Coburn JW, Foley J, et al. Effects of oral calcium carbonate on control of serum phosphorus and changes in plasma aluminum levels after discontinuation of aluminum-containing gels in children receiving dialysis. *J Pediatr.* 1986;108:767–770.

40. Malberti F, Maurizio S, Francesco P, et al. Efficacy and safety of long-term treatment with calcium carbonate as a phosphate binder. *Am J Kidney Dis.* 1988;12:487–491.

41. Williams B, Vennegoor M, O'Nunan T, et al. The use of calcium carbonate to treat the hyperphosphataemia of chronic renal failure. *Nephrol Dial Transplant.* 1989;4:725–729.

42. Slatopolsky E, Weerts C, Lopez-Hilker S, et al. Calcium carbonate as a phosphate binder in patients with chronic renal failure undergoing dialysis. *N Engl J Med.* 1986;315:157–161.

43. Slatopolsky E, Weerts C, Norwood K, et al. Long term effects of calcium carbonate and 2.5 mEq/L calcium dialysate on mineral metabolism. *Kidney Int.* 1989;36:897–903.

44. Kawanishi K, Tuschiya T, Namba S, et al. Clinical application of low calcium peritoneal dialysis. *ASAIO Trans.* 1991;37:M404–M406.

45. Meric F, Yap P, Bia MJ. Etiology of hypercalcemia in hemodialysis patients on calcium carbonate therapy. *Am J Kidney Dis.* 1990;16:459–464.

46. Moriniere P, Boudailliez B, Hocine C, et al. Prevention of osteitis fibrosa, aluminum bone disease and soft-tissue calcification in dialysis patients: a long-term comparison of moderate doses of oral calcium ± Mg (OH)$_2$ vs Al(OH)$_3$ ± 1 alpha vitamin D$_3$. *Nephrol Dial Transplant.* 1989;4:1045–1054.

47. Sheikh MS, Maguire JA, Emmett M, et al. Reduction of dietary phosphorus absorption by phosphorus binders: a theoretical, in vitro and in vivo study. *J Clin Invest.* 1989;83:66–73.

48. Mai ML, Emmett M, Sheikh MS, et al. Calcium acetate, an effective phosphorus binder in patients with renal failure. *Kidney Int.* 1989;36:690–695.

49. Emmett M, Sirmon MD, Kirkpatrick WA, et al. Calcium acetate control of serum phosphorus in hemodialysis patients. *Am J Kidney Dis.* 1991;27:544–550.

50. Hess B, Binswanger U. Long-term administration of calcium acetate efficiently controls severe hyperphosphataemia in hemodialysis patients. *Nephrol Dial Transplant.* 1990;5:630–632.

51. Schaefer K, Scheer J, Asmus G, et al. The treatment of uraemic hyperphosphataemia with calcium acetate and calcium carbonate: a comparative study. *Nephrol Dial Transplant.* 1991;6:170–175.

52. Delmez JA, Tindira CA, Windus DW, et al. Calcium acetate as a phosphorus binder in hemodialysis patients. *J Am Soc Nephrol.* 1992;3:96–102.

53. Cushner HM, Copley JB, Lindverg JS, et al. Calcium citrate, a non aluminum-containing phosphate-binding agent for treatment of CRF. *Kidney Int.*

1988;33:95–99.

54. Coburn JW, Mischel MG, Goodman WG, et al. Calcium citrate markedly enhances aluminum absorption from aluminum hydroxide. *Am J Kidney Dis*. 1991;17:708–711.

55. Domingo JL, Gomez M, Llobet JM, et al. Influence of some dietary constituents on aluminum absorption and retention in rats. *Kidney Int*. 1991;39:598–601.

56. Cook JD, Passenko SA, Whittaker P. Calcium supplementation: effect on iron absorption. *Am J Clin Nutr*. 1991;53:106–11.

57. Hallberg L, Brune M, Erlandsson M, et al. Calcium: effect of different amounts on non heme-and-heme-iron absorption in humans. *Am J Clin Nutr*. 1991;53:112–119.

58. Fine KD, Santa Ana CA, Porter JL, et al. Intestinal absorption of magnesium from food and supplements. *J Clin Invest*. 1991;88:396–402.

59. O'Donovan R, Baldwin D, Hammer M, et al. Substitution of aluminum salts by magnesium salts in control of dialysis hyperphosphataemia. *Lancet*. 1986;1:880–882.

60. Shah GM, Winer RL, Cutler RE, et al. Effects of a magnesium-free dialysate on magnesium metabolism during continuous ambulatory peritoneal dialysis. *Am J Kidney Dis*. 1987;10:268–275.

61. Schiller LR, Santa Ana CA, Sheikh MS, et al. Effect of the time of administration of calcium acetate on phosphorus binding. *N Engl J Med*. 1989;320:1110–1113.

62. Kobrin SM, Goldstein SJ, Shangraw RF, et al. Variable efficacy of calcium carbonate tablets. *Am J Kidney Dis*. 1989;14:461–465.

63. Delmez JA, Slatopolsky E. Hyperphosphatemia: its consequences and treatment in patients with chronic renal disease. *Am J Kidney Dis*. 1992;19:303–317.

64. Delmez JA, Slatopolsky E. Renal osteodystrophy: pathogenesis and treatment. *Kidney*. 1990;22:1–8.

65. Hruska KA. Requirements for calcium, phosphorus, and vitamin D. In: Mitch WE, Klahr S, eds. *Nutrition and the Kidney*. Boston, Mass: Little, Brown and Co; 1988:104–130.

66. Parfitt AM. Soft tissue calcification in uremia. *Arch Intern Med*. 1969;124:544–556.

67. Yamamoto M, Igarashi T, Muramatsu M, et al. Hypocalcemia increases and hypercalcemia decreases the steady-state level of parathyroid hormone messenger RNA in the rat. *J Clin Invest*. 1989;83:1053–1056.

68. Ginsberg DS, Kaplan EL, Katz AI. Hypercalcemia after oral calcium carbonate therapy in patients on chronic hemodialysis. *Lancet*.

1973;1:1271.

69. Massry SG, et al. Intractable pruritus as a manifestation of 2° hyperparathyroidism in uremia: disappearance of itching following subtotal parathyroidectomy. *N Engl J Med*. 1968;279:697.

70. De Luca HF, Krisinger J, Darwish H. The vitamin D system: 1990. *Kidney Int*. 1990; 29(suppl):S2–S8.

71. Sherrard DJ, Coburn JW, Bickman AS, et al. A histologic comparison of 1,25(OH)$_2$–vitamin D treatment with calcium supplementation in renal osteodystrophy. In: Norman AW, Schaefer K, Coburn JW, et al, eds. *Vitamin D: Biochemical and Clinical Aspects Related to Calcium Metabolism*. Berlin, Germany: De Gruyter; 1977:719–721.

72. Sherrard DJ, Brickman AS, Coburn JW, et al. Skeletal response to treatment with 1,25-dihydroxyvitamin D in renal failure. *Contrib Nephrol*. 1980;18:92–98.

73. Slatopolsky E, Weerts C, Thielan J, et al. Marked suppression of secondary hyperparathyroidism by intravenous administration of 1,25-dihydroxycholecalciferol in uremic patients. *J Clin Invest*. 1984;74:2136–2143.

74. Slatopolsky E, Lopez-Hilker S, Delmez J, et al. The parathyroid-calcitriol axis in health and chronic renal failure. *Kidney Int*. 1990; 29(suppl):S41–S47.

75. Delmez JA, Tindira C, Groom P. Parathyroid hormone suppression by intravenous 1,25-dehydroxyvitamin D. A role for increased sensitivity to calcium. *J Clin Invest*. 1989;83:1349–1355.

76. Costa EM, Feldman D. Homologous upregulations of the 1,25(OH)$_2$ vitamin D receptor in rats. *Biochem Biophys Res Commun*. 1986; 137:742–747.

77. Tsukamoto Y. Oral 1,25(OH)$_2$D$_3$ pulse therapy. *JBMM*. 1991;9:54–57.

78. Akiba T, Ando R, Shioyama K, et al. Intermittent high-dose oral 1,25-dihydroxyvitamin for secondary hyperparathyroidism in hemodialysis patients. *JBMM*. 1991;9:287–293.

79. Gonzalez E, Bander S, Thielan B, et al. Comparison of intravenous and pulse oral calcitriol for suppression of PTH in patients on hemodialysis (abstr). *Am Soc Nephrol*. 1991.

80. Brown AJ, Ritter CS, Finch JL, et al. The noncalcemic analogue of vitamin D, 22-oxacalcitriol, suppresses parathyroid hormone synthesis and secretion. *J Clin Invest*. 1989;84:728–732.

81. Brown AJ, Finch JL, Lopez-Hilker S, et al. New active analogues of vitamin D with low calcemic activity. *Kidney Int*. 1990;519:22–27.

82. Urena P, Basile C, Brateau G, et al. Short term effects of parathyroidectomy on plasma bio-

chemistry in chronic uremia. *Kidney Int.* 1989;36:120–126.

83. Llach F. Parathyroidectomy in chronic renal failure: indications, surgical approach and the use of calcitriol. *Kidney Int.* 1990;29(suppl): S62–S68.

84. Delmez JA, Slatopolsky E. What are the most common errors in the management of renal osteodystrophy? *Semin Dial.* 1989;2:148–152.

13. ATTAINING NUTRITION GOALS FOR HYPERLIPIDEMIC AND OBESE RENAL PATIENTS

Epidemiologic studies, dietary intervention trials, and studies in experimental animals provide strong evidence that saturated fat and cholesterol restriction can improve plasma lipid levels.[1] Recently, the effects of other dietary constituents in the management of plasma lipid levels have been established. In particular, monounsaturated fatty acids and soluble fibers favorably affect plasma lipid levels. Omega-3 (ω-3) fatty acids are hypotriglyceridemic and antithrombotic. Dietary modifications can result in a 15% to 20% reduction in plasma total cholesterol (TC).

The National Choelesterol Education Program[2] recommends that fat make up less than 30% of total calories, with saturated fat less than 10% of total calories, polyunsaturated fat 10% or less, and monounsaturated fat the balance (10% to 15%) of fat calories. Cholesterol intake should be less than 300 mg/d. The challenge lies in incorporation of these recommendations with the many dietary restrictions already imposed on renal patients.

There is no consensus as to specific intervention therapy for hyperlipidemia associated with renal failure. No previous studies have directly addressed two important issues: (1) whether hyperlipidemia in renal failure should be reduced to slow renal disease progression, and (2) whether the hyperlipidemia of ESRD should be treated to reduce cardiovascular morbidity and mortality.

It should be recognized that abnormal lipid metabolism is a universal finding in patients with renal disease. Members of the medical community who have ignored this problem must now reassess the need for intervention. Accumulating evidence suggests that abnormal lipid metabolism may stimulate degenerative vascular disease, which in turn promotes renal destruction. Investigators are now exploring intensively both the extent of lipid involvement in progressive kidney disorders and the effect of modification of the hyperlipidemia on the rate of renal deterioration.[3]

Hyperlipidemia in Renal Disease

Deranged lipid metabolism is detectable early in the course of progressive renal failure and persists throughout. Some of the lipid disturbances identified in uremic patients include hypertriglyceridemia in most, reduced high density lipoprotein cholesterol (HDL-C) levels in uremic and hemodialysis patients, and elevated total cholesterol levels in patients under-

This chapter originally appeared, in a slightly altered form, in: *Renal Nutrition: Report of the Eleventh Ross Roundtable on Medical Issues.* Columbus, Ohio: Ross Laboratories; 1991:26–33. Used by permission.

going continuous ambulatory peritoneal dialysis (CAPD) and transplantation.[4–6] Lipoprotein lipase, hepatic lipase, and lecithin-cholesterol acyltransferase levels are depressed in uremic patients.[4] Additionally, the altered carbohydrate metabolism associated with renal failure has been implicated as a cause of the lipid abnormalities. The concurrent hyperinsulinemia and peripheral insulin resistance contribute to the development of hypertriglyceridemia. Of the two mechanisms implicated in hypertriglyceridemia—increased production and impaired removal—the latter emerges as the primary cause.[5]

Predialysis and Hemodialysis

For 15 years, Maschio et al[7] followed a large population of patients with early renal failure and long-term dietary protein restriction. These patients were maintained on a diet containing approximately 35 kcal/kg, 0.6 g of protein per kilogram, and 700 mg of phosphate per day. Approximately 50% of total calories was provided by carbohydrate and 40% by fat with a polyunsaturated to saturated (P:S) ratio of 2.0, and the cholesterol content averaged 300 mg/d. Throughout the study, these patients demonstrated no significant changes in serum cholesterol levels, the means of which were at the upper limit of normal, or in serum triglyceride (TG) levels, the mean values of which were only slightly elevated. Maschio and associates[7] also noted that if this diet successfully inhibits renal functional deterioration, it may prevent some of the metabolic abnormalities leading to decreased catabolism of lipoprotein. Low protein diets supplemented with essential amino acids of their keto analogs do not seem to influence serum lipid abnormalities in patients with advanced renal failure.[8]

Most treatment for altered lipid metabolism in renal failure has focused on elevated serum TG levels, which may be compounded by dietary considerations. Because diets for renal failure are often restricted in protein, potassium, phosphorus, sodium, and fluids, it is difficult to satisfy a patient's energy needs without prescribing large intakes of purified sugars, which may enhance TG production. The dietary study by Sanfelippo and colleagues[9] in nondialyzed uremic patients found that a 15% reduction in carbohydrate intake produced a significant reduction in the serum TG turnover rate, and other research has shown that increasing dietary P:S fatty acid ratios ameliorates the lipid abnormalities in uremic patients treated with maintenance dialysis.[10,11]

Studies have shown that treating chronically uremic patients who have elevated serum TG levels with L-carnitine lowers these levels, presumably by facilitating fatty acid oxidation.[12–15] Most of the cases of carnitine deficiency in renal failure have been described in patients treated with maintenance hemodialysis or CAPD.

Fish oil supplementation also has reduced lipid profiles in uremic and hemodialysis patients. Hamizaki and coworkers[16] reported that in hyperlipidemic hemodialysis patients, serum TG and total cholesterol levels and diastolic blood pressure decreased after administration of fish oil concentrate.

Elevated serum TG levels constitute a weak risk factor for cardiovascular disease, and studies have not evaluated whether lowering them in chronically uremic patients will improve morbidity and mortality. Serum total cholesterol levels are usually normal in CRF. If the serum cholesterol level is elevated, Kopple and Hirschberg[17] recommend a diet providing 50% of total calories from carbohydrate, with an emphasis on complex carbohydrate; the rest of nonprotein calories should come from fat, with a P:S ratio of 1.0 and emphasis on monounsaturated fatty acid sources. If the serum TG level increases, the serum carnitine level is measured. If the serum carnitine level is low and TG levels do not respond to carnitine therapy, carbohydrate, primarily from complex carbohydrate sources, should be reduced to 35% of total calories. The fat content should be raised to supply the rest of the calories by emphasizing monounsaturated fatty acid sources, with the P:S ratio remaining at 1.0. A trial with ω-3 fatty acids also should be considered.

High fiber foods should be incorporated with caution, because many of these foods are also high in potassium and phosphorus. A high fiber diet also requires increased fluid consumption to avoid constipation, and this would be contraindicated for patients with a fluid restriction. The quantity of soluble fiber intake required to realize such a small reduction in serum cholesterol level could result in more important metabolic abnormalities, such as hyperkalemia and metabolic bone disease. High fiber foods also are higher in protein of low biological value, particularly that from starches; consequently, their use is limited in a protein-controlled diet requiring 60% protein of high biological value.

Compliance with these modifications in dietary lipid and carbohydrate intake is often difficult for patients. Unless serum TG levels are quite abnormal, adherence to the appropriate protein, phosphorus, sodium, and potassium intake should be emphasized. Dietary lipid and carbohydrate intake should be modified only if the patient is adhering well to the protein and mineral prescription and is able to tolerate further restrictions in the diet, or if the patient's lipid levels are quite elevated. Because these dietary modifications often reduce the palatability of the diet, the patient must be monitored closely to ensure that energy intake does not decrease and calorie malnutrition does not develop.

In the nephrotic syndrome, plasma albumin levels decrease, leading to synthesis of apoprotein B by the liver and suppression of low density lipoprotein-receptor synthesis, both of which result in the characteristic severe hypercholesterolemia. Consequently, dietary therapy, although a valuable adjunct to treatment, will not normalize serum cholesterol levels in most nephrotic patients, and drug therapy will be required.[4]

Continuous Ambulatory Peritoneal Dialysis

CAPD is associated with a number of metabolic abnormalities, including lipid abnormalities such as hypertriglyceridemia, increased levels of very low density lipoprotein cholesterol (VLDL-C), and decreased HDL-C levels; carbohydrate abnormalities resulting from the absorption of large quantities of glucose; protein losses consisting of albumin and amino acid losses; and a propensity to obesity.[18] Few long-term studies of lipid metabolism in CAPD patients have been conducted, but some available data indicate that hypertriglyceridemia worsens in a significant proportion of patients treated with CAPD within 2 to 3 months of the initiation of this form of therapy.[18] This complication has been attributed to the large quantities of glucose (150 to 200 g/d) absorbed from the dialysate, stimulating endogenous VLDL-C production by the liver. Prospective studies have found that patients whose plasma TG level initially increases remain hypertriglyceridemic and continue to have elevated VLDL-C levels and reduced HDL-C levels while treated with CAPD.[19] Other studies have shown, however, that TG levels return to baseline in about 1 year, suggesting an adaptation to the peritoneal dialysis dextrose load.[20]

Because energy in the form of glucose is constantly absorbed from the peritoneal cavity, CAPD patients can receive between 500 and 800 kcal/d in addition to their oral dietary intake. In many, this increased intake results in weight gains of up to 5 kg within several months after initiation of treatment.[19] Although salt and fluid intake need not be restricted in many patients undergoing CAPD, obese and hypertriglyceridemic patients may require individual guidelines for sodium and fluid intake to avoid using the hypertonic exchanges. Obesity is a complication, particularly if large quantities of 4.25% glucose dialysate must be used to achieve adequate ultrafiltration. Until a noncaloric osmotic agent becomes readily available, undesirable weight gain among some CAPD patients will remain a problem. Ingestion of a diet containing carbohydrate in excess of caloric needs results in obesity and increased adipose tissue and further compounds lipid abnormalities.

In light of the continuous absorption of glucose from dialysate, the diet recommended to CAPD patients limits dietary sources of concentrated sweets and emphasizes complex carbohydrates, which provide 35% of total calories. This regimen requires dietary counseling because compliance at this level of carbohydrate restriction is difficult. The remainder of the nonprotein calories should be provided as fat with a P:S ratio of 1.0 and an emphasis on monounsaturated fatty acids. A trial of ω-3 fatty acids also can be considered. A calorie intake of 25 to 30 kcal/kg/d is recommended for stable maintenance patients. If repletion or weight gain is indicated, caloric intake should increase to 35 to 40 kcal/kg/d. For obese patients, calories should be restricted to 20 to 25 kcal/kg/d. None of these recommendations include kilocalories contributed by the glucose in the dialysate. In the obese patient, the conflicting problems of providing 1.2 to 1.5 g of protein per kilogram per day and reducing caloric intake produce a further complication.

Transplantation

It is estimated that more than two thirds of renal transplant recipients may have hyperlipidemia, depending on when lipid profiles are examined.[21] Unlike the isolated hypertriglyceridemia of CRF and dialytic therapy, lipid profiles change after transplantation, with a rise in cholesterol concentration alone or in combination with TGs. Type IIb hyperlipidemia is at least as common as type IV, and HDL-C levels often return to normal. A number of factors may be responsible for the hyperlipidemia, including cyclosporine and steroid therapy, underlying renal dysfunction, basal hyperinsulinism with glucose intolerance, antihypertensive drug therapy, and obesity.[22]

Posttransplantation obesity is a common phenomenon. Among the multiple factors favoring this weight gain are the sudden increase in the sense of well being following a successful transplant procedure, with concomitant food splurging; the high-calorie intake typically prescribed in the initial postoperative days; freedom from the dietary constraints associated with the treatment of progressive renal failure and dialysis; stimulation of appetite by high doses of steroids; metabolic bone disease that limits the mobility needed for exercise; and the relatively sedentary life-style and low energy expenditure to which patients have become accustomed during their period of renal insufficiency.[22]

Usually, most weight is gained (an average of 25 lb) in the first 6 to 12 months following successful transplantation, and the rate of weight gain subsequently levels off. This obesity has undesirable effects on blood pressure, glucose metabolism, and hyperlipidemia, increasing the likelihood of accelerating atherosclerosis. For these reasons, transplantation candidates should be told about the posttransplantation risks of obesity and encouraged both to limit their total caloric intake by avoiding simple carbohydrate and added fats and to initiate a program of exercise to maintain a desirable body weight. As in all weight control programs, motivation is paramount to success. Any modality of renal replacement therapy a patient selects requires his or her initiative and cooperation. Unfortunately, the rate of compliance with low calorie diets is poor, and exercise programs may not be possible for many patients. Clinical observations have indicated that patients who return to employment and lead active, productive lives are better able to control their stimulated appetite and weight gain.

In a recent study of cadaveric kidney transplant recipients, 46 obese patients were matched with 50 nonobese control patients and analyzed retrospectively for mortality, morbidity, and graft survival.[23] Obesity was defined as a body mass index greater than 30. Only 13 of the 46 obese patients were defined as morbidly obese. Significant differences were found between obese and nonobese patients in mortality (11% vs 2%), immediate graft function (38% vs 64%), 1-year graft survival (66% vs 84%), wound complications (20% vs 2%), intensive care unit admissions (10% vs 2%), reintubations (16% vs 2%), and new-onset diabetes (12% vs 0%). These results suggest that significant weight reduction is indicated in obese patients before renal transplantation.[23]

Fortunately, irrespective of cause, transplant-associated hyperlipidemia often is amenable to dietary therapy, as evidenced in studies by Disler et al[22] and Shen et al.[24] The usefulness of fish oil for patients with transplants also has been a subject of recent investigation.[25] Hyperlipidemic kidney transplant recipients consuming a 3-g dose of ω-3 fatty acids over a 3-month period experienced a significant (34%) reduction in serum TG and VLDL-C levels, with no significant changes observed in total cholesterol or low density lipoprotein cholesterol levels.

Dietary guidelines for the stable transplant patient generally correspond to the National Cholesterol Education Program guidelines: Limit cholesterol to 300 mg daily; consume fewer than 30% of calories from fat, with saturated fatty acid intake limited to 10%; consume at least 50% of calories from carbohydrate, with an emphasis on complex carbohydrate and fiber; restrict consumption of concentrated sweets; and consume total calories appropriate to attain ideal weight. Research also indicates that ω-3 fatty acids at a dose of 3 g daily can be safely recommended for and tolerated by kidney transplant patients with elevated serum TG levels not amenable to traditional diet therapy.[24]

Conclusion

Since atherosclerotic plaque develops over many years, risk factors for atherogenesis should be modified early in the course of CRF. Management strategies for uremic patients can be patterned after recommendations for the general population. Lipid profiles should be checked early in the course of CRF and regularly thereafter. The cornerstone of therapy remains diet modification. Although large diet trials have not been performed in uremic patients, several small studies[9–11] indicate that diet management may be effective in ameliorating the lipid abnormalities seen in uremia.

References

1. American Heart Association Nutrition Committee. Dietary guidelines for healthy American adults: a statement for physicians and health professionals. *Circulation.* 1986;74:1465A.

2. Report of the National Cholesterol Education Program Expert Panel on detection, evaluation, and treatment of high blood cholesterol in adults. *Arch Intern Med.* 1988;148:36.

3. Avram MM. Cholesterol and lipids in renal disease. *Am J Med.* 1989;87:1N-2N.

4. Chan MK, Varghese Z, Moorhead JF. Lipid abnormalities in uremia. *Kidney Int.* 1981;19:625.

5. Ibels LS, Simons LA, King JU, et al. Studies on the nature and cause of hyperlipidemia in uremia, maintenance dialysis and renal transplantation. *Q J Med.* 1975;44:601.

6. Cattran DC, Fenton SA, Wilson DR, et al. Defective triglyceride removal in lipidemia associated with peritoneal dialysis and hemodialysis. *Ann Intern Med.* 1976;85:29.

7. Maschio G, Oldrizzi L, Rugiu C, et al. Serum lipids in patients with chronic renal failure on long-term, protein-restricted diets. *Am J Med.* 1989;87:5.

8. Attman PO, Bustafson A, Alaupovic P, et al. Effect of protein-reduced diet on plasma lipids, apolipoproteins, and lipolytic activities in patients with chronic renal failure. *Am J Nephrol.* 1984;4:92.

9. Sanfelippo ML, Swenson RS, Reaven GM. Reduction of plasma triglyceride by diet in subjects with chronic renal failure. *Kidney Int.* 1977;11:54.

10. Tsukamoto Y, Okubo M, Yoneda T, et al. Effects of a polyunsaturated fatty acid-rich diet on serum lipids in patients with chronic renal failure. *Nephron.* 1982;31:236.

11. Dornan IL, Gokal R, Pearce JS, et al. Long-term dietary treatment of hyperlipidemia in patients treated with chronic hemodialysis. *Br Med J.* 1980;281:1044.

12. Bertoli M, Battistella PA, Vergani MS, et al. Carnitine deficiency induced during hemodialysis and hyperlipidemia: effect of replacement therapy. *Am J Clin Nutr.* 1981;34:1496.

13. Borum PR. Carnitine. *Annu Rev Nutr.* 1983;3:233.

14. Vacha GM, Giorcelli G, Siliprandi N, Corsi M. Favorable effects of L-carnitine treatment on hypertriglyceridemia in hemodialysis patients: decisive role of low levels of high-density lipoprotein cholesterol. *Am J Clin Nutr.* 1983;38:532.

15. Caruso U, Cravotto E, Tisone G, et al. Long-term treatment with L-carnitine in uremic patients undergoing chronic hemodialysis: effects on the lipid pattern. *Curr Ther Res.* 1983;33:1098.

16. Hamizaki T, Nakazawa R, Tateno S, et al. Effect of fish oil rich in eicosapentaenoic acid on serum lipids in hyperlipidemic hemodialysis patients. *Kidney Int.* 1984;26:81.

17. Kopple JD, Hirschberg RR. Requirements for protein, calories, and fat in the predialysis patient. In: Mitch WE, Klahr SK, eds. *Nutrition and the Kidney.* Boston, Mass: Little, Brown and Co; 1988;131–153.

18. Morrison G. Metabolic effects of continuous ambulatory peritoneal dialysis. *Annu Rev Med.* 1989;40:163.

19. Lameire N, Matthys D, Matthys E, et al. Effects of long-term CAPD on carbohydrate and lipid metabolism. *Clin Nephrol.* 1988;30:S53.

20. Lindholm B, Norbeck HE. Serum lipids and lipoproteins during continuous ambulatory peritoneal dialysis. *Acta Med Scand.* 1986;220:143–152.

21. Cattran DC, Steiner G, Wilson DR, et al. Hyperlipidemia after renal transplantation: natural history and pathophysiology. *Ann Intern Med.* 1979;91:554.

22. Disler PB, Goldberg RB, Kuhn L, et al. The role of diet in the pathogenesis and control of hyperlipidemia after renal transplantation. *Clin Nephrol.* 1981;16:29.

23. Holley JL, Shapiro R, Lopatin WB, et al. Obesity as a risk factor following cadaveric renal transplantation. *Transplantation.* 1990;49:387.

24. Shen SY, Lukens CW, Alongi SV, et al. Patient profile and effect of dietary therapy on post-transplant hyperlipidemia. *Kidney Int.* 1983;24:S147.

25. Pagenkemper JJ, DiMarco NM, Hull AR, et al. The management of hypertriglyceridemia and hypercholesterolemia by omega-3 fatty acids in renal transplant patients. *CRN Q.* 1989;13:9.

14. Nutrition Management of the Patient With Urolithiasis

Urolithiasis is a common and often recurrent disorder that frequently causes significant morbidity as well as intermittent loss in productivity in susceptible persons. In societies that have shifted toward an industrial focus, the location of calculi has shifted from the bladder to the upper urinary tract. The incidence of upper urinary tract stones is increasing, particularly in the highly industrialized areas of western Europe and North America.[1,2]

A number of theories have been proposed to explain the epidemiology of urolithiasis, particularly calcium urolithiasis. The incidence tends to vary with patient age, sex, and racial group. Two major factors are probably inherited anatomic or biochemical predisposition and environmental influences such as climate, geographic location, occupation, dietary pattern, and the volume of fluid intake and urine excretion.

Causes of Urolithiasis

Most calculi are formed in the kidney and result from an organic matrix that contains variable amounts of calcium, oxalate, and phosphate. A small proportion of calculi are composed of cystine or uric acid or have a core of one of these substances surrounded by calcium oxalate. About 80% of calculi seen in North America are calcium-containing stones. In the majority of cases they are idiopathic, consisting predominantly of calcium oxalate crystals. Nutrition management tends to have its greatest impact on calcium urolithiasis, so the discussion that follows will focus on this disorder.

Persons in whom kidney stones form experience a shift in the body's homeostatic balance, allowing occurrence of a number of disordered processes that favor the formation of calculi. The goal of medical and nutrition therapy is the restoration of homeostatic control, aimed at providing a normalized urine composition and the inhibition of further calculi formation.

The formation of kidney stones is dependent on the following factors, which occur simultaneously: (1) retention of particles that promote crystal formation and growth, (2) increased supersaturation of the urine with organic salts, and (3) decreased levels of naturally occurring inhibitors of crystal formation.[3-5]

The impact of diet on the alteration of urine composition and the formation of kidney stones is significant and well recognized.[5-11] Dietary habits that tend to increase the risk of future stone formation in susceptible people include inadequate fluid consumption and excessive intake of sodium, calcium, oxalate, and animal protein products, particularly those from flesh protein sources.[7-12] *Table 14.1* illustrates the relationship between urinary risk factors and dietary components.

Table 14.1
Correlation of Urinary Risk Factors to Dietary Components

Urinary Risk Factors	Significant Dietary Intake Factors
High sodium	Salt and sodium
High calcium	Salt and sodium, protein, calcium, fiber, vitamin D
High oxalate	Oxalate, protein, vitamin C
High uric acid	Protein, purine
Low urine volume	Fluid

Patient Evaluation

Urolithiasis generally begins as a surgical problem involving an already formed stone, which frequently causes the patient a great deal of pain and suffering. Referral of patients for medical diagnosis and individualized therapy aimed at the prevention of future stone formation tends to occur after surgical intervention.

Nutrition advice on the modification of dietary risk factors is an important part of prevention of future stone formation. Indications for patient referral to the dietitian should include the following disorders: (1) multiple calculi, (2) recurrent calculi, and (3) abnormalities of urine chemistry that are potentially responsive to diet modification.

Screening to determine which patients will benefit from nutrition intervention by a qualified dietitian should ideally be completed by staff nephrologists or urologists. Referral to the dietitian frequently occurs after surgery or lithotripsy, at a time when the patient is comfortable, free from pain, and ready to absorb educational information. Intervention, data on stone composition, and serial laboratory information on blood and urine chemistry should be reviewed for each patient before dietetic evaluation.

It is important to become familiar with the evaluation of parameters that confirm the accuracy of 24-hour urine collections. Urine creatinine and creatinine clearance are particularly significant. Inaccurate collections make it impossible to evaluate accurately the results given for excretory products. It is also important to consider urine volume in relation to the concentration of ionic substances excreted.

Information obtained from a 24-hour diet recall and a food frequency recall are correlated with metabolic and stone composition data. An individualized education plan should be prepared and discussed with the patient. Follow-up 24-hour urine collections and blood work should be arranged about 1 month after diet modification to determine compliance with advice given and impact on urine composition.

Patient progress on the medical and nutrition regimen should be monitored through follow-up appointments with the nephrologist and additional referrals to the dietitian as required. Intermittent monitoring of therapy is important because medical intervention provides a prophylactic, rather than a curative, mode of treatment for recurrent urolithiasis.

Nutrition Considerations in Calcium Urolithiasis

Nutrition advice on the modification of the following risk factors is an important part of preventive management.

Fluid Intake

Maintenance of a high fluid intake is important in reducing the risk of recurrent urolithiasis. In a recent paper by Embon, Rose, and Rosenbaum,[13] a low urine volume secondary to chronic dehydration because of occupation or the avoidance of drinking water was found to be the most significant risk factor for urinary stone formation in susceptible people.

An adequate fluid intake is encouraged to ensure a minimum urine output of about 2 L per day. During normal activity, approximately 3 L of fluid must be consumed to enable the production of 2 L of urine.[8,12,14] Persons with additional gastrointestinal losses or losses through perspiration need to increase fluid consumption further.

An increase in urine output permits a decrease in the concentration of ionic particles and the saturation level of various salts, thereby diluting the effect of potential lithogenic substances. Fluids should be taken in divided doses throughout the day, with about 50% of the total volume coming from water.[8,12] It has been reported that the prevention of new stone formation can be achieved in about 60% of patients with idiopathic calcium urolithiasis if they consistently comply with advice on adequate fluid intake.[14]

Sodium Intake

Hypercalciuric patients who reduce their intake of dietary sodium typically have a concurrent decrease in the urinary calcium excretion.[10,15] Patients with recurrent calcium stones and hypercalciuria tend to be more sensitive than healthy control subjects to the hypercalciuric action of dietary sodium.[16] A high sodium intake may contribute to calcium stone formation through the enhanced renal excretion of calcium and by the enhancement of urine supersaturation with calcium salts.[8,9,15]

A moderate restriction in sodium intake to about 100 to 150 mEq (2300 to 3500 mg) per day might be helpful for patients with hypercalciuria. The North American habit of consuming frequent meals at fast-food restaurants and the regular use of packaged convenience foods and sodium-rich snack products can have a significant impact on sodium excretion.

Care must be taken not to overrestrict sodium in some people, however, since aggressive restriction of this element can sometimes adversely affect thirst, resulting in reduced fluid intake and inadequate urine volume.

Calcium Intake

Severe dietary restriction of calcium is unlikely to be beneficial in reducing the frequency of new stone formation in patients with recurrent urolithiasis. A negative balance in calcium along with secondary hyperoxaluria are potential outcomes if dietary calcium is too severely restricted.[10]

A moderate restriction in dietary calcium is indicated when the patient is motivated and when the appropriate metabolic disorder has been identified. Calcium restriction is not indicated in patients with idiopathic hypercalciuria who have normal intestinal absorption of this element; however, an excessive intake should be avoided.[8] Subjects with absorptive hypercalciuria are ideal candidates for the use of a mildly restricted calcium regimen (800 mg/d). A limit of 1200 mg/d for pregnant and lactating women and 1200 to 1500 mg/d for postmenopausal women has been suggested as well.[9]

Patients being maintained on calcium-restricted regimens need adequate education and intermittent monitoring. Dairy products should be permitted in limited quantity, depending on individual metabolic parameters, stone composition, and the results of diet intake history. Dietary restriction of calcium must always be accompanied by simultaneous restriction in oxalate consumption; otherwise, free oxalate present in the intestine will diffuse across the membrane, causing an increase in urinary oxalate excretion.

Oxalate Intake

Dietary oxalate has a significant effect on urinary oxalate excretion.[17,18] Small increases in oxalate excretion can significantly affect urinary supersaturation with calcium oxalate crystals. Hyperoxaluria is probably the most important risk factor (after a low urine volume) for calcium oxalate stone formation.[7,13,19] Of interest, the role of hypercalciuria in the formation of calcium stones seems secondary compared to the influence of hyperoxaluria.[19]

Serial 24-hour urine values for oxalate do not always indicate significant elevation. It is therefore important to be aware of stone composition. If 24-hour urine values are consistently normal for oxalate but stone composition data indicate calcium oxalate crystals, then dietary advice on oxalate control is indicated.

Overall, urinary oxalate levels tend to be higher in patients with recurrent urolithiasis.[18] The sustained hyperoxaluria found in patients with recurrent calculi might be explained by the following factors. These patients might ingest an excess of dietary oxalate, absorb a greater proportion of normal dietary oxalate intake, or have a metabolic defect leading to increased oxalate synthesis.[7,10,20]

Concurrent hyperoxaluria with hyperuricosuria was found to be more common than hyperoxaluria on its own in one study.[21] Hyperuricosuria might be an important additional risk factor for calcium oxalate urolithiasis.[21]

Approximately 10% to 15% of the oxalate excreted in urine comes from dietary sources, with the remainder arising from endogenous metabolism. The portion of dietary oxalate that is absorbed depends on its bioavailability (the portion available for intestinal absorption).[8,22]

Dietary oxalate restriction should be undertaken simultaneously with regimens restricted in calcium, to prevent the stimulus of increased oxalate excretion that occurs when dietary calcium is controlled. Foods believed to be major sources of oxalate in the diet are listed in *Table 14.2.*[23] Comprehensive data from tables on food sources of oxalate and its bioavailability are presently limited. As a result, inconsistencies in the education of patients on oxalate-restricted regimens are frequent.

Protein Intake

In healthy people, a diet that is high in animal protein increases the urinary excretion of calcium, oxalate, and uric acid. This shift in urinary parameters has been found to occur immediately after a protein meal and is sustained for as long as protein intake remains high.[10]

Calcium stone formation has been correlated with an abnormal urine composition in which increased calcium, oxalate, and uric acid along with decreased urine pH and the inhibitor substance citrate all act to increase the probability of future stone formation.[5,8,19,24] Epidemiologic evidence suggests a relationship between calcium urolithiasis and dietary protein intake.[5,19,24] Animal protein sources seem to have a greater impact than vegetable protein sources on increasing urinary risk factors.[25,26]

Table 14.2
Foods High in Oxalate Content (More Than 10 mg per ½-Cup Serving)[23,33,34]

Beans
   String, wax
    Legume types (including
      baked beans canned in tomato sauce)
Beets
Blackberries
Carob powder
Celery
Chocolate/cocoa
   other chocolate drink mixes
Concord grapes
Dark leafy greens
   Spinach
    Swiss chard
    Beet greens
    Endive, escarole
    Parsley
Draft beer
Fruitcake
Eggplant
Gooseberries
Grits (white corn)
Instant coffee (more than 8 oz/d)
Leeks
Nuts, nut butters
Okra
Peel: lemon, lime, orange
Raspberries (black)
Red currants
Rhubarb
Soy products (tofu)
Strawberries
Summer squash
Sweet potatoes
Tea
Wheat germ

The mechanisms by which dietary protein intake leads to hypercalciuria have been suggested as follows: (1) The acid load in a diet high in animal protein can cause bone resorption and a decrease in renal tubular calcium reabsorption[27,28]; and (2) a high protein diet increases the glomerular filtration rate, which also increases the amount of calcium filtered into the tubule.[28] In one study, a distinct linear relationship was found between dietary protein intake and urinary calcium excretion, with the slope of the relationship being greater for patients with recurrent urolithiasis than for the control population.[10] These data prompted a hypothesis that patients with recurrent calculi are more sensitive to the calciuric action of protein, since any incremental increase in protein consumption resulted in a proportionately greater increase in calcium excretion.[10] Studies performed by Iguchi and coworkers[29] have also shown that the ingested amount of total protein influences urinary calcium excretion much more than does calcium intake.[29]

Long-term balance studies in rats suggest that the hypercalciuric action of dietary protein is greatest when sulfur-containing amino acids such as methionine provide a large part of the protein load.[10] Further studies suggest that the hypercalciuric effect of dietary protein intake correlates well with the urinary excretion of sulfate. In fact, urinary sulfate is felt to be a good index of protein-induced calciuria.[10,30,31]

Hyperoxaluria, although correlated with dietary protein intake, does not tend to be enhanced by the sulfur-containing amino acids (methionine) but does respond to glycine loading.[30]

An elevation in urinary uric acid excretion has been found to also occur in conjunction with a high protein intake.[10] The hyperuricosuria observed in patients with hypercalciuria and recurrent calculi is associated with a particularly severe form of urolithiasis and is the consequence of an excess consumption of dietary purine, not an abnormality in purine metabolism.[32]

The mechanisms by which dietary protein intake increases the risk of recurrent urolithiasis still need further study. An increase in knowledge of amino acid metabolism as it applies to patients with recurrent urolithiasis may provide additional answers. For the present it is probably reasonable to advise a decrease in animal protein consumption (1.0 g/kg or less), particularly from flesh and muscular protein sources, which are rich in purine content and will significantly influence uric acid excretion. The North American habit of consuming generous portions of flesh protein products probably has a significant influence on uric acid excretion in susceptible people.

Summary

The nutrition management of persons with recurrent calcium urolithiasis requires an individualized approach to the establishment of long-term goals. Diet therapy should be instituted only after careful consideration of serial metabolic evaluation of blood and urine parameters, along with stone analysis data. Interval monitoring of patient progress provides an opportunity for the identification and correction of clinical problems associated with the establishment of long-term goals. Many working in the field of nephrology will find the nutrition management of this group of patients to be a challenging experience.

References

1. Andersen DA. Environmental factors in the aetiology of urolithiasis. In: Cifuentes, Delatte L, Rapado A, Hodgkinson A, eds. *Urinary Calculi.* Basel, Switzerland: Karger; 1973.

2. Hodgkinson A, Marshall RW. Changes in the composition of urinary tract stones. *Invest Urol.* 1975;13:131.

3. Smith LH. Pathogenesis of renal stones. *Mineral Elect Metab.* 1987;13:214.

4. Robertson WG, Peacock M, Hephurn PJ, Marshall DH, Clark PB. Risk factors in calcium stone disease of the urinary tract. *Br J Urol.* 1978;50:449.

5. Robertson WG, Peacock M, Hodgkinson A. Dietary changes and the incidence of urinary calculi in the U.K. between 1958 and 1976. *J Chron Dis.* 1979;32:469.

6. Smith LH, Van Den Berg CJ, Wilson DM. Nutrition and urolithiasis. *N Engl J Med.* 1978;298:87.

7. Robertson WG. Diet and calcium stones. *Mineral Elect Metab.* 1987;13:228.

8. Pak CYC, Smith LH, Resnick MI, Weinerth JL. Dietary management of idiopathic calcium urolithiasis. *J Urol.* 1984;131:850.

9. Smith CL, Davis M, Berkseth RO. Dietary factors in calcium nephrolithiasis. *J Renal Nutr.* 1992;2:146-153.

10. Goldfarb S. Dietary factors in the pathogenesis and prophylaxis of calcium nephrolithiasis. *Kidney Int.* 1988;34:544.

11. Iguchi M, Umekawa T, Ishikawa Y, et al. Clinical effects of prophylactic dietary treatment on renal stones. *J Urol.* 1990;144:229.

12. Pak CYC, Sakahaee K, Crowther C, Brinkley L. Evidence justifying a high fluid intake in treatment of nephrolithiasis. *Ann Intern Med.* 1980;93:36.

13. Embon OM, Rose GA, Rosenbaum T. Chronic dehydration stone disease. *Br J Urol.* 1990;66:357.

14. Hosking DH, Erickson SB, Van Den Berg CJ, Wilson DM, Smith LH. The stone clinic effect in patients with idiopathic calcium urolithiasis. *J Urol.* 1983;130:115.

15. Muldowney FP, Freaney R, Moloney MF. Importance of dietary sodium in the hypercalciuric syndrome. *Kidney Int.* 1982;22:292.

16. Wasserstein AG, Stolley PD, Soper KA, Goldfarb S, Maislin G, Agus Z. Case-control study of risk factors for idiopathic calcium nephrolithiasis. *Mineral Elect Metab.* 1987;13:85.

17. Finch AM, Kasidas GP, Rose GA. Urine composition in normal subjects after oral ingestion of oxalate-rich foods. *Clin Sci.* 1981;60:411.

18. Hodgkinson, A. Evidence of increased oxalate absorption in patients with calcium-containing renal stones. *Clin Sci Med.* 1978;54:291.

19. Robertson WG, Peacock M. The cause of idiopathic calcium stone disease: hypercalciuria or hyperoxaluria? *Nephron.* 1980;26:105.

20. Marganella M, Bianco O, Martini C, Petrarulo M, Vitale C, Linari F. Effect of animal and vegetable protein intake on oxalate excretion in idiopathic calcium stone disease. *Br J Urol.* 1990;63:348.

21. Laminski NA, Meyers AM, Kruger M, Sonnekus MI, Margolius LP. Hyperoxaluria in patients with recurrent calcium oxalate calculi: dietary and other risk factors. *Br J Urol.* 1991;68:454.

22. Brinkley L, McGuire J, Gregory J, Pak CYC. Bioavailability of oxalate in foods. *Urology.* 1981;17:534.

23. Kasidas GP, Rose GA. Oxalate content of some common foods: determination by an enzymatic method. *J Human Nutr.* 1980;34:255.

24. Robertson WG, Heyburn PJ, Peacock M, Hanes FA, Swaminathan R. The effect of high animal protein intake on the risk of calcium stone formation in the urinary tract. *Clin Sci.* 1979;57:285.

25. Robertson WG, Peacock M, Heyburn PJ, et al. Should recurrent calcium oxalate stone formers become vegetarians? *Br J Urol.* 1979;51:427.

26. Breslau NA, Brinkley L, Hill KD, Pak CYC. Relationship of animal protein-rich diet to kidney stone formation and calcium metabolism. *J Clin Endocrinol Metab.* 1988;66:140.

27. Licata AA. Acute effects of increased meat protein on urinary electrolytes and cyclic adenosine monophosphate and serum parathyroid hormone. *Am J Clin Nutr.* 1981;34:1779–1784.

28. Sutton RAL, Wong NLM, Dirks JH. Effects of metabolic acidosis and alkalosis on sodium and calcium transport in the dog kidney. *Kidney Int.* 1979;15:520–533.

29. Iguchi M, Kataoka K, Kohri K, Yachiku S, Kurita T. Nutritional risk factors in calcium stone disease in Japan. *Urol Int.* 1984;39:32.

30. Tschope W, Ritz E, Schmidt-Gayk H, Knebel L. Different effects of oral glycine and methionine on urinary lithogenic substances. *Proc EDTA.* 1983;20:407.

31. Tschope W, Ritz E. Sulfur-containing amino acids are a major determinant of urinary calcium. *Mineral Elect Metab.* 1985;11:137.

32. Coe FL, Moran E, Kavalich AG. The contribution of dietary purine overconsumption to hyperuricosuria in calcium oxalate stone formers. *J Chron Dis.* 1976;29:793.

33. Pennington JAT. *Bowes and Church's Food Values of Portions Commonly Used.* Philadelphia, Pa: JB Lippincott; 1989.

34. Ney DM, Hofmann AF, Fischer C, Stubblefield N. *The Low Oxalate Diet Book for the Prevention of Oxalate Kidney Stones.* San Diego, Calif: The University of California; 1981.

APPENDIXES

A. Nutrition Care of the Hospitalized Patient With Renal Failure

Malnutrition is a continuum that begins when the patient fails to eat enough to meet his or her needs or has a medical condition that prevents normal utilization of nutrients and progresses through a series of functional changes that precede any changes in body composition. Traditional markers of malnutrition lose their specificity in the sick adult.[1] The hospitalized population with renal failure, therefore, poses special nutrition-related problems. The presentation of multiple needs requires treatment of the whole patient in whom kidney failure is a component and not the sole or main focus. The following overview explores the importance of nutrition care for this population and includes suggested guidelines for its provision.

Malnutrition in Renal Failure

"Wasting" syndrome has been documented for patients with renal failure. Causes include the catabolic effects of intercurrent illnesses, endocrine disorders, poor dietary intake, uremic toxins, and impaired metabolic functioning of the kidney. Hospitalization may make the patient more susceptible to this syndrome because of imposition of new factors and/or exacerbation of existing problems.

A study performed in 1980 showed a 19% incidence of protein-energy malnutrition in hemodialyzed patients.[2] It is believed that at least one third of all dialysis patients have evidence of protein undernutrition.[3]

An international study of 224 continuous ambulatory peritoneal dialysis (CAPD) patients from six centers documented 8% with severe malnutrition and almost 33% with mild to moderate malnutrition, with a higher incidence among diabetic patients. Females showed a trend toward more anorexia, greater weight loss from muscle wasting, and a greater decrease in albumin. The decline in males was more gradual.[4]

Dietitians need to be cognizant of the effects of hospitalization on the dialysis population, which is already at risk. It may take months for a patient to regain lost nutritional status in the acute care setting. Nutrition intervention may not always raise serum albumin concentration, but it may stabilize the level of malnutrition and help prevent further decline in status.

Effect on Patient Outcome

Malnutrition and wasting contribute to increased susceptibility to infection, impaired wound healing, decreased strength and vigor, poor rehabilitation, and decreased quality of life. It is associated with increased morbidity and mortality in dialysis patients. CAPD patients show correlations between malnutrition and an increased rate of peritonitis and length of hospital stay. Because low serum albumin levels may be specifically related to morbidity and mortality, nutrition intervention is vital to patient outcome.[3]

Screening for Nutrition Problems

The following screening factors must be evaluated to form comprehensive care plans that address the multifaceted needs of the hospitalized patient with renal failure.

DIAGNOSIS AND PAST MEDICAL HISTORY

Primary reason for admission—Type of surgery, gastrointestinal bleeding, orthopedic problems, or stroke alter the patient's status.

Related medical problems—Diabetes mellitus, severe congestive heart failure, cancer, pancreatitis, AIDS, and pulmonary disease add additional nutrition concerns.

Renal failure history—Acute or chronic status, the cause, and treatment modality all affect the need for nutrients.

PHYSICAL DATA

Height—Amputations should also be delineated.

Weight history—Includes admission weight, usual weight, recent weight changes, and estimated dry weight. Special considerations when weight is obtained are designation of weight before or after dialysis, with or without peritoneal dialysate indwelling, and with or without a prosthesis worn (can weigh 3 to 6 lb).

RECENT INTAKE HISTORY VERSUS COMPLETE DIET HISTORY

Appetite factors—Dialysis treatment schedules that interfere with mealtimes, volume of peritoneal dialysis fluid, bad taste in the mouth, aversion to red meat, smell alterations, medication effects, and mental status can all influence intake and lead to a lack of appetite.

Eating problems—The patient's ability to chew and swallow, dry mouth, mouth sores, and need for feeding assistance all need to be considered.

Diet before admission—The patient's knowledge of his or her diet and previous degree of compliance influence acceptance of the current diet.

Eating habits—The patient's usual meal schedule altered while in the hospital, ethnic preferences in food choices, and psychological factors have impact on intake.

Gastrointestinal problems—Nausea, vomiting, diarrhea, constipation, heartburn, hiccups, and reflux esophagitis can all affect appetite and/or intake.

Conditions Placing the Patient at Further Risk

The presence of serious high fevers, dermal ulcers (stages III and IV), or recent surgical procedures may cause hypermetabolic states in patients with CRF. Altered mental status may also influence the patient's ability to take in adequate nutrition.

Formulation of the Nutrition Care Plan

Assessment of the appropriateness of the diet order is essential. This involves coordination of information based on the type of renal failure and its treatment plans, modifications for any superimposed illness, and the patient's nutritional status. Each situation must be fully assessed, with diet orders individualized per need. Liberalization of the diet is an option to be considered to promote optimal intake. The dietitian is the patient's advocate and may need to discuss diet orders with the physician in a constructive manner to accomplish desired goals.

Implementation of the diet encompasses more than numerical calculations. Aspects to consider are texture modifications, the patient's food preferences, use of calorie boosters, and possible need for protein supplementation. Careful attention may avert the need for more aggressive intervention later.

Monitoring includes an awareness of oral intake, examination of intake and output records, assessment of tube feeding tolerance (when used), updates of laboratory results, keeping of weight records, and constant review of medical progress and plans.

Reassessment is performed according to need. Plans and goals are always subject to change because the patient is not in a static state.

To be effective, the dietitian needs to communicate regularly with the patient and his or her family, friends, and/or caregivers, as well as with the physicians and allied health care team; each provides vital information. Contact with the outpatient dietitian (if the patient is already undergoing dialysis) can provide background material and enable coordination of care at discharge. Nutrition care does not exist in a vacuum and should be seen as an integral part of the patient's overall treatment in the hospital.

References

1. Jejeebhoy MBBS, Detsky AS, Baker JP. Assessment of nutritional status. *JPEN J Parenter Enter Nutr.* 1990;14(suppl):257S–259S.

2. Bansal VK, Popli S, Pickering J, et al. Protein-calorie malnutrition and cutaneous anergy in hemodialysis maintained patients. *Am J Clin Nutr.* 1980;33:1608–1611.

3. Blagg CR. Importance of nutrition in dialysis patients. *Am J Kidney Dis.* 1991;17:458–461.

4. Young GA, Kopple JD, Lindholm B, et al. Nutritional assessment of continuous ambulatory peritoneal dialysis patients: an international study. *Am J Kidney Dis.* 1991;17:462–471.

B. Helpful Hints for Common Patient Problems

Loss of Appetite or Changes in Taste

Poor appetite and/or altered taste sensation may occur in the dialysis patient as a result of inadequate dialysis therapy, severe diet restrictions, specific medications, anxiety, weakness, or depression. Manipulation of the dialysis prescription, medication, and/or dietary regimen may be helpful in many cases of inadequate intake. If depression or anxiety persists for a long period, however, the patient should be referred to appropriate health care professionals.

The following information can be used to counsel patients on methods of improving altered taste or appetite loss:

■ Appetite is a learned response triggered by food intake; therefore, food intake is important to maintain a desire for food.

■ Modular supplements of protein and carbohydrate may be added to foods to provide nutrients without changing the flavor significantly.

■ Protein-containing foods, especially meat, may taste better when served cold at room temperature or in a sauce or casserole.

■ Easy-to-chew foods may be better tolerated (eg, hamburger or ground meat [vs roasts or steak] and casseroles)

■ Food odors should be minimized. Encourage patients to barbecue or grill meats outside if possible or leave the house while food is being prepared. Placing lids on pots and operating the kitchen vent hood while cooking can reduce odors.

■ Patients should be encouraged to eat in a relaxed atmosphere. Eating should be postponed during an acute upset and resumed later.

■ Liquids served during meals should be avoided if early satiety is a problem. Liquids should be taken 1 hour before or after a meal to reduce the feeling of fullness.

■ A bad taste in the mouth can be reduced by using mouthwash, brushing the teeth and tongue, chewing gum, or sucking lemon wedges, hard candy, or small amounts of ice before meals.

■ Small frequent meals should be encouraged despite lack of appetite. Six small meals instead of three large meals is usually recommended for anorexia and/or early satiety.

■ Patients' food preferences should be encouraged in the diet, within the limitations of the diet prescription.

■ Seasonings, herbs, and spices can be added to improve the aroma and taste of foods.

■ Lactose-free commercial supplements may be better tolerated than solid food at times. These need to be used within the fluid and dietary prescription.

■ Patients should be encouraged to eat nutrient-dense foods before foods such as salads and broth.

Nausea and Vomiting

Persistent nausea and vomiting may be a problem in patients with renal disease. The following recommendations may help in alleviating these symptoms:

■ Before rising in the morning, eat unsalted crackers, hard candy, or other dry carbohydrate foods. Eat these while still in bed.

■ Take fluid feedings only if previous dry feedings have been tolerated.

■ Eat promptly when hunger is first felt.

■ Avoid highly seasoned foods.

■ As tolerance for food increases, fats and fluids may be gradually added and time between meals increased until three to four meals per day are reestablished.

■ Effective medications are available to counteract slow gastric emptying, as well as nausea; thus, a consultation with the physician may be necessary if nausea and vomiting persist.

■ Nausea and vomiting during a hemodialysis treatment may be lessened by eating a light meal 2 hours before or waiting to eat until after the treatment.

Constipation

Factors contributing to constipation include intake of phosphate-binding medications, restriction of fluid, reduced dietary intake of fiber, lack of exercise, use of antidepressant and antihypertensive medications, and surgery.

Various sources recommend intakes as high as 25 to 50 g of dietary fiber per day to prevent constipation in healthy persons. When high fiber diets are prescribed for dialysis patients, the potassium content of some high fiber foods such as fruits and vegetables must be considered. Serum potassium levels should be checked frequently until the diet becomes routine and there is no evidence of hyperkalemia. Also, high fiber foods can be rich sources of phosphorus, thus commercially available fiber supplements may be recommended to attain increased fiber goals (*Table B.1*).

Excessive Interdialytic Fluid Weight Gains

Desirable interdialytic weight gains vary from patient to patient and facility to facility. It is important to establish a patient's fluid allowance as soon after the initiation of dialysis as possible and to follow the patient's weight gains regularly to assess if further instruction or adjustment of the fluid allowance is indicated. Fluid overload can lead to shortness of breath, hypertension, congestive heart failure, and pulmonary edema. In addition, large shifts of fluid can result in nausea, vomiting, muscle cramps, and hypotension during hemodialysis.

During instruction of the patient and reinforcement of the fluid allowance, the following guidelines and hints may be helpful.

1. Avoid high sodium foods.
2. Drink when thirsty, only in limited amounts.
3. Anything liquid at room temperature should be counted as fluid, such as ice, ice cream, gelatin, and fruit ices.

Table B.1
Some Commercially Available Fiber Supplements

Product	Fiber (g)	Potassium (mg)	Kilocalories	Phosphorus
Fiberall				
1 rounded tsp	3.4	60	6	NA
FiberMed				
2 wafers	10.0	110	120	NA
Metamucil	3.4	31	1–30	Trace
1 package regular				
(not effervescent)				
Unifiber	3.0	0.8	0.4	NA
1 tbsp				
Fibrad	7.0	15	5	NA
1 tbsp				

NA, data not available.

Adapted with permission from: Burgess MB, Littlefield D. Effect of wheat bran supplementation on colonic function and serum mineral levels in chronic renal failure and hemodialysis patients. *Dial Transplant.* 1987;16:184.

4. Plan ahead to spread allowed fluids over the course of the day.
5. Measure the amount of fluid that regularly used cups and glasses contain so that intake can be regulated more easily. Use small cups and glasses for beverages if possible.
6. Measure ice allotment for the day and store in a special container in the freezer. Most people find ice more satisfying than the same amount of water since it stays in the mouth longer.
7. Try putting lemon juice in ice cubes. Use about half a lemon for each tray of ice. Lemonade and other allowable fruit juices can be frozen into small juice bars in an ice cube tray.
8. Rinse mouth with water or chilled mouth wash (but do not swallow).
9. Try eating allowed fruits and vegetables ice cold or frozen (eg, strawberries and grapes).
10. Try hard candies, chewing gum, and sliced lemon wedges to moisten the mouth.
11. When thirsty, try eating something like bread and margarine before taking fluids. Food may alleviate the dry mouth as liquids do.
12. Try to keep as active as possible to prevent preoccupation with the desire for liquids as well as to encourage perspiration.
13. Weigh every morning and evening and adjust fluid intake to have a fluid weight gain of only 1 to 2 lb or 1 kg/d.
14. Be advised that 1 pint or 2 cups of retained fluid will equal 1 lb of fluid weight gain.
15. If wandering far from the recommended fluid allowance, measure and keep a written list of fluid intake for a few days to get back on track.

Reducing the Potassium Content of Foods*

By using the principle of dialysis on food preparation, it is possible to reduce the potassium content of those vegetables usually restricted in the renal diet. This method, however, does not eliminate the potassium; the patient should be instructed about the judicious intake of "dialyzed" vegetables.

For potatoes, carrots, beets, and rutabagas[1]:
- Peel and slice 1/8-in thick. Place in water.
- Soak for at least 2 hours in warm water by using 10 times the amount of water to the amount of vegetables.
- Rinse and cook for 5 minutes in five times the amount of water.
- Cooked vegetables can then be frozen in individual portion sizes and prepared later in a variety of ways.
- In one study in which different leaching times and cooking methods for potatoes only were compared, it was suggested that french fry–cut potatoes were not reduced significantly in potassium for an average serving size (100 g) once the leached product was fried. Also, results showed that preparation in a microwave oven may not be a suitable method of cooking potatoes for potassium-restricted diets.

For greens (kale, mustard, or spinach), lima beans, squash, mushrooms, and cauliflower[1]:
- Place frozen greens in a sieve or strainer and allow to thaw at room temperature. Drain.
- Rinse fresh or frozen vegetables in warm water.
- Soak and cook as above.

Reference

1. McVeigh ER, Hemstock JE. The effect of leaching and cooking method on the potassium content of potatoes. *CRN Q.* 1990;14:15.

*Adapted from Tsaltas TT. *Am J Clin Nutr.* 1969;22:490–493.

C. Overview of the Management of Anemia in End-Stage Renal Disease

One of the complications associated with renal disease is normocytic, normochromic, hypoproliferative anemia. It is primarily the result of insufficient production and release of erythropoietin from the kidneys.[1,2] Through genetic engineering, recombinant human erythropoietin (rHuEPO) is available for the treatment of the anemia associated with renal failure.[3]

Recombinant human erythropoietin therapy is currently used in all phases of renal failure and in all modes of ESRD treatment. Predialysis patients frequently are treated with rHuEPO therapy to correct anemia when the hematocrit falls below 30 mg%.[4] The erythropoietin is given by means of subcutaneous injection in this population and is reported to lead to increased appetite and improved sense of well being.[5]

For both hemodialysis and peritoneal dialysis patients, rHuEPO can be administered subcutaneously. Studies have shown that rHuEPO is more effective when given subcutaneously because it allows for a more gradual sustained rise in circulating erythropoietin levels than with intravenous administration.[6] However, because of patient convenience, rHuEPO is often given intravenously to hemodialysis patients during the dialysis treatment.

In addition to using this drug for predialysis and dialysis patients, rHuEPO may also be used in renal transplant patients.[7] If a transplant patient's kidney is not functioning well, anemia can develop. For these patients, rHuEPO is administered primarily through subcutaneous routes.

Administration of rHuEPO stimulates red blood cell production, resulting in a rise in hematocrit. With the increase in number of red blood cells being generated, the body's use of iron significantly increases.[8] If sufficient iron is not available, red cell production will be hindered and the rise in hematocrit may slow or stop. To maximize the benefit of rHuEPO, therefore, good iron status must be maintained.

For patients treated with rHuEPO therapy, it is recommended to monitor both ferritin and percentage of transferrin saturation regularly. Ferritin indicates how much iron is in storage, whereas the percentage of transferrin saturation indicates how much iron is available for use by the bone marrow for erythropoiesis. Some patients are unable to mobilize iron from storage fast enough, resulting in relative or functional iron deficiency even though ferritin is normal or high. In general, it is recommended to keep the ferritin level above 100 ng/mL and the percentage transferrin saturation above 20%.[9]

Almost all patients treated with rHuEPO require iron supplementation to maintain an adequate iron status. Iron supplementation can be given orally and intravenously. Oral iron supplementation is generally started first. The usual dose is 100 to 300 mg of elemental iron per day as tolerated. Iron salts such as sulfate, fumarate, and gluconate are most frequently used. Oral iron preparations should be taken between meals, away from phosphate binders, because phosphate binders bind iron. Although it is well recognized that ascorbate increases iron absorption, one must be wary of recommending ascorbate supplements to be taken with iron because of the potential for oxalosis.[10]

Even with the use of oral iron, many patients receiving rHuEPO require periodic administration of intravenous iron dextran to maintain adequate iron status. Usually, if a patient's percentage saturation falls below 20%, iron dextran is administered. Recommended iron dextran administration is 100-mg doses at five to ten doses, for a total iron load of 500 to 1000 mg.[9] It is important for iron status to be closely monitored and recommendations made for iron administration to ensure the patient is using rHuEPO, thereby reducing the severity of anemia.

In addition to monitoring iron status, it is important to evaluate overall nutritional and biochemical status of patients receiving rHuEPO therapy. With the general improvement in sense of well being and improved appetite, dietary intake can increase.[11,12] Elevated serum potassium and phosphorus levels have been documented in patients treated with rHuEPO therapy.[11,13] Two factors considered to play a role include increased dietary intake and reduced dialyzer clearance. The dialysis prescription may require minor adjustment to compensate for these factors.

Along with elevated potassium and phosphorus levels, rises in blood pressure can also be seen with rHuEPO therapy secondary to increased peripheral vascular resistance and increased blood viscosity. Careful monitoring and counseling regarding sodium and fluid restrictions is important because of their relationship to blood pressure control in many patients.

Finally, evaluation of the patient's dietary intake to ensure adequate calorie, protein, and folic acid intake is necessary because erythropoietin is used most effectively in the presence of adequate calories, protein, and folic acid.[14]

References

1. Eschbach JW, Adamson JW. Recombinant human erythropoietin: implications for nephrology. *Am J Kidney Dis.* 1988;11:203–209.

2. Eschbach JW, Mladenori J, Garcia JF, et al. The anemia of chronic renal failure in sheep: response of erythropoietin-rich plasma in vivo. *J Clin Invest.* 1984;74:434–441.

3. Lin FK, Suggs S, Lin CH, et al. Cloning and expression of the human erythropoietin gene. *Proc Natl Acad Sci USA.* 1985;82:7580–7585.

4. Eschbach JW, Adamson JW. Guidelines for recombinant human erythropoietin therapy. *Am J Kidney Dis.* 1989;14(suppl):2–8.

5. Brown CD, Kieran M, Zhao ZH, et al. Treatment of azotemic, anemic patients with human recombinant erythropoietin (rHuEPO) raises whole blood viscosity proportional to hematocrit. *Kidney Int.* 1988;33:184.

6. Egrie JC, Eschbach JW, McGuire T, et al.

Pharmacokinetics of recombinant human erythropoietin (rHuEPO) administered to hemodialysis patients. *Kidney Int.* 1988;33:262.

7. Sun CH, Paul W, Ward HJ, et al. Erythropoiesis and radioimmunoassayable recombinant human erythropoietin (rHuEPO) in renal transplant (Tx) recipients. *Kidney Int.* 1988;33:452.

8. Eschbach JW, Egrie JC, Downing MR, et al. Correction of the anemia of end-stage renal disease with recombinant human erythropoietin. *N Engl J Med.* 1987;316:73–78.

9. Van Wyck DB. Iron management during recombinant human erythropoietin therapy. *Am J Kidney Dis.* 1989;14(suppl):9–13.

10. Ono K. Secondary hyperoxalemia caused by vitamin C supplementation in regular hemodialysis patients. *Clin Nephrol.* 1986;26:239.

11. Combs HL. The impact of recombinant human erythropoietin induced correction of anemia

on nutritional status of hemodialysis patients. Thesis, University of Washington; 1988.

12. Quinn-Cefaro R, Lundin AAP, Delano RG. Subjective benefits of recombinant human erythropoietin in hemodialysis patients. *Dial Transplant.* 1990;18:444–446.

13. Eschbach JW, Abdulhadi MH, Browne JK, et al. Recombinant human erythropoietin in anemic patients with end-stage renal disease. *Ann Intern Med.* 1989;111:992–1000.

14. VanBeber AD, Peraglie C, Smith RD, et al. The effect of recombinant human erythropoietin therapy in anemic kidney patients: a nutritional emphasis. *J Renal Nutr.* 1992;2:96–104.

D. Pregnancy and Dialysis: A Discussion and Case Review

Historically, few pregnancies have been reported for patients with CRF and undergoing dialytic therapy. Of those reported, few have resulted in delivery of a viable fetus.

Since the approval of recombinant human erythropoietin (rHuEPO) to treat the anemia associated with CRF, it appears the incidence of pregnancy in this population may be increasing. The rationale for this occurrence may be due to the fact that many women with CRF report a return of regular menses.

Pregnancies for women with CRF tend to have been discovered at an average of 16.5 weeks' gestation.[1] Symptoms of pregnancy, such as bloating, abdominal distention, and nausea, especially without a noted interruption in a regular menstrual cycle, are similar to those of CRF and are often overlooked. It is hoped that return of regular menses will allow pregnancies to be discovered earlier so that these women may receive optimal prenatal management sooner.

The concerns for a pregnant woman who also has CRF are greater than for those who possess normal renal function. Blood pressure control, management of anemia, uremia, additional nutrition needs, and a high incidence of preterm labor are a few. A team approach to patient care involving the physician, nurse, social worker, and dietitian must be emphasized for the woman with CRF who elects to proceed with a pregnancy.

The following presentation profiles the case of a pregnant hemodialysis patient. Some observations and aspects of management in her care are discussed. Considerations for the renal dietitian involved with assessment and management of pregnant patients with CRF are identified in this review.

Case Review

DC, a 33-year-old woman, began undergoing hemodialysis in February 1990. The cause of her renal failure was unknown. The patient's past medical history included hypertension, head trauma, seizures, and some alcohol use. Data prior to initiation of dialysis were as follows:

Anthropometric
    Height, 5 ft 5 in.
    Weight, 110 lb (50 kg)
    Usual weight, 126 lb (57.3 kg)
    Ideal weight, 125 lb (56.8 kg)

Laboratory

Na$^+$/K$^+$, 145/6.1 mEq/L

BUN/creatinine, 180/30.4 mg/dL

Ca^{++}-P, 6.2/10.5 mg/dL

Albumin, 4.3 g/dL

Total cholesterol, 210 mg/dL

Hemoglobin, 6.5 g/dL

Hematocrit, 20%

Caloric needs were estimated by using the calculation of actual weight (kilograms) × 40, because the patient weighed less than ideal body weight, and protein needs were estimated by using actual weight (kilograms) × 1.2 (see chapter 4). Nutrient goals were 2000 kcal and 60 g of protein per day.

Renal vitamins, phosphate binders, and other appropriate medications for anemia and hypertension were also prescribed. Hemodialysis was tolerated well, and the patient was immediately referred to the transplantation team to initiate a workup for cadaveric renal transplantation. This was completed, and she was added to the waiting list while continuing to receive regular hemodialysis treatments for a total of 12 h/wk in the outpatient dialysis center.

Routine blood chemistry values and diet reviews revealed the patient to have a generally good appetite and to be gradually gaining dry weight, while maintaining acceptable serum laboratory values and interdialytic weight gains between 4 and 7 lb.

In October 1990, DC presented to the high-risk obstetrics clinic, where ultrasound confirmed a viable pregnancy. Her estimated delivery date was determined to be March 22, 1991.

A multidisciplinary team conference was subsequently scheduled and included physicians and nurses from both the obstetric and nephrology departments, the renal social worker, renal dietitian, and a pharmacist from the home infusion company used by the dialysis unit.

Data at the time of the multidisciplinary meeting included:

Anthropometric

Estimated dry weight (EDW), 116 lb (53 g)

Laboratory (predialysis)

Na$^+$/K$^+$, 137/4.1 mEq/L

BUN/creatinine, 56/9.6 mg/dL

Ca^{++}-P, 8.9/2.9 mg/dL

Albumin, 3.0 g/dL

Total cholesterol, 206 mg/dL

Glucose, 74 mg/dL

Ferritin, 68 ng/mL

Hemoglobin, 6.1 g/dL

Hemotacrit, 18.6%

The plan for patient care was discussed and included the following:

■ Dialysis treatment time was increased to 15 h/wk (in the inpatient dialysis unit) to keep the predialysis BUN concentration at 50 to 60 mg/dL.[1]

■ Diet was liberalized to "regular"

■ MA 97 forms were to be processed for potential intradialytic parenteral nutrition if intakes revealed persistent inadequate ingestion of protein or kilocalories.

- Vitamin and mineral supplementation now included[2]:
    two renal vitamins per day (prenatal vitamins were discontinued)
    20 mg $ZnSO_4$ per day
    325 mg $FeSO_4$ twice a day
    Three $CaCO_3$ tablets three times a day (actual dose unknown)
    0.25 µg calcitriol per day
- Other medications included nifedipine and rHuEPO
- A blood transfusion was given because of severe anemia
- A 24-hour urine collection was requested
- Kilocalorie and protein intakes were monitored by verbal recall
- The earliest elective delivery date was determined to be January 26, 1991 (at 32 weeks' gestation)

Estimated caloric intake at the time of the meeting was 2454 kcal/d, and estimated protein intake was 90 g/d. Nutrition needs for pregnancy were now estimated on ideal body weight to ensure optimal goals. They were calculated as follows: ideal body weight (kilograms) × 35 + 300 kcal/d (RDA for pregnancy) and ideal weight (kilograms) × 1.2 + 10 g/d (RDA for pregnancy).[3] (Also see chapter 4.) Goals were 2295 kcal and 78 g protein per day.

In late November 1990, DC was admitted to the hospital with preterm labor and polyhydramnios (an excess of amniotic fluid). She was given medications, including terbutalene sulfate, intravenous ritodine hydrochloride, indomethacin, and magnesium sulfate, in efforts to control the polyhydramnios and contractions. After the first day of hospitalization, the contractions ceased, but she remained in the hospital for observation until a standard pelvic examination was performed. Medications containing magnesium were discontinued when found to be unsuccessful because they pose a risk to a person with CRF who does not adequately excrete excess magnesium.

On December 6, 1990, ultrasound revealed normal fetal growth at 24 weeks' gestation. However, by December 12, the obstetric physicians decided that DC required fetal Doppler monitoring because of her history of preterm labor and continued polyhydramnios. She was subsequently admitted to another university hospital. Data just before transfer were as follows:

Anthropometric
    EDW, 123 lb (56 kg)
Laboratory (predialysis)
    Na^+/K^+, 138/3.4 mEq/L
    BUN/creatinine, 29/5.1 mg/dL
    Ca^{++}-P, 8.2/1.8 mg/dL
    Albumin, 3.6 g/dL
    Glucose, 100 mg/dL
    Total cholesterol, 290 mg/dL
    Ferritin, 130 ng/mL
    Hemoglobin, 8.0 g/dL
    Hemotacrit, 23.3%

After transfer she continued on her recently revised dialysis schedule of 4 hours five times per week and had her "regular" diet carried over as well. Some of her medications remained the same, such as terbutaline sulfate to prevent preterm labor and indomethacin for polyhydramnios, while others were adjusted for various reasons. The nifedipine was increased further relative to the status of her blood pressure, and methyldopa was added.

Hypertension was a significant concern for DC at this time. This is a common problem during pregnancy in a woman with CRF and is a danger primarily to the mother.[1] At the same time, with frequent dialysis and the new antihypertensive regimen, extreme care had to be taken to avoid hypotension, which is a danger especially to the fetus and can also promote premature uterine contractions. The rHuEPO therapy was also "on hold" at this time, because of DC's severe hypertension and the possibility that this medication could aggravate the condition. Iron supplementation continued, however, as had been prescribed before the transfer. An additional 1 mg of folate was added to the daily regimen, although this was probably not necessary because the patient had been receiving 2 mg/d by way of the renal vitamins.

Other medications included continuation of the recent addition of sodium phosphate preparation because of low phosphorus levels and a decrease in calcium carbonate supplementation. This change in calcium supplementation may not have been a "true" decrease based on the dosage of elemental calcium the patient was *actually* taking. Her serum calcium level remained essentially unchanged with only one tablet containing 500 mg elemental calcium three times a day (not specified with meals). It is important to keep in mind that with a low serum albumin concentration, "corrected" calcium must be calculated, and with more frequent dialysis, calcium absorption from the dialysate must be considered. Serum calcium and phosphorus levels should be monitored carefully. In retrospect, this patient may have tolerated increased calcium dosage if it was ensured that she was taking this medication *between* meals because of already low serum phosphorus levels.

Shortly after transfer, the gestational age was reevaluated and found to be 24 weeks and 3 days on December 15 (previously thought to be 24 weeks on December 6). Also, on December 16, DC was transferred to the labor and delivery floor because of continued preterm labor and the need for amniocentesis because of polyhydramnios. A total of 1000 mL of amniotic fluid was drained, and contractions ceased shortly after transfer. Soon after these events, a fetal monitor was used continuously in this patient, even during dialysis. A nurse from the obstetric floor accompanied the patient to each dialysis treatment in the dialysis unit.

DC continued to report eating well, but "calorie count" evaluations were initiated the second week of her admission to ensure adequate intakes. After 2 weeks of hospitalization at the second hospital, data were as follows:

Anthropometric
    EDW, 125.4 lb (57 kg)
Laboratory (predialysis)
    Na^+/K^+, 130/4.9 mEq/L
    BUN/creatinine, 76/7.0 mg/dL
    Ca^{++}-P, 8.3/3.3 mg/dL
    Albumin, 2.7 g/dL
    Glucose, 61 mg/dL

Nutrient intake was now estimated at 2050 kcal and 82 g of protein per day. The sodium phosphate was discontinued because of improved serum phosphorus levels. DC's interdialytic weight gains continued at an average of 1 to 2.5 kg, with one excessive gain of 3.4 kg over the Christmas holidays. She selected high sodium menu items at times but continued to avoid added salt. She was advised to avoid some of these high sodium foods when weight gains were on the higher side of her average range.

Serum laboratory values were significant for increasing BUN, decreasing albumin levels, and one elevated 2-hour postprandial blood glucose level. The low serum albumin despite apparent adequate kilocalorie and protein intake is a normal finding during pregnancy, with an overall decrease of about 1 g/dL.[4] The cause of this finding is not really known.

The elevated postprandial glucose level was felt to be because of the terbutaline therapy, and the obstetric physicians felt the patient should be placed on a "no concentrated sweets" diet. DC was cooperative with this change and agreed to use the saccharin packets provided on her meal trays sparingly relative to the ability of this substance to cross the placental barrier in human beings.[5]

By January 2, 1991, DC had increased her daily intakes to an average of 2500 kcal and 90 g protein, on the basis of "calorie count" evaluations. These were, of course, an approximation because of the subjectivity of those observing and recording meal portions consumed. Additional data were as follows:

Anthropometric
    EDW, 127.6 lb (58 kg)
Laboratory (predialysis)
    Na^+/K^+, 130/5.4 mEq/L
    BUN/creatinine, 87/7.2 mg/dL
    Ca^{++}-P, 8.1/3.4 mg/dL
    Albumin, 2.5 g/dL
    Glucose, 55 mg/dL
    Hemoglobin, 6.4g/dL
    Hematocrit, 19.0 %

As noted, the BUN level continued to rise, and serum albumin level continued to decrease. The EDW was not changed from that of December 29. The patient's glucose level was actually below normal, but she was not symptomatic for hypoglycemia. DC agreed to a blood transfusion on January 2, 1991, after much deliberation. This was her fourth transfusion during the course of pregnancy.

On January 5, 1991, DC underwent dialysis, and shortly thereafter began developing shortness of breath, hypertension, and uterine contractions. Because of the presence of pulmonary edema, it was decided that day that a cesarean section should be performed. A 2 lb 8 oz baby boy was delivered at approximately 29 weeks' gestation. DC was transferred to the surgical intensive care unit for observation, and the baby was transferred to the neonatal intensive care unit where he was initially intubated.

When DC was visited for the first time after her cesarean section, she appeared to be suffering from severe postpartum depression. On January 10, 1991, she underwent dialysis for the last time at the hospital to which she had been transferred. She appeared to be less depressed at this time and reported having held her baby, who was now extubated. Her new EDW was being established, and brief instructions were given to her concerning the return to her advised prepregnancy medication schedule and diet regimen with potassium, sodium, and fluid restrictions. Adequate calorie and protein intakes were emphasized, however, because of her recent surgery. DC resumed her usual 12 hour per week hemodialysis schedule in her initial outpatient dialysis facility. She was returned to the cadaveric renal transplant waiting list when she was determined to be medically stable. In early February 1991, her baby was discharged to home from the neonatal intensive care unit.

Additional Observations and Comments

Urea kinetics were not performed for this patient, and were initially thought to be a possible added parameter to monitor the adequacy of dialysis, as well as nutritional status for the next pregnant hemodialysis patient. When these were measured for another pregnant hemodialysis patient, the Kt/V (see chapter 2) and protein catabolic rate (PCR) showed a dramatic increase. The PCR did not correlate with oral intakes initially, and it has been speculated that this may be because of excessive urea production by the fetus; thus, the increased urea generation observed. Because appropriate Kt/V values are still being evaluated even for the nonpregnant population undergoing dialysis, the use of this parameter during pregnancy may not be feasible to evaluate dialysis adequacy. Therefore, dialysis time and diet needs are presently decided upon arbitrarily by the nephrologist and dietitian, respectively. Frequent intake evaluations are suggested in efforts to ensure adequate protein and calorie intake.

One further difficult assessment during the course of pregnancy is the evaluation of EDW. There is a fine line between (1) avoidance of hypotension during dialysis and the promotion of preterm labor and injury to the fetus and (2) the risk of the mother's suffering the consequences of hypertension and pulmonary edema. More frequent dialysis is prescribed during pregnancy, in part to avoid the need for excessive ultrafiltration (and resultant hypotension) during each treatment. The health care team, especially the nurse and dietitian, need to work closely regarding observation of the patient's nutrient intake and tolerance of dialysis. Weight gain grids for normal pregnancy were used as a guide for EDW change, and DC remained at the lower end of the normal curve. Perhaps in the future a grid for weight gain curves for women with CRF during the course of pregnancy will be developed as more data for this population become available.

Few data are also available for micronutrient requirements in the pregnant dialysis patient. General water-soluble vitamin replacement needs continue, but additional supplementation to assist fetal growth is also required. A maternal vitamin and mineral supplement was compared with a renal multivitamin; each was compared with recommended dietary allowances for vitamins during pregnancy. With possible dialysate vitamin losses taken into consideration, it was concluded that vitamin needs could be met with two renal vitamins in combination with additional active vitamin D (calcitriol), calcium, iron, and zinc daily. Questions still remain about the needs for other trace minerals and vitamins such as selenium, biotin, pantothenic acid, and iodine, which are available in the prenatal vitamin and mineral supplement but not in the renal vitamins.

Additionally, as noted, this patient's serum total cholesterol level increased during pregnancy. All aspects of lipid metabolism are altered during pregnancy in general and are believed to be because of anabolic fat storage in early pregnancy and maternal adipose tissue catabolism in the third trimester as the fetus increases the use of glucose and amino acids.[6] No intervention for hypercholesterolemia is therefore felt to be necessary.

Last, the issue of breast-feeding by mothers with CRF has been raised. For this patient, who was undergoing hemodialysis at a different facility from where her baby was hospitalized, this option was not practical. Because lactation will increase caloric and protein needs, breast-feeding may only be feasible concerning the mother's general health and well being if the baby is able to be discharged after birth simultaneously with the mother. Breast milk composition may need to be analyzed in this population to check for appropriate nutrient content and lack of uremic toxins. Perhaps breast-feeding in conjunction with formula feeding will be the best option, especially for women undergoing hemodialysis.

This presentation and discussion have involved the care of a woman being treated with hemodialysis. Pregnancies in women undergoing peritoneal dialysis have been reported as well, and the renal dietitian is referred to the appropriate references and suggested readings that follow.

References

1. Hou SH, Grossman SD. Pregnancy in chronic dialysis patients. *Semin Dial.* 1990; 3:224–229.

2. Brookhyser J. The use of parenteral nutrition supplementation in pregnancy complicated by end-stage renal disease. *J Am Diet Assoc.* 1989;89:93–94.

3. Recommended Dietary Allowances. 10th ed. *J Am Diet Assoc.* 1989;89:1748.

4. Hytten FE. Nutrition and metabolism. In: Hytten F, ed. *Clinical Physiology in Obstetrics.* Oxford, England: Blackwell Scientific Publications; 1988:177.

5. London RS. Saccharin and aspartame. Are they safe to consume during pregnancy? *J Reprod Med.* 1988;33:17–20.

6. Moore TR, Hollingsworth DR. Diabetes and pregnancy. In: Creary RK, Resnik R, eds. *Maternal-Fetal Medicine: Principles and Practice.* Philadelphia, Pa: WB Saunders; 1990:935.

Suggested Readings

Amoah E, Arab H. Pregnancy in a hemodialysis patient with no residual renal function. *Am J Kidney Dis.* 1991;17:585–587.

Dunbeck D, et al. Peritoneal dialysis patient completes successful pregnancy. *ANNA J.* 1992;19:269–272.

Elliott JP, et al. Dialysis in pregnancy: a critical review. *Obstet Gynecol Surv.* 991;46:319–324.

Ferris T. Pregnancy and chronic renal diseases. *Kidney* 1986;19:1–3.

Frohling PT, Birnbaum M, Halle H, Lindenau K. Successful pregnancy of a woman with advanced renal failure on nutritional treatment. *Nephron.* 1986;44:195–197.

Gaudier FL, Santiago-Delpin E, Rivera J, Gonzales Z. Pregnancy after renal transplantation. *Surg Gynecol Obstet.* 1988;167:533–543.

Gratter U, Peleg D, et al. Successful pregnancies in women on regular hemodialysis treatment. *Isr J Med Sci.* 1990;26:266–270.

Grossman SD, Hou S, Moretti M, Saran M. Nutrition in the pregnant dialysis patient. *J Renal Nutr.* 1993;3:56–66.

Harum P, DeVelasco R, Pellegrini E, Garcia-Estrada H, Robbins ML. Nutrition in a pregnant hemodialysis patient. *CRN Q.* 1987;11:10–14.

Hou SH. Pregnancy in women with chronic renal failure. *N Engl J Med.* 1985;312:836–839.

Hou SH. Frequency and outcome of pregnancy in women on dialysis. *Am J Kidney Dis.* 1994; 23:60–63.

Jakobi P, Ohel G, et al. Continuous ambulatory peritoneal dialysis as the primary approach in the management of severe renal insufficiency in pregnancy. *Obstet Gynecol.* 1992;79:808–810.

Orsini-Negroni J, Guiam-Gruta C, Long R, et al. Nursing management of the pregnant hemodialysis patient. *ANNA J.* 1990;17:451–455.

Owen WF. Peritoneal dialysis in a pregnant woman with chronic renal failure. *Semin Dial.* 1990;3:249–251.

Redrow M, Cherem L, Elliott J, et al. Dialysis in the management of pregnant patients with renal insufficiency. *Medicine.* 1988;67:199–208.

Rizzoni G, Ehrich JH, et al. Successful pregnancies in women on renal replacement therapy: report from the EDTA registry. *Nephrol Dial Transplant.* 1992;7:279–287.

Souqiyyeh MZ, Huraib SO, Saleh AG, Aswad S. Pregnancy in chronic hemodialysis patients in the Kingdom of Saudi Arabia. *Am J Kidney Dis.* 1992;19:235–238.

E. Hyperdietism: Its Prevention, Control, and Relation to Compliance in Dialysis Patients

The following article is intended to describe potential pitfalls encountered when dealing with a complicated medical treatment such as the renal diet. The article carries a warning for the professional, who must be aware of the symptoms of hyperdietism both in themselves as well as in the persons most affected by the condition—their patients. The article in no way advocates disregard for the dietary principles and management of patients with ESRD. It encourages individuality, creativity, and realism when practicing the art of diet instruction.

Hyperdietism is defined as a physical and emotional state resulting from a rigid, complicated, and unpalatable diet, conceived by a nephrologist and perpetuated by a renal dietitian—neither of whom is required to adhere to it! Typical symptoms include: depression, anxiety, confusion, hostility, and failure to eat.

Why should we be concerned about hyperdietism? At the present time, when we are confident that the life of a patient with ESRD can be extended and that we can even offer a choice of modality of treatment, there seems to be greater emphasis on the quality of life being extended.

The plight of patients with this condition is a sad one. Life-styles have been severely altered; disease and treatment have resulted in many deprivations; physical capabilities are usually limited, and, consequently, capacity to work is often markedly decreased.

Sexual activities have become greatly diminished, if not completely absent. It has become necessary to take multiple medications and spend a large percentage of time dialyzing. One of the few remaining pleasures in life is food. Although this also must be restricted, by preventing and controlling hyperdietism, food can be made one thing patients can enjoy with as few limitations as possible. This certainly can help improve their quality of life.

This view is supported in the literature, which concurs that food and fluid limitations create considerable psychological stress and greatly detract from the quality of life.[1] Indeed, food seems to have become an obsession with many patients[2] who are preoccupied with the subject, frequently talking about it and often having elaborate dreams about it.[1] Perhaps this explains the high degree of fussiness about hospital trays, anxiety that a tray might not be received, and explosiveness when some food item is missing or is not the one selected.

Dietary compliance is also a subject of increased attention. It, too, is closely related to hyperdietism in that the symptoms of this state all lead to noncompliance. Compliance with dietary restrictions is probably the most difficult part of the whole medical regimen because it affects long-standing personal habits and alters life-style.

Adapted with permission from Gardner J. Hyperdietism. *Dial Transplant.* 1981; 10:57.

Studies show that dietary compliance of renal patients is poor, with less than 25% of the patient population meriting a *good* compliance rating.[3,4] Another study shows only 39% as simply "compliant" as opposed to "noncompliant,"[5] and still another, a rating of *bad* compliance in 40% of patients.[6]

There seems to be little correlation between compliance and age, sex, socioeconomic status, education, and marital status.[7] However, reports of a far better compliance rate exist among married patients living with a spouse and children.[8] Other studies show that education, strong family support, and the ability to work have positive correlations with dietary compliance,[9–13] while IQ or intelligence was found to be unrelated.

Depression, one of the hyperdietism symptoms, significantly decreases compliance; one study reveals that 53% of renal patients are moderately to severely depressed.[3] Increased aggression, certainly akin to hostility, another symptom, is found in virtually all patients as they react to their restrictions. Noncompliance with the diet may be the reaction of some patients who are more likely to act our their aggression.[3] At any rate, it seems appropriate to examine the dietary regimens in use, the methods of instruction, the relationships with patients, and the degree of flexibility in the hope of preventing and controlling hyperdietism.

In efforts to practice such prevention and control, the following suggestions are made:
1. Restrict only the nutritional elements necessary for that individual patient at that particular time.
2. Keep diet instructions simple.
3. Develop and maintain a good relationship with the patient.
4. Be flexible.

The literature shows that the greater the complexity of the diet, the poorer the compliance, especially when dietary restrictions are combined with the many medications and other aspects of treatment necessary for the ESRD patient.[2,3,7,12] Certainly, a potential problem exists when we know that several elements will need to be restricted by diet sooner or later, that numerous medications are almost always indicated, and that some sort of dialysis is imminent.

A partial solution to this problem may be the restriction of only those elements necessary for that individual patient at any particular time. In other words, the use of a highly individualized diet, based on very current chemistries, clinical symptoms, and the physical and nutrition assessment of the patient would seem to be preferable to a pat renal diet that automatically restricts sodium, potassium, phosphorus, protein, and fluids. Many patients present with symptoms and chemistries that initially require only a protein and sodium restriction. It seems unduly confining to impose other restrictions at that time, even though we are reasonably certain they will eventually be indicated. By forestalling any unnecessary restrictions, we can give the patient time to adjust to a fewer number of limitations, decrease confusion, and possibly increase compliance.

Perhaps another approach to help solve the problem is to make the restrictions as moderate as possible. For example, a 1000-mg sodium restriction is difficult for a patient to follow, especially after discharge from the hospital. A more realistic approach might be a 2000-mg sodium restriction or, if the blood pressure and degree of edema will allow, a no-added-salt diet.

Potassium may be monitored closely, but usually a restriction is not instituted until the serum level is 5.5 mEq/L or greater. Recent research has shown that potassium deficiency has been associated with hypertension in humans as well as in experimental rats.[14] It might then be reasoned that potassium should not be restricted unless necessary, since lowering potassium intake might increase the hypertension so prevalent in renal patients. Supporting this concept are two other reports indicating that increased potassium intake results in significantly lower blood pressure.[15,16]

Traditionally, the writing of the diet order has been strictly the province of the physician, but more recently, especially in the renal area, diet orders are often written in consultation with the dietitian. It is often felt that any member of the health care team who has access to the laboratory data and is aware of the patient's clinical symptoms and medical background, has not only the right, but the obligation to institute a discussion of the diet order with staff, especially if there is a chance that a less restrictive diet might serve the patient well.

The concept of restricting only elements that require limitation at one particular time results in frequent changes in the diet order. This is certainly good medical practice, but it can be a real challenge for the dietitian. There may be a subtle advantage here, however. In the process of explaining a diet change to the patient, there is an opportunity to point out the close relationship of the diet to the patient's changing physical condition, thereby demonstrating the importance of the diet as a form of therapy.

The next step in an antihyperdietism program is to present the diet instruction in a simple form to alleviate the symptoms of anxiety, confusion, frustration, and perhaps even failure to eat. Although the generally accepted method of diet instruction is with a carefully calculated plan, limiting several elements at once is confusing to most patients, and they may not understand such an involved format. It is easier for patients to understand that they may have regular bread but not salted crackers than it is for them to understand that they are allowed three salted starches and five unsalted starches in the diet plan. Patient advocates, psychologists, and behavioral scientists support the philosophy of simplicity as a means toward compliance.[11,12,17] Even though there is conflicting evidence on the relationship of education to compliance,[1,6] common sense would indicate there is little hope of a patient following instructions that leave him or her totally confused.

Part of the confusion may result from too much dietary information being presented at one time. This may only serve to overwhelm the patient.[12] The idea is to instruct the patient on only one limitation at a time. Several short sessions are better than one long one.

The protein restriction is usually first, since the patient, once he or she has an interest in food again, may be curious about the limited amount of food being served, especially the small servings of meat. For this instruction, a diet sheet employing simple exchange groups based on protein content alone may be used. The patient who is reasonably adept at simple arithmetic and who prefers to figure his or her own protein intake for the day should be taught to do so. Most patients seem to prefer a sample meal plan based on their protein restriction and individual eating patterns. Sometimes though, even this seems to confuse them. Just trying to convince them to limit the size of their servings of meat may be a better approach. Another point of emphasis is the importance of consuming that small amount of high-quality protein, and the sample meal plan is always designed with a high percentage of protein of high biological value.

In most cases, protein is restricted on a temporary basis after dialysis is initiated. By the time a patient has been treated with hemodialysis for a month, the protein restriction can be lifted. Generally, diets now are not protein-restricted at all once a patient begins dialysis. There are a few patients whose protein intakes are too high even with no restriction. Kinetic modeling and conscientious monitoring of monthly chemistries identifies these patients, and appropriate protein reduction is advised. Patients on peritoneal dialysis, especially chronic ambulatory peritoneal dialysis, often must be encouraged to increase their levels of dietary protein to compensate for the protein loss in the peritoneal fluid exchange.

If the patient's diet order also contains a sodium restriction, which is often the case, it is best to try to let a few days elapse after the protein instruction before discussing the sodium. At this time, instruction may be given by using a protein content sheet that is also modified for sodium. This diet sheet points out the high sodium foods to be avoided as well as the limitation of table salt.

When a potassium restriction is necessary, discuss this limit at a different time if possible. Stress that the most dangerous time for high serum potassium levels is during that longer-than-usual interval between dialysis treatments. In addition to the high potassium fruits and vegetables to be avoided, other high potassium foods such as nuts and chocolate are listed, and the total amount of meat per day is limited. A serious effort should be made to make the patient understand that potassium is water soluble, and directions for the special preparation of vegetables for cooking should be given. A list of all fruits and vegetables classified according to potassium content (with the lowest being listed first) may be distributed. This enables the patient to determine the potassium level of any fruit or vegetable that may have escaped discussion.

Even though some studies indicate that there is no correlation between the knowledge of one's illness and compliance,[7] efforts to explain to the patient in the simplest possible way the reasons for the various restrictions are suggested. This philosophy has been supported by Campbell and Campbell, who have included in their *Factors of Noncompliance* the failure of the staff to communicate the purpose of the treatment adequately.

The timing of the diet instruction is also of utmost importance. The dietitian must be sensitive to the patient's physical and mental condition, and no diet instruction should be undertaken while there is any evidence of nausea, vomiting, or the lethargy and confusion associated with uremia. Emotional readiness must be considered as well. If the patient is experiencing a great deal of anger, fear, or depression after receiving news that dialysis is imminent, he or she is not ready to accept detailed diet instruction. In many cases, diet instructions for the hospitalized patient must be simple, clear, concise, and well-timed. More detailed information can be given later. Presenting the diet in this simplified way (in small doses, with a brief rationale, at an appropriate time) makes it more understandable and increases patients' confidence in their ability to cope with it. This, too, is a factor associated with compliance[7] and must certainly decrease anxiety and frustration.

The quality of the relationship between the health care provider and the patient is of great importance in establishing communication, reducing hostility, and increasing compliance. Dietitians have an advantage in establishing rapport because they deal with food, which has an emotional connotation with love and concern. It has been said that "food feeds the psyche as well as the body."[18] If dietitians can provide a favorite food for a patient with an almost nonexistent appetite or work some ethnic dish into a meal plan, they may have a head start toward establishing a good relationship with that patient. Trust and genuine caring are essential. Food is one good door-opener for communication. Often, patients who are not yet ready to talk about their situations or feelings can be drawn into a conversation about breakfast, and the barriers may start to come down.

A satisfying, warm relationship between physician and patient over a long period has been shown to increase compliance.[2,7] This certainly must be true of other members of the health care team as well. Those of us dealing with ESRD patients have an opportunity to build and maintain warm relationships.

However, it is overly idealistic to believe that a warm, satisfying relationship can be established between the staff member and every patient. Studies have suggested that rapport is better when the patient and the therapist are of the same ethnic group.[19] This arrangement is usually impractical. Our chances of establishing good relationships with patients of different ethnic backgrounds will be enhanced by learning more about these cultures and increasing our understanding of them. We must realize that food habits are deeply embedded in culture and are very difficult to change.[17]

There will be other instances when a good provider-patient relationship just does not happen. This should not cause concern. If the dietitian cannot adequately relate to a certain patient, finding a nurse or a social worker who can may reinforce the diet instruction.

Family support is considered one of the most important factors in achieving good compliance.[5,11] Strong support may be essential to adjustment, and family members, especially a spouse, need the same positive attitudes and attributes as the patient if the patient is to do well.[10] Assistance from family members with the diet, especially the fluid restriction, is associated with increased compliance.[10] The dietitian should include family members in a developing relationship. This could improve the relationship and teach others in the family more about the diet and its importance. Very often it is a family member, not the patient, who buys the groceries and prepares the food. This person needs appropriate instruction. However, it does not seem wise for the patient to delegate all the responsibility for his diet to a family member and become passive about it. It is the patient's diet, and every effort to understand it should be made. Family members should not have to police the actions of the patient, nor should they feel they have failed if the patient refuses to comply.

A great deal of compassion and patience are sometimes called for in maintaining a good patient-provider relationship. Listening to frequent complaints about hospital food and dietary restrictions can be very trying. It may be helpful to realize that the diet is sometimes the scapegoat, and that the patient is really lashing out at the situation.

Flexibility is essential. Cheating or abandoning all the dietary principles we have struggled to make understood is not advocated. However, if the patient has been significantly impressed with the importance of the diet and the reasons for the restrictions, perhaps compromises on small portions of usually forbidden foods on special occasions can be made. Of course, it must be stressed that this compromising must not take place often or there will be serious consequences. Our sympathetic attitude and recognition of the patient's need to be "normal" may increase his or her general compliance and decrease hyperdietism.

References

1. Blackburn SL. Dietary compliance of chronic hemodialysis patients. *J Am Diet Assoc.* 1977;70:31.

2. Francis V, Korsch BM, Morris MJ. Gaps in doctor-patient communications: patients' response to medical advice. *N Engl J. Med.* 1969;280:535–540.

3. Kaplan De-Nour A, Czaczkes JW. The influence of patients' personalities on adjustment to chronic dialysis: a predictive study. *J Nerv Ment Dis.* 1976;162:323–333.

4. Skoutakis VA, Arcchida SR, Marinez DR, et al. Role effectiveness of the pharmacist in the treatment of hemodialysis patients. *Am J Hosp Pharmacol.* 1978;35:62–65.

5. Procci WR. Hemodialysis patients and dietary abuse. *Psychomatics.* 1978;19:16–24.

6. Kaplan De-Nour A, Czaczkes JW. Adjustment to chronic hemodialysis. *Isr J Med Sci.* 1974;10:498–503.

7. Marston M. Compliance with medical recommendations: a review of the literature. *Nurs Res.* 1970;19:312.

8. Procci WR. Psychological factors associated with severe abuse of the hemodialysis diet. *Gen Hosp Psychiatry.* 1981;3:111–118.

9. O'Brien ME. Effective social environment

and hemodialysis adaptation: a panel analysis. *J Health Soc Behavior.* 1980;21:360.

10. Cummings JW. Hemodialysis—the pressures and how the patients respond. *Am J Nurs.* 1970;70:70–76.

11. Miller JW, St. Jeor ST. Compliance with renal diets: a review and analysis. *Dial Transplant.* 1980;9:968.

12. Campbell J, Campbell A. Chronic illness and its effect on dietary compliance. *CRN News.* 1979;3:3–8.

13. Winokur MZ, Czaczkes JW, Kaplan De-Nour A. Intelligence and adjustment to chronic hemodialysis. *J Psychosom Res.* 1973;17:29–34.

14. McCarron A. Calcium and magnesium in human hypertension. *Ann Intern Med.* 1983; 98:800–805.

15. Fregly MJ. Estimates of sodium and potassium intake. *Ann Intern Med.* 1983;98:792–799.

16. MacGregor GA. Dietary sodium and potassium intake and blood pressure. *Lancet.* 1983;1:750–753.

17. Schoolwerth A, Engle J. Calcium and phosphorus in the diet therapy of uremia. *J Am Diet Assoc.* 1975;66:460–464.

18. McCarron A. Dietary calcium in human hypertension. *Science.* 1982;217:267–269.

19. Biller DC. A patient's point of view: diet in chronic renal failure. *J Am Diet Assoc.* 1977;71:633–635.

20. Williams SR. *Nutrition and Diet Therapy.* St. Louis, Mo: CV Mosby;1983:264.

21. Whatley IW. Significance of racial and ethnic issues in providing effective care in a renal unit. *Dial Transplant.* 1980;9:909.

22. Griffiths MS. The influence of race on the psychotherapeutic relationship. *Psychiatry.* 1977; 10:27–40.

F. Forms and Documentation

This appendix provides suggested guidelines for documenting nutrition care for renal patients. The specific format of documentation will depend on each facility's criteria, reasons for nutrition intervention, and the individual dietitian's documentation style. At the time of this writing, medical review criteria screens developed by an expert panel appointed by the Health Care Financing Administration (HCFA) in 1988 (to facilitate the provision of quality care to dialysis patients) are not in final form. However, the Council on Renal Nutrition (CRN) has had input regarding the nutrition components of these screens, and these as well as reports from pilot audits will be reviewed by the expert HCFA panel before final criteria screens are developed. A dietitian's checklist based on these screens was developed by Pat Ellis, MS, RD, chairperson of the CRN Quality Assurance Committee, 1990–1991, and is used by many renal dietitians to form the basis for documentation (*Figure F.1*).

Diet History and Nutrition Assessment

A diet history form is often used to collect information from initial interviews with the patient and/or the patient's family. (See chapter 2, Nutrition Assessment in Chronic Renal Failure.) This information might include intake and activity patterns; previous diet counseling; factors influencing food intake and compliance; and medical, physical, and social needs affecting nutrition. An additional assessment and recommendation section may also be included on this form, especially if it is to become part of the patient's medical chart (*Figure F.2*). Each facility's policies will determine whether specific forms may be part of the patient's medical record. Many dietitians prefer to keep the diet history in their own files for periodic review and develop a separate form for the initial nutrition assessment, which is placed in the chart.

Figure F.1
Medical Review Criteria—Dietitian's Checklist

	Yes	No	Passed by Exception	Comments

Blood Pressure
HD ≤100 mm Hg,
   6 of 12 treatments
PD ≤100 mm Hg, 5 of 6 visits
Peds ≤99%ile/age,
   10 of 12 mo
			A. Diet instruction
			B. Dry weight reassessed
			C. Meds reassessed
			D. Tx Rx changed
			E. Psychosocial review
			F. Noncompliance	

Metabolic Control Potassium HD <6.5 mEq/L, 2 of 3 mo PD <6.0 mEq/L, 2 of 3 times			A. Diet instruction B. HD bath changed C. Tx Rx changed D. Psychosocial review E. K$^+$ binding resin	
Nutritional Status Albumin HD >3.5 g/dL, 2 of 3 mo PD >3.0 g/dL, 2 of 3 mo CAPD >3.0 g/dL, 2 of 3 mo Peds >3.0 g/dL, 2 of 3 mo			A. Nephrotic syndrome B. Liver disease C. Recent hosp within 1 week D. Peritonitis within 6 weeks E. Debilitating illness F. Economic deprivation G. RD intervention	
No Weight Loss >5% in 3 months			A. 1st 3 mo of dialysis B. Recent PD transfer C. Failed transplant within 3 mo D. Debilitating illness E. MD/RD OKd weight loss F. RD intervention	

Peds Increased Head
   Circumference <36 mo
   of age
			No exceptions	

Renal Osteodystrophy Phosphorus Adults 3.5–6.0 mg/dL, 2 of 3 mo Peds 3.0–6.5 mg/dL, 2 of 3 mo <10 years old no aluminum			A. Medications adjusted B. Diet, meds reviewed C. Psychosocial review No exceptions	
Calcium 8.5–11.5 mg/dL, 2 of 3 mo Peds 9.0–11.5 mg/dL in 2 of 3 mo			A. Non-renal bone Dx B. Meds adjusted C. Diet, meds reviewed D. Psychosocial review E. Hypoalbuminemia F. PTHx within 6 mo	
Alkaline Phosphatase <2× normal or <50% increase in 6 mo			A. Non-bone cause B. Fracture C. Medications adjusted D. Diet, meds reviewed	
Parathyroid Hormone Peds <2× normal 1 of 2 quarters				

Based on current HCFA Medical Review Criteria Guidelines. CRN QA Committee.

Figure F.2
Diet History/Nutrition Assessment

Patient name _____ Phone _____

Address_____

Age _____Sex M F   Date of Birth _____ Ethnicity _____Marital Status S M W D

Relevant Medical History

    Cause of CRF_____

    Past medical history_____

    _____

    Disabilities/impairments_____

    Medications (relevant)_____

    Laboratory values (date)_____

    BUN _____ Creat _____ Na _____ K _____ CO_2 _____ Ca_____ PO_4_____

    Alk phos _____ PTH ____ Alb _____ Chol _____ Trig _____ Al _____

    Hct _____ Fe _____ TIBC _____ % Transferrin saturation _____ Ferritin _____

    Other _____

Social Data

    Employment status _____ Occupation _____

    Education _____ Reading/writing skills _____

    Insurance coverage/other services_____

    Use of tobacco _____ Alcohol _____ Other drugs _____

    Current Diet Rx_____

Interviewee: Patient_____ Family member_____ Other _____ (Name)

  1. Current appetite: Excellent_____ Good_____ Fair_____Poor_____

  2. Recent change: Incr._____ Decr._____ Reason_____

  3. Current height_____Weight_____Historical_____(Date)_____ IBW_____

  4. Activity: Sedentary_____Moderate_____Very active_____

             Regular exercise_____

  5. Previous diet instruction: Rx_____

  6. Difficulty with previous diet_____

  7. Family members/others in household_____

  8. (Who) shops/cooks?_____ Instructed on diet? Yes_____No_____

  9. Adequate kitchen facilities: Yes_____ If no, describe_____

10. Vitamins: No_____ If yes, type/brands_____

11. Minerals: No_____ If yes, type or name_____

12. Food supplements, "diet" or "herbal products"_____

13. Food allergies/intolerance_____

14. Difficulty swallowing or chewing: Yes_____ No_____

15. Dentures: Yes_____No_____Condition of teeth_____

16. Digestion difficulty/intestinal disorders_____

17. Recent or chronic: Nausea_____Vomiting_____

               Diarrhea_____Constipation_____

18. Cultural influences_____

19. Favorite foods_____

20. Food dislikes_____

(Continued)

Figure F.2—continued
Diet History/Nutrition Assessment

21. Do you use salt? In cooking_____ At table_____ None_____
22. Salt substitute? Yes_____ No_____ Other seasonings (name)_____
    _____
23. Do you use sugar substitute (artificial sweeteners)? Yes_____ No_____
24. Meals eaten away from home: How often?_____
    Where?_____
25. Different routine on weekends? No_____ If Yes, what?_____
    _____

Typical Meal Pattern (Recall)
Breakfast: Time _____ Lunch: Time _____ Dinner: Time _____

Snacks: Time(s)

Food Frequency Checklist (How Often Consumed)

D = daily	W = weekly	M = monthly	No. of servings
Milk: sk/2%/wh	Piz/tom sauce dshs		Butter/marg
Ice cream/pud/yogurt	Casseroles		Salty snacks
Cheese: reg/other	Soup: cn/dry/HM		Candy: choc/other
Eggs	Cereal: hot/cold		Sugar/sweets
Fish/shellfish	Pasta/rice		Fruit: fresh/cn'd
Red meat	Breads/starches		Juice: fresh/cn'd
Poultry	Baked goods		Coffee/tea
Cold cuts/hot dogs	Potato		Soda pop: reg/diet
Bacon/sausage/ham	Veg. cooked		Alcohol
Frozen entrees	Veg. raw/salad		Ice
Canned meats/meals	Oil/sld. drsg.		Water

Assessment Recommendations
Estimate of current daily intake: Calories _____ Protein _____
    Na _____ K _____ Ca _____ P _____ Fluid _____
Type of dialysis: Hemo _____ PD _____ Initiation date: _____
Estimate of needs: Calories _____ Protein _____ Na _____
    K _____ P _____ Fluid _____

Current problems:

Teaching needed:

Recommendations/plan:

Medical Review Criteria—Dietitian's Checklist*

The checklist in Figure F.1 may be used for developing documentation and quality assurance guidelines for the renal dietitian. The criteria under each screen can be incorporated into documentation in the progress notes of the patient's medical chart or onto forms that may be placed in the chart (*Figures F.3* and *F.4*). The HCFA Medical Review Criteria also contain screens on anemia and urea kinetics, which the dietitian may also wish to use for nutrition assessment of the patient. Figures F.1, F.3, and F.4 contain monitoring parameters from these screen categories as well.

At the time of this writing, there are still concerns regarding some of the allowed exceptions on these HCFA screens. For instance, under the blood pressure screen, diet instruction, if documented, would pass an audit using these criteria even if no other medical modifications were made. Because hypertension is not always related or responsive to dietary sodium and/or fluid control, the HCFA expert panel will need to review how often this exception has been used to pass the blood pressure screen.

Another area of concern is the use of diet review included as an exception to abnormal alkaline phosphatase values. Dietary intervention does not directly affect this biochemical parameter, and the direct effect of diet on osteodystrophy is included in the calcium and phosphorus sections of the screen.

Last, the acceptable serum albumin level for a peritoneal dialysis patient may be changed to 3.5 from the current norm of 3.0, which indicates a potential nutritionally compromised state.

The renal dietitian is therefore encouraged to keep up to date regarding the status of the HCFA screens. The criteria used for nutrition documentation may need to be altered on the basis of modifications of the screens.

Figure F.3
Nutrition Progress Notes/Laboratory Review*

Patient_____Facility_____

Metabolic Control

Date	BUN	Creat	K+	Glu	Chol	Trig	KrU	Kt/V	URR

Comments:_____

Goals:_____

(Continued)

* Adapted from Medford S. Medical review criteria: dietitians' criteria. *J Renal Nutr.* 1992;2:77–78.

Figure F.3—continued
Nutrition Progress Notes/Laboratory Review

Renal Osteodystrophy

Date	Ca^{++}	PO$_4$	Ca $\times$ PO$_4$	Alk phos	Alum	PTH

Comments:_____

_____

Goals:_____

_____

Nutritional Status

Date	Alb	PCR/kg	EDW	Appetite	GI complaints

Comments:_____

_____

Goals:_____

_____

Anemia

Date	Hgb	Hct	Iron	TIBC	Transferrin	% Sat	Ferritin	EPO dose

Comments:_____

_____

Goals:_____

_____

Blood Pressure and Fluid Control

Date	PreD BP	PostD BP	Avg. fluid wt gain

Comments:_____

_____

_____

Goals:_____

_____

_____

Prepared by Peggy Wright Harris, RD, Shreveport Regional Dialysis Center, Shreveport, La. Used by permission.

Figure F.4
Interdisciplinary Note

Name _____Date _____

Dialysis Rx_____Time_____Frequency_____Dialyzer_____BFR_____

	PROB #	NO	YES	ENTER STATUS/COMMENTS
1. DIALYSIS				
Excessive ID weight gain/DW change				
Complications during dialysis				
Hypotension				
Muscle cramps				
Nausea and vomiting				
Headaches				
Missed or shortened dialysis				
Other				
2. ACCESS				
S/S infection				
Infiltration				
Recirculation %				
Aneurysms				
Adequate BFR				
Resticks				
Thrombosis (clotted)				
3. ANEMIA				
Hct/Hgb				
EPO dose				
No. transfusions				

(Continued)

Figure F.4—continued
Interdisciplinary Note

4. OSTEODYSTROPHY				
Bone/joint pain				
Other				
5. HYPERTENSION				
6. CAD ANGINA REQUIRING TX				
New/symptomatic arrhythmia				
7. GASTROENTEROPATHY				
Increased S/S				
8. PERIPHERAL VASCULAR DISEASE				
Ulcers (specify)/other				
9. INCREASED RETINOPATHY				
10. NEUROLOGICAL				
Increased neuropathy				
Confusion/disorientation				
11. RESPIRATORY STATUS				
12. MEDICATION REVIEW				
13. HOSPITALIZATION (specify)				
14. OTHER NEW PROBLEMS (specify)				
Signature:				Date:

15. NUTRITIONAL PARAMETERS	PROB #	OK	ABNL	ASSESSMENT/ INTERVENTION
Dry weight/kcal intake				
ID weight gain/fluid status				
Potassium				
BUN/albumin				
PCR/NPCR				
Calcium/adjusted				
Phosphorus/product				
Alk phos/PTH				
Ferritin				
Transferrin saturation %				
UKM:(Kt/V)				

OTHER NUTRITIONAL PROBLEMS/COMMENTS:

Signature: _____ Date: _____

16. PSYCHOSOCIAL PROBLEMS	NO CHANGE	STATUS AND/OR INTERVENTION
Living situation		
Support system		
Psychosocial status		
Compliance		
Treatment modality		
Rehabilitation status		
Life-style changes		
Other comments		

Signature: _____ Date: _____

ACTIVE PROBLEMS/CARE PLAN REVIEWED
_____MD _____RN _____RD _____MSW

Adapted from "Interdisciplinary Progress Note" form prepared by Satellite Dialysis Centers, Inc., Menlo Park, Calif. Used by permission.

Nutrition Progress Notes/ Laboratory Review and Interdisciplinary Note

A progress or monitoring form may be useful in reviewing a patient's laboratory results and subsequent nutritional intake and medications. Intervention as stated on the Dietitian Checklist (see Figure F.1) can be documented in the "Comments" section on these forms. The forms may be designed to include only nutrition documentation (see Figure F.3) or to include notations by the nurse and social worker as well as information from the dietitian (see Figure F.4). An assessment of the patient's compliance and understanding of the diet may also be incorporated along with the plan for follow-up nutrition intervention to attain desirable goals. Monitoring is simplified by having clearly stated, measurable goals and specific target dates for completion. These forms are examples of those that would be placed directly into the medical chart so that all renal team members may keep informed about the patient's progress. Figure F.3 has been designed to include categories from the HCFA Medical Review Criteria Screens and may be used to compile data for more than 1 month at a time if desired. Comments and goals can then be dated for each month's review of laboratory results.

Nutrition Assessment/Review

In some facilities, laboratory data, nutrition assessment, and input may be summari; quarterly, with only necessary nutrition intervention documented more frequently. This fc (*Figure F.5*) can be utilized for this purpose, or in addition to regular monthly documentatior a quarterly, semiannual, or annual nutrition review. It has also been designed to include sim categories as those included in the HCFA Medical Review Criteria Screens.

Figure F.5
Nutrition Assessment/Review

Name of facility_____

( ) Quarterly   ( ) Semiannual   ( ) Annual

Name_____

Date _____ Date of last assessment_____

Metabolic Control

   Dialysis regimen

      Hemo_____ CAPD_____ CCPD_____

      Dialyzer_____ QB_____ Dialysate_____

      Frequency_____ Length of time_____

   Kinetic modeling

   Kt/V_____URR_____

   Pertinent serum laboratory values

      BUN_____

      K^+_____

      Glucose_____

      Chol_____Trig_____

   Pertinent oral medications

      Kayexalate_____

      K^+ supplement_____

      Lipid-lowering agents_____

      Insulin/OHA_____

   Problems_____

   Plans/goals

_____

_____

_____

Renal Osteodystrophy

   Dialysis regimen

      Ca^{++} bath _____ IV Calcijex _____Deferoxamine_____

      Date of last PTH_____ Results_____

Pertinent serum laboratory values
    Ca^{++}_____
    PO_4_____
    Alk Phos_____
    $Ca \times PO_4$_____
    Serum aluminum_____
Pertinent oral medications
    Ca^{++} supplements_____
    Vitamin D therapy_____
    Al^+ binder_____
    Ca^{++} binder_____
Problems_____
Plans/goals

_____
_____
_____

Nutritional Status
Nutrient intake
    Enteral supplements_____
    IDPN therapy_____
    Appetite_____
    Evaluation of intake_____
    Understanding/attitude about diet_____

_____
Weight status
    EDW_____ Lost_____ Gain_____ % Wt change_____ IBW_____
Pertinent serum laboratory values
    Alb_____ PCR_____
Pertinent oral medications
    Vitamin supplements_____
    Others_____
Problems_____
Plans/goals

_____
_____
_____

(Continued)

Figure F.5—continued
Nutrition Assessment/Review

Anemia
　Dialysis regimen
　　EPO therapy_____ IV iron_____
　Pertinent serum laboratory values   TIBC_____
　　Hgb_____ Hct_____
　　Fe_____ Ferritin_____
　　Transferrin_____ % sat_____
　Pertinent oral medications
　　Iron supplements_____
　　Others_____
　Problems_____
　Plans/goals_____

Blood Pressure and Fluid Control
　Diastolic blood pressure
　　PreD BP_____ PostD BP_____ Avg fluid wt gain_____
　Pertinent oral medications_____
　Problems_____
　Plans/goals_____
　_____

_____

Adapted from Nutritional Assessment/Review Form - prepared by Peggy Wright Harris, RD, Shreveport Regional Dialysis Center, Shreveport, La. Used by permission.

Nutrition Referral Sheet (Interagency Transfer Form)

A nutrition referral sheet is useful to provide communication between dietitians when a patient is transferred from one dialysis unit to another or to another type of health care facility (*Figure F.6*). For instance, this form may be useful when a dialysis patient is transferred for transplant evaluation, when a patient is moved into a nursing home or retirement facility, or for a patient who is on an extended vacation and receiving long-term treatment at another facility. Useful information may include transfer diet order, description of method of instruction, assessment of patient's knowledge and compliance with the diet, specific diet-related problems, a copy of the meal plan, and the referring dietitian's name and phone number so that further information may be obtained if it is desired.

Figure F.6
Nutrition Referral Sheet (to be completed by the dietitian)

Name _____

Height _____ Estimated "dry" weight _____Ideal "dry" weight (per ht/wt charts)_____

Weight change past yr _____ Approximate urine vol _____

Current treatment   Hemodialysis   Peritoneal   Frequency/wk _____

Transfer diet order:

      ____g protein

      ____g sodium   Fluid restriction _____

      ____g potassium   Calories_____

      ____g phosphorus   Other (please specify)_____

Diet instruction given: Yes ___ No ___ Person(s) instructed _____

Instructional materials used:

Does patient have written copy of complete diet? Yes _____No _____

Patient's knowledge of diet is: Very good _____ Good _____ Fair _____ Poor _____

  Does patient need review of diet? Yes _____ No _____

  If yes, which aspects?_____

Comments about patient's knowledge of diet and specific follow-up needed
_____

Specific diet-related problems before transfer

                                      Resolved (date)   Unresolved

1._____   _____   _____

2._____   _____   _____

3._____   _____   _____

Comments about these specific problems_____
_____

Social/nutrition information

Age _____   Marital status: S   M   D   SEP   W

Occupation _____Currently employed _____ Unemployed _____

Person preparing meals:

  Has this person received appropriate diet instruction?   Yes _____ No _____

Service agencies involved

      _____ VNA   Phone number _____

      _____ Homemaker   Phone number_____

      _____ Other   Phone number _____

Comments (eg, sample meal plan, suggested exchanges, or any other pertinent information)
_____
_____
_____

Referring dietitian's signature_____

                  Phone number_____

                  Referring dialysis facility_____

                  Date_____

Do not write below this line - to be completed by dietitian in referred facility

Date referral reviewed _____

Patient interviewed: Yes _____ No _____

Comments: _____
_____

Dietitian's signature:_____
_____

Reviewed and adapted for use by the Council on Renal Nutrition of New England, August 18, 1989.

Frequency of Documentation

The question may arise as to the "required" frequency of nutrition documentation. There are federal and state guidelines as well as individual facility guidelines. The renal dietitian is referred to the *Federal Register* June 3, 1976;41(108) and October 19, 1978;43(203) for "general" federal regulations regarding renal nutrition care. Each facility should have a copy of these items as well as Joint Commission on Accreditation of Healthcare Organizations (JCAHO) requirements for nutrition care. State guidelines, on the other hand, differ across the country. Contacting state surveyors has enabled some local renal dietitian organizations to clarify these guidelines. The HCFA Medical Review Criteria Screens mentioned previously in this section may also be used in the formulation of renal nutrition documentation. The renal dietitian should check with his or her facility head nurse or administrator for updated screens as they are available.

Initial documentation is generally performed either within 48 hours of admission for inpatients (JCAHO standards) or within 30 days of initiation of chronic outpatient dialysis treatments (federal regulations). This should include the patient's present status, the dietitian's impression of how work on the stated goals will affect the present status, and a plan summarizing the short-term goals and methods or strategies to be used to achieve the goals. Ongoing progress notes (either recorded in the progress note section of the chart or on a monitoring form) serve as good monitoring tools to assess progress of nutritional plans and goals. These are frequently performed on a monthly or quarterly basis after review of blood chemistry values and perhaps after patient reviews by the entire health care team. Also, whenever a diet prescription is changed or requested or nutrition counseling is performed, a brief notation in the chart is helpful for effective team follow-up and continuity of care. Additional documentation may coincide with long-term care plans developed in conjunction with other health care team members. Many facilities conduct an annual review of their overall care for each patient. This may be an appropriate time to document the accomplishment of nutritional goals and to outline changes and ongoing goals for nutrition care.

The forms in this section regarding documentation of nutrition care for the renal population will not be available at every facility. They are offered only as guidelines or suggestions to inform practitioners of what is being done across the country. It may be necessary to develop forms and guidelines that meet specific patient and facility needs.

G. Disaster Diet Information for Hemodialysis Patients

The following guidelines are intended for use in the event a natural disaster occurs and dialysis becomes unavailable in the local area. You may have to miss dialysis and your well-being may be dependent upon your ability to adjust to a very restricted diet. You will be on this diet for just a few days, until you can dialyze.

Food previously stored in your refrigerator and/or freezer will stay fresh for several days if the appliances are opened only for meal preparation. It is best to eat refrigerator-stored foods first. Additional foods in your kitchen may extend the time that you can be self-sufficient.

If you have a food supply for disaster preparedness, plan to rotate food to guarantee freshness.

It is hoped that these diet guidelines will never be necessary. However, by preparing for a disaster in advance, your nutritional well-being will be assured.

Recommendations

1. It is very important that you eat, but select foods wisely and limit fluid intake.
2. Limit protein intake to one half your current intake. For example, if you eat two eggs for breakfast, decrease to one. If you eat 3 ounces of meat each meal, decrease to 1 to 2 ounces of meat per meal.
3. Restrict fluid intake to approximately one half your current intake. If you routinely abuse your fluid intake, then you will need to cut back even more.
4. Limit intake of foods containing large percentages of liquid (eg, cooked cereals and pastas, fruits, vegetables, and pudding).
5. Avoid foods that are liquid at room temperature (eg, fruit-flavored gelatin, ice cream, sherbet, and ice).
6. Use salt-free foods whenever possible.
7. Avoid all foods with high potassium content. Be more careful than before in limiting kind and quantity of fruits and vegetables eaten.
8. Medications: Plan ahead and always have at least 1 week's supply of all your medications readily available to you.
9. As an added precaution, keep an extra copy of your diet with your food supplies.
10. Persons with diabetes may want to have sugar, honey, or juice available for low blood sugar reactions.

Suggested Emergency Food List

This food list is purposely much stricter than the "normal" renal diet to provide safe suggestions until dialysis is available.

Milk — 1/3 cup per day

Meat and protein — 2–3 ounces per day
  Canned meat — salt free
  Chicken
  Salmon
  Tuna

Fruit — 2 servings per day
  Canned applesauce, cherries, peaches,
    pears, plums, pineapple

Beverages — limit intake
  Powdered juice mixes
  Soda pop
  Fruit juice

Fats — 6 or more servings per day
  Salt-free salad dressings
  Margarine
  Oils

Vegetables — 2 servings per day
  Canned carrots, corn, green beans, peas

Breads and cereal/pasta — 2–4 servings
    per day
  Dry cereals
  Pasta and rice
  Breads
  Crackers, salt-free and grahams
  Cookies
  Wafers

Sweets (if you do not have diabetes)
    — any amount
  Sugar
  Hard candy
  Gumdrops
  Jelly beans
  Jam
  Jelly
  Marshmallows

H. Guidelines for Estimating Renal Dietitian Staffing Levels

In December 1983, the Council on Renal Nutrition (CRN) Executive Committee formally recognized the lack of any practical, realistic tool for estimating renal dietitian staffing levels. Renal dietitians from across the country had expressed frustration as they struggled to estimate the hours needed to provide quality nutrition care for the ESRD population. The continuing changes in federal regulations and reimbursement for dialysis services, with their potential negative effect on quality patient care, added to the frustration. The CRN prioritized the project of developing a method for estimating renal dietitian staffing levels and an ad hoc committee was established.

The committee drew upon CRN member input and previous studies addressing renal dietitian staffing levels and formulated the following criteria as essential for any method of estimating staffing levels.
1. The method must be as objective as possible.
2. The method must be realistic and practical.
3. The method must consider all ESRD programs and patient differences that complicate nutrition care.

The original document was adapted from "An Approach to Patient/Social Worker Staffing" and was approved by the National Kidney Foundation (NKF) in December 1983.[1]

After 4 years of experience with the guidelines, the committee reconvened to revise the document. Revisions included clarification of instructions and format, inclusion of outpatient and pre-ESRD programs as separate categories, and expansion of the nutrition functions.

A second revision was completed in 1992 by a subcommittee of the CRN of Northern California/Nevada. This revision expanded nutrition functions (NFs, or job responsibilities) to represent current renal practice and to recognize the important role nutrition has been shown to play in the care of renal patients. The NFs were compiled from numerous references and CRN historical files.[2-16] Estimated time values were assigned to the patient-direct-

Renal Dietitian Staffing Levels Ad Hoc Committee: Nancy Spinozzi, RD, chairperson, Childrens' Hospital, Boston, Massachusetts; Kathryn Norwood, MS, RD, Chromalloy American Kidney Center, St Louis, Missouri; Mary Kay Hensley, RD, St. Margaret's Hospital, Hammond, Indiana; Sandra Smith-DeTar, RD, Chabot Dialysis, Hayward, California; Jessie Pavlinac, MS, RD, Oregon Health Sciences Center University, Portland, Oregon.

1992 Revision Committee: Sandra DeTar, RD, Chabot Dialysis, Hayward, California; Linda McCann, RD, Satellite Dialysis Centers, Menlo Park, California.

With review and approval by the original ad hoc committee, the 1992 CRN Executive Committee, CRN of Northern California/Nevada, the NKF Public Policy Committee, Scientific Advisory Board, and the Board of Directors. This appendix has been adapted from the Council on Renal Nutrition of the National Kidney Foundation Guidelines for estimating renal dietitian staffing levels. *J Renal Nutr.* 1993;3:84–92.

ed NFs, with 10 points being equivalent to 1 hour of work. These estimated time values were based on the time it takes a qualified renal dietitian to complete specific tasks, as documented by Northern California renal dietitians with a range of experience from 2 to 20 years. Also, new patients, who require additional time, were separated from patients receiving ongoing care. Administrative or professional (indirect) NFs or job responsibilities were separated from NFs that relate directly to patients. Because the amount of time spent on administrative and professional activities varies greatly, clinicians are asked to estimate the time they spend per week on non-patient-related NFs and to add that amount of time at the end of their calculations. A brief time study may be necessary to validate time estimations for indirect NFs and increase the credibility of the estimations.

Each aspect of the formula should be approached realistically. For example, NFs should be considered only when they are mandated and regularly performed. The number of patients must be determined by counting only those patients who routinely receive the specific nutritional care listed in each area. The goal of these guidelines is to adequately estimate the time required to maintain quality nutrition services while recognizing the financial constraints that have been placed on ESRD facilities.

It is imperative that both the dietitian and program director or supervisor agree on job responsibilities and participate in working through all aspects of the formula to obtain useful information.

The following formula should be used to estimate renal dietitian staffing levels.

$$\frac{\text{Program factor (PF)} \times \text{number of patients}}{\text{nutrition function ratio (NFR)}} \times 40 + \text{hours/week of indirect NFs}$$

Each component of the formula must be arrived at separately. A worksheet is provided at the end of this document to facilitate the calculations.

Dietitians who have responsibilities for more than one major program setting should work through the formula for each program setting separately (ie, transplant clinic patients and outpatient dialysis patients would be two different program settings). It is essential that those working with the formula use their clinical judgment and common sense.

Determining the Program Factor

The PF represents the type of ESRD program setting for which a dietitian is responsible as well as the patient acuity factors that require additional work, time, and/or expertise from the dietitian. PF categories include:
1. Chronic Outpatient Dialysis Programs
2. ESRD Programs—Hospitalized
   a) Newly diagnosed patients, not yet undergoing dialysis
   b) Patients beginning dialysis treatment
   c) Inpatient dialysis patients
   d) Acute renal failure patients
3. Pre-ESRD outpatient programs
4. Transplant programs
   a) Hospitalized transplant patients
   b) Outpatient or clinic transplant recipients

5. Pediatric programs
    a) Hospitalized, outpatient, and clinic patients
To Calculate the PF:
1. Decide which category outline in the next section best describes your program setting(s). Program settings that require additional time and/or expertise are weighted accordingly.
2. Decide which additional factors listed with the chosen category further define the patient population. An increment of 0.10 is added for each factor that adds to the complexity of care and time needed to care for the patient. You may count the same patient more than once in this area if the patient has more than one complicating factor. The program factor could increase by a fraction if a full 0.10 is not warranted (eg, if only 13% of the patient population is older than 70 years, add 0.05 instead of 0.10). *Note:* The first additive factor listed refers to patients who have at least two ongoing nutrition problems that require prudent monitoring or at least monthly counseling (ie, serious noncompliance with potassium, fluid, phosphorus restrictions; at risk for malnutrition with low serum protein levels and weight loss; or receiving some form of nutrition support).
3. Total the baseline program factor and any additional factors that are applicable to the patient population. The total is your PF. Record this on your worksheet.

Categories

1. *Chronic outpatient dialysis programs*, PF = 0.40. Add:
    0.10 if 25% or more of the patient population has at least two nutrition problems that affect medical status or require ongoing counseling and documentation.
    0.10 if 25% or more of the patient population has diabetes or has a history of diabetes with current complications.
    0.10 if you provide 10% or more of your patients with nutrition services when they are hospitalized.
    0.10 if 25% or more of the patient population is 70 years of age or older.
    0.10 if 25% or more of the patient population is 18 years of age or younger.
    0.10 if 25% of the patient population does not speak English or is illiterate.
    0.10 if 25% of the patient population lacks essential family support and/or community services (living alone, in a nursing home, or needing home help).
2. *ESRD programs—hospitalized*, PF = 0.40. Add:
    0.10 if 25% or more of the patient population has at least two nutrition problems that affect medical status or require ongoing counseling and documentation.
    0.10 if 25% or more of the patient population has diabetes or has a history of diabetes with current complications.
    0.10 if 25% or more of the patient population is 70 years of age or older.
    0.10 if 25% or more of the patient population is 18 years of age or younger.
    0.10 if 25% of the patient population does not speak English or is illiterate.
    0.10 if 25% of the patient population lacks essential family support and/or community services (living alone, in a nursing home, or needing home help).
3. *Pre-ESRD outpatient programs,* PF = 0.40. Add:
    0.10 if 25% or more of the patient population has at least two nutrition problems that affect medical status or require ongoing counseling and documentation.
    0.10 if you provide 10% or more of your patients with nutrition services when hospitalized.

0.10 if 25% or more of the patient population has diabetes or has a history of diabetes with current complications.

0.10 if 25% or more of the patient population is 70 years of age or older.

0.10 if 25% or more of the patient population is 18 years of age or younger.

0.10 if 25% of the patient population does not speak English or is illiterate.

0.10 if 25% of the patient population lacks essential family support and/or community services (living alone, in a nursing home, or needing home help).

4. *Transplant programs,* PF = 0.40. Add:

0.10 if 25% or more of the patient population has at least two nutrition problems that affect medical status or require ongoing counseling and documentation.

0.10 if 25% or more of the patient population has diabetes or a history of diabetes with current complications.

0.10 if 25% or more of the patient population is 70 years of age or older.

0.10 if 25% or more of the patient population is 18 years of age or younger.

0.10 if 25% of the patient population does not speak English or is illiterate.

0.10 if 25% of the patient population lacks essential family support and/or community services (living alone, in a nursing home, or needing home help).

5. *Pediatric programs,* PF = 0.50. Add:

0.10 if 25% or more of the patient population has at least two nutrition problems that affect medical status or require ongoing counseling and documentation (poor growth, special feedings, or formulas included).

0.10 if 25% or more of the patient population has diabetes or has a history of diabetes with current complications.

0.10 if you provide 10% or more of your patients with nutrition services when hospitalized or regular nutrition services in the outpatient clinic after discharge from the hospital.

0.10 if 25% or more of the patient population is 2 years of age or younger.

0.10 if 25% of the patient or family population does not speak English or is illiterate.

0.10 if 25% of the patient population lacks essential family support and/or community services (single parent family with financial needs, institutionalized, or in foster care).

Determining the Number of Patients

In deciding on the number of patients to count, estimate only those patients for whom a dietitian will be providing nutrition care on a regular basis. Do not count patients who are seen briefly once or twice a year (ie, stable transplant or pre-ESRD patients) as you would patients seen weekly or monthly. Those patients you see infrequently can be counted as fractions (eg, 40 stable transplant patients seen twice yearly would count as approximately 6.5 patients because they are seen one sixth the number of times of a patient who is seen monthly). Dietitians who are involved with more than one program setting should calculate each program setting separately. Beware of counting the same patient twice in this section.

1. *Chronic outpatient dialysis programs.*

■ Average number of patients counseled per month using statistics from the past 6 months.

■ Stable patients who are seen infrequently should be counted together with other patients as "whole" patients (eg, home patients who come to clinic but do not require counseling every month would not be counted the same as in-center patients who are seen at least monthly).

2. *ESRD programs—-hospitalized.*

■ Average number of patients with new diagnoses or patients beginning dialysis per month.

■ Average number of unstable, hospitalized chronic patients followed per month.

■ Average number of acute renal failure patients followed per month.

■ Add these numbers together, being careful not to count the same patient twice.

3. *Pre-ESRD outpatient programs.*

■ Average number of patients who receive full diet instruction and at least monthly follow-up in clinic settings.

■ Stable patients who are seen infrequently should be counted together with other patients as "whole" patients.

4. *Transplant programs.*

■ Average number of hospitalized transplant patients followed per month.

■ Average number of patients receiving monthly follow-up or requiring rehospitalization per month.

■ Stable patients who are seen infrequently should be counted together with other patients as "whole" patients.

5. *Pediatric programs.*

■ Average number of patients or families counseled per month.

■ Stable patients who are seen infrequently should be counted together with other patients as "whole" patients.

Nutrition Functions

The following pages list NFs that are performed in providing nutrition services to the ESRD population and its supportive components (ie, family, staff, community, facility administration). The functions performed are determined by federal regulations, state inspection agencies, networks, and the dietitian in collaboration with the facility management. Only those NFs that are performed regularly as described should be counted.

The NFs have been divided into direct and indirect functions. Direct NFs are those that are performed directly with patients or require patient contact. They are divided into three sections, on the basis of the population in which they are performed (ie, new patients, Section 1; all patients, Section 2; some patients, Section 3). They have been assigned point values on the basis of the time it takes a qualified renal dietitian to perform the NFs. The time estimates and testing of the guidelines were provided by the CRN of Northern California/Northern Nevada (experience range, 2 to 20 years).

Remember that each 10 points is equivalent to approximately 1 hour of work. Forty points is equivalent to 4 hours of work or one full NF (from the old guidelines). Use of the point system allows for a more accurate reflection of the time spent on each function without having to use fractions (eg, 10 points rather than 0.25 NF). If an NF is not performed regularly enough to consider it to have full point value, it may be considered as a fraction of the full assigned point value. Points may be weighted accordingly if you perform the task more or less frequently than indicated or if you do not perform all of the tasks described.

Indirect NFs are those that do not require direct patient or family contact (ie, professional, administrative, teaching responsibilities.) Determination of the time spent on indirect

NFs requires the dietitian to estimate the time spent each week to fulfill mandated job responsibilities. This time is considered absolute and is added to the formula calculations after all the other steps have been completed.

Determining Direct NFs

Section 1. NFs performed on new patients.
1. Gathering information on the nutrition history, including review of the medical record; laboratory values; usual eating habits and meal pattern; activity level; status of urine output; previous instruction; understanding of the disease; social, emotional, economic, and family resources; and performance of anthropometric measurements. *10 points*
2. Preparing a formal, written nutrition assessment on the basis of information obtained from the nutrition history, including documentation of nutrition problems, the patient's current nutrition needs, and a recommended diet prescription. *20 points*
3. Developing a nutrition care plan outlining appropriate, prioritized treatment options and goals of management, providing oral and written patient diet instruction, and follow-up (inpatient or outpatient). *20 points*
4. Follow-up of nutrition assessment or instruction, including documentation of patient intake, satisfaction, comprehension of and compliance with the nutrition care plan, recommendations for modification, and reinstruction on diet modification, if appropriate. *10 points*

Determine the average number of new patients per month by calculating the average number of admissions per month over the past 6 months. Total the number of points above based on which functions you routinely perform on each new patient. Partial points may be given if you do not perform all of the tasks described. Multiply the total NF points times the average number of new patients per month. Write the total on the worksheet under item 3.

Section 1 total_____

Example: Average new patients per month = 3. All of the above functions are routinely performed = 60 points. 3 × 60 = 180. (This would be the number you write in on the worksheet under item 3 on the worksheet.)

Section 2. NFs performed on all patients.
5. At least quarterly performance of urea kinetic modeling, including data collection, calculation, evaluation of results with written and/or verbal communication with other team members for the purpose of development and/or revision of nutrition care plans or dialysis prescriptions. *3 points* (Determining percentage urea reduction with evaluation of results and communication to the care team = *1 point.*)
6. At least monthly participation in a structured team care planning meeting, providing specific information regarding patients' nutritional status (progress and problems) and contributing to the development or revision of the renal care team's patient care plan. *1 point*
7. At least weekly participation in bedside rounds with medical, surgical, or renal services and/or regular collaboration and communication with the same. *0.5 point*
8. At least monthly documentation in the medical record (progress notes), including review of laboratory data (including status of anemia or bone disease) and the care plan; telephone follow-up with home patients, chronic care facilities, or schools; performance of calorie counts, dietary recalls, review of medical records. *1.5 points*

Determine your average monthly census over the past 6 months. Add the total points based on the above functions you routinely perform on all patients and multiply by the average number of patients. Write that total on your worksheet under item 3.

Section 2 total_____

Example. Average number of patients per month = 80. For no. 5 = 3 points; 6 = 1 point; 7 = not done = 0; 8 = 1.5 point. Total points = 5.5 × 80 = 440. (This would be the number you record under item 3 on the worksheet.)

Section 3. NFs performed on some patients

9. At least monthly medication (calcitriol, rHuEPO) monitoring usually done under a unit protocol and including review of laboratory findings, medication changes, documentation, and patient instruction and follow-up. *1 point per patient;* number of patients __ × 1 = __

Example: 40 patients are followed on at least a monthly basis; 40 × 1 = 40 points.

10. At least monthly monitoring of patients receiving nutrition support, including intradialytic parenteral nutrition (IDPN), total parenteral nutrition (TPN), and tube feeding. This includes chart review for criteria acceptance, provider arrangements, patient instruction, staff in-service, patient evaluation, and documentation. *3 points per patient;* number of patients ___ × 3 = ___

Example: An average of four patients receive IDPN, and one patient receives tube feeding per month; 5 × 3 = 15 points.

11. At least monthly communication or consultation with a transfer facility (ie, other hospitals, dialysis unit, nursing home, home health agency) regarding patient's nutrition needs, progress, and/or care plan. *2 points per patient per month;* number of patients ___ × 2 = ___

Example: Five patients whose monthly laboratory results and/or progress must be reported by telephone or in writing to a nursing home; 5 × 2 = 10 points.

12. Monthly performance of home visits to patients for nutrition assessment and monitoring. *10 points per patient per month;* number of patients _____ × 10 = _____

Example: You make one home visit per month; 1 × 10 = 10 points.

Total all the points of the above functions and record the total under item 3 on the worksheet.

Section 3 total _____

Example: 40 + 15 + 10 + 10 = 75 points would be recorded under item 3 on the worksheet.

Determining the NFR

The NFR has one of seven values based on the adjusted number of NFs performed. The ratios were originally adapted from "A Method for Developing Staffing Recommendations for Renal Dietitians," by Lyn Piercy, RD, San Francisco, Calif. The ratios were adjusted for both the current revisions in determining nutrition functions and when applied to the formula for estimating the number of patients per full-time equivalent (FTE) of dietitian time when the appropriate NFs are considered.

NFR = 90 if the adjusted NF is <5
= 85 if the adjusted NF is 6–8
= 70 if the adjusted NF is 10–13
= 60 if the adjusted NF is 14–17
= 50 if the adjusted NF is 18–21
= 40 if the adjusted NF is ≥ 22

Record the NFR on your worksheet.

Determining Indirect NFs

This section requires that you estimate the number of hours per week that you spend on each function. Accuracy can be enhanced with a brief time study.

13. Development and/or revision of nutrition education materials to be used in the hospital or facility. Average hours per week = _____

Example: Estimate that you complete one project per year that takes an average of 20 hours. Divide the yearly time by 52, to get 0.4 hours per week.

14. In-service education on renal nutrition for hospital or facility staff or regular teaching or lecturing on renal nutrition to students, professional colleagues, and/or lay personnel outside the hospital or facility. Average hours per week = _____

Example: 1 hour per month is spent teaching as described above. Divide 1 hour by 4 weeks per month to get 0.25 hours per week.

15. Regular education and supervision of students (eg, dietetic interns, medical students) regarding the nutrition care of ESRD patients. Average hours per week = _____

Example: If 45 minutes per week are spent lecturing students, the average time spent is 0.75 hours per week.

16. Participation in menu planning, budget development, product evaluation, meeting with vendors, purchasing, and so forth. Average hours per week = _____

Example: If 3 hours per quarter are spent reviewing menus for hospital foodservice, divide 3 hours by 12 weeks per quarter to get 0.25 hours per week.

17. Participation in the administrative activities and mechanisms of the hospital or facility that relate to short- and long-term planning and program development (eg, committee work). Average hours per week = _____

Example: You attend a 1-hour management meeting per week, for 1 hour per week.

18. Working with the community and its agencies to develop necessary programs; identifying community resources to meet patient and family needs, such as investigating home health services and/or community resources appropriate for patients' nutrition needs (eg, location of low sodium food products, enteral supplements, meals-on-wheels programs); general consultation with home services or community agencies. Average hours per week = _____

Example: You spend 1 hour per month calling drug stores and suppliers to update information about available products. One hour divided by 4 weeks per month = 0.25 hours per week. (There are actually 13 weeks per quarter and 4.3 weeks per month.)

19. Responsibility for representing the hospital or facility or discipline to community, state, or national groups carrying out programs that relate to or benefit ESRD patients or the ESRD community (eg, Networks, NKF, CRN). Average hours per week = _____

Example: You represent your facility 6 work days of 8 hours each per year at local CRN meetings and attend a 1-hour NKF meeting per month (12 hours) for a total of 60 hours per year, divided by 52 weeks per year = 1.15 hours per week.

20. Regular participation in the formal regulatory review process of the hospital or facility related to JCAHO Medical Review Board, state government, and or the Network. Average hours per week = _____

Example: If you spend 2 hours per year on JCAHO-related activities, divide 2 by 52 for approximately 0.04 hours per week.

21. Ongoing development, revision, and/or field testing of continuous quality improvement (CQI) programs; participating in CQI performance and review. Average hours per week = _____

Example: If you spend 4 hours per quarter, divide by 12 weeks per quarter for 0.33 hours per week.

22. Regular ongoing supervision of at least one full-time nutrition care provider involved in direct patient care activities, and/or responsibility for coordinating renal nutrition services within the hospital or facility. Average hours per week = _____

Example: You spend 3 hours per week meeting with employees to direct their activities and 5 hours per year to prepare and administer their annual evaluation. Three hours plus 4 divided by 52 = 3.1 hours per week.

23. Any additional responsibilities not included in the above (eg, travel time between facilities, continuing education responsibilities, research) required on a regular, ongoing basis and significant to the mission or function of the renal program. Average hours per week = _____

Example: You cover two dialysis units on 3 days of your 5-day work week and spend 15 minutes on those 3 days commuting between the units; $3 \times 15 = 45$ minutes or 0.75 hours per week.

Total the hours from nutrition functions 19 through 23. This total should be added to your worksheet at item 9 to give you the hours per week you need to cover your current job responsibilities.

Note: It is suggested that dietitians with minimum experience (1 to 2 years) should be allowed more time than this formula allows as they learn the complex aspects of renal practice.

Figure H.1 Worksheet

1. Determine program factor (PF) _____
2. Determine number of patients_____
3. Determine the direct nutrition functions (NFs)
   Section 1 (new patients)_____
   Section 2 (all patients)_____
   Section 3 (some patients)_____
   Total direct NF points_____
4. Divide total direct NF points by 40 to determine the adjusted direct NF points_____
5. Determine the nutrition function ratio (NFR) using the adjusted direct
   NF points_____
6. Calculate the formula:
$$\frac{PF \times \text{number of patients}}{NFR} = \underline{\hspace{2cm}} \text{ FTE}$$
7. Solving the equation above gives you the estimated staffing ratio for direct patient care_____FTE
8. Determine hours per week by multiplying the FTE times 40 hours
   _____hours per week
9. Add the hours per week of indirect NFs to get total hours per week
   _____hours per week

References

1. An approach to patient-social worker staffing. *NKF-CNSW Newsletter.* 1984;9:15.

2. 41 (108) *Federal Register* 406, 423.

3. Liddle VR. Standards for nutritional care in the end stage renal disease treatment setting. *CRN Q.* 1983;7:21–22.

4. Lohr KN, ed. *Institute of Medicine, Medicare: A Strategy for Quality Assurance.* Washington, DC: National Academy Press; 1990:1,2.

5. Network No. 3 Renal Dietitians (CRN of Northern California/Northern Nevada). Criteria for standards of practice in ESRD. *CRN News.* 1977;2:5.

6. Identification of clinical dietetic practitioner's time use for the provision of nutrition care. *J Am Diet Assoc.* 1981;79:708.

7. Schmitt J. Peer review of the renal dietitians' tasks. *Dial Transplant.* 1989;18:513.

8. Network Coordinating Council No. 2. Medical care evaluation study on renal nutrition assessment. Seattle, Wash: Federal Facility Survey; June 1981.

9. Dahl L. Minimum criteria for dietitian involvement in the care of ESRD patients. *CRN News.* 1981;5:24.

10. Duello K. Network No. 9 staffing recommendations for renal dietitians. *CRN News.* 1979;3:16.

11. Recommendations for optimizing the role of the renal dietitian. *CRN News.* 1979;3:6.

12. *Knowledge and Performance Requirements for Entry-Level Dietitians.* Chicago, Ill: The American Dietetic Association; 1991.

13. *Interpretive Guidelines for Federal Requirements—End stage renal disease.* Rev. 218, H-31-32. Sausalito, Calif: Network 17, Transpacific Renal Network.

14. Liddle VR. CRN dietitian/patient staffing questionnaire. *CRN News.* 1981;5:25–26.

15. Wilkins K, Schiro K, eds. *Suggested Guidelines for Nutrition Care of Renal Patients.* 2nd ed. Chicago, Ill: The American Dietetic Association;1992.

16. Piercy L. A method for developing staffing recommendations for renal dietitians. *CRN Q.* 1983;7:15–17.

I. Funding for ESRD Nutrition Services

Since the earliest demonstration projects on dialysis were conducted in the 1960s, nutrition counseling has been recognized by the federal government as an integral part of ESRD therapy. Federal regulations identifying the conditions for participation of dialysis units require a qualified dietitian for nutrition assessment and long-term care of the dialysis patient. Each dialysis unit is paid a *composite rate* of reimbursement for each treatment performed and must cover the costs of nursing care, supplies, basic laboratory tests, and psychosocial and nutrition services. Nutrition services, therefore, cannot be billed separately or in addition to the dialysis treatment.

Nutrition counseling for the patient before dialysis or transplantation can be billed as fee-for-service in conjunction with the nephrologist's office visits. Success in obtaining third-party reimbursement for predialysis patients is similar to that of other forms of outpatient nutrition counseling. Medicare generally does not reimburse for these services; however, Medicaid may do so, depending on state guidelines. Individual policies determine reimbursement by private health insurance companies.

Oral nutrition supplements are considered oral medication by Medicare and are not covered for either predialysis or dialysis patients. Coverage by Medicaid and/or private health insurance companies depends on state or policy provisions, respectively. Some states may provide grant programs that fund medications *and* nutrition supplements needed by dialysis patients. Also, some local organizations provide grants for these supplements. It is recommended that the renal dietitian work closely with the renal social worker regarding issues of financial support for nutrition products utilized in this population.

J. Professional Organizations for Renal Dietitians

Renal Dietitians, a Dietetic Practice Group of The American Dietetic Association (RPG)

In addition to caring for patients with renal disease, the RPG is concerned with the professional needs and interests of the renal dietitian, including salary surveys, employment concerns, current legislation, and specialization. This group publishes a quarterly newsletter entitled *Renal Nutrition Forum*. This newsletter includes a feature article that concerns renal disease and/or renal nutrition, an information sharing section, legislative highlights, and news of note, which summarizes recent renal nutrition articles. The RPG sponsors scientific sessions related to renal nutrition at the annual ADA meeting as well. For more information on the RPG, contact the Division of Practice, The American Dietetic Association, 216 W Jackson Blvd, Suite 800, Chicago, IL 60606-6995, or phone 800/877-1600. Membership in an ADA practice group is limited to ADA members.

Council on Renal Nutrition (CRN)

The CRN was formed under the umbrella of the National Kidney Foundation (NKF) to unite renal dietitians working toward common goals on its behalf. All CRN members receive the *Journal of Renal Nutrition*, a quarterly publication that includes current research and practice in a variety of areas in renal nutrition, as well as *The Kidney*, a newsletter that includes current research on various causes of kidney disease.

In many areas of the United States and in a few areas in Canada, local CRN affiliates hold regular meetings for the purpose of sharing ideas and continuing education. An annual CRN meeting is held each fall in conjunction with the scientific sessions of the NKF and the American Society of Nephrology. This three-day meeting as well as an annual spring clinical nephrology meeting are sponsored by NKF. For more information on CRN, contact the National Kidney Foundation, 30 E 33rd St, New York, NY 10016, or phone 800/622-9020.

K. Medication and Manufacturer Reference Index

The following medications appear throughout the text in this manual. They are listed in alphabetical order and referenced by manufacturer.

Medications

Aldactone (49)
Aldomet (29)
Alka-Mints (30)
Alka-Seltzer (30)
Alternagel (22)
Alu-Cap (52)
Alu-Tab (52)
Amphojel (61)
Apresoline (12)
Arthritis Pain Formula (59)
Ascriptin (40)
Basaljel (61)
Bufferin (9)
Bumex (41)
Calan (49)
Calci-Chew (38)
Calcijex (1)
Calci-Mix (38)
Calcium carbonate (43)
Calcium gluconate (43)
Calcium lactate (56)
Calcium phosphate (34)
Caltrate 600 (25)
Capoten (9)
Carafate (27)
Cardizem (27)
Catapres (7)
Chromagen (46)

Citracal (31)
Cordarone (61)
Crystodigin tablets (26)
Danocrine (45)
Deca-Durabolin (32)
Deltasone (54)
Desferal (12)
Dialume (40)
Dicarbosil (50)
Digoxin (43)
Dilantin (34)
Donnagel (39)
Durabolin (32)
Duraquin (34)
Edecrin (29)
Epogen (2)
Equilet (31)
Feosol (50)
Feostat (17)
Feratab (53)
Fergon (60)
Fero-Gradumet (1)
Ferro-Sequels (25)
Ferrous gluconate (26)
Ferralet (31)
Fiberall (12)
Fiber Med (37)
Fibrad (42)

Fleet Phospho-Soda (16)
Fumerin (24)
Gaviscon (27)
Gelusil (34)
Hemaspan (6)
Hemocyte (55)
Hydrocortone (29)
Inderal (61)
InFeD (47)
Irospan (14)
Kaolin (43)
Kaopectate (54)
Kayexalate (45)
K-Lyte (9)
K-Phos Neutral (4)
Lanoxicaps (10)
Lanoxin (10)
Lasix (20)
Loniten (54)
Lopressor (18)
Maalox (40)
Massengil (50)
Medrol (54)
Metamucil (36)
Minipress (35)
Mol-Iron (48)
Mylanta (22)
Mysoline (61)

NeoCalglucon (44)
Nephro-Calci (38)
Nephro-Fer (38)
NeutraPhos (3)
Neutraphos-K (3)
Niferex (11)
Nipride (41)
Nitro-Bid (27)
Nitro-Dur Patch (23)
Nu-Iron (28)
OsCal (27)

Phos-Lo (8)
Phosphajel (61)
Phillips' Milk of Magnesia (51)
Posture (59)
Prednisolone (19)
Prednisone (19)
Procardia (35)
Procrit (33)
Quinaglute Dura-Tabs (5)
Reglan (39)
Riopan (59)

Rocaltrol (41)
Rolaids (57)
Slow Fe (13)
Tabron (34)
Tenormin (21)
Titralac (52)
Trinsicon (58)
Tums (50)
Vasotec (29)
Visken (44)
Zaroxolyn (15)

Manufacturers

1. Abbott Laboratories, North Chicago, IL
2. Amgen, Inc., Thousand Oaks, CA
3. Baker Norton Pharmaceuticals, Inc., Miami, FL
4. Beach Pharmaceuticals, Tampa, FL
5. Berlex Laboratories, Wayne, NJ
6. Bock Pharmaceutical Company, St. Louis, MO
7. Boehringer Ingelheim Pharmaceuticals, Inc., Ridgefield, CT
8. Braintree Laboratories, Braintree, MA
9. Bristol-Myers Squibb Company, Princeton, NJ
10. Burroughs Wellcome, Research Triangle Park, NC
11. Central Pharmaceuticals, Inc., Seymour, IN
12. Ciba Consumer Pharmaceuticals, Woodbridge, NJ
13. Ciba Pharmaceutical Company, Summit, NJ
14. The Fielding Pharmaceutical Company, Inc., Maryland Heights, MO
15. Fisons Corporation Prescription Products, Rochester, NY
16. C. B. Fleet Company, Lynchburg, VA
17. Forest Pharmaceuticals, Inc., St. Louis, MO
18. Geigy Pharmaceuticals, Ardsley, NY
19. Geneva Pharmaceuticals, Inc., Broomfield, CO
20. Hoechst Roussel Pharmaceuticals, Inc., Somerville, NJ
21. ICI Pharmaceuticals, Wilmington, DE
22. Johnson & Johnson—Merck Consumer Pharmaceuticals Co., Ft. Washington, PA
23. Key Pharmaceuticals, Inc., Kenilworth, NJ
24. Laser, Inc., Crown Point, IN
25. Lederle Laboratories, Wayne, NJ
26. Eli Lilly and Company, Indianapolis, IN
27. Marion Merrell Dow, Inc., Kansas City, MO
28. Mayrand Pharmaceutical, Inc., Greensboro, NC
29. Merck & Co., Inc., West Point, PA
30. Miles, Inc. Consumer Healthcare Products, Elkhart, IN
31. Mission Pharmaceutical Company, San Antonio, TX
32. Organon, Inc., West Orange, NJ

33. Ortho Pharmaceutical Corporation, Raritan, NJ
34. Parke-Davis, Morris Plains, NJ
35. Pfizer Labs Division, New York, NY
36. Procter & Gamble, Cincinnati, OH
37. The Purdue Frederick Company, Norwalk, CT
38. R & D Laboratories, Inc., Marina del Rey, CA
39. A.H. Robins Company, Inc., Richmond, VA
40. Rhone-Poulenc Rorer Pharmaceuticals, Inc., Collegeville, PA
41. Roche Laboratories, Nutley, NJ
42. Ross Laboratories, Division of Abbott Laboratories, Columbus, OH
43. Roxane Laboratories, Inc., Columbus, OH
44. Sandoz Pharmaceuticals Corporation, East Hanover, NJ
45. Sanofi Winthrop Pharmaceuticals, New York, NY
46. Savage Laboratories, Melville, NY
47. Schein Pharmaceuticals, Inc., Roslyn, NY
48. Schering-Plough, Kenilworth, NJ
49. G.D. Searle & Co., Chicago, IL
50. SmithKline Beecham Consumer Brands, Pittsburgh, PA
51. Sterling Health Division of Sterling Winthrop, Inc., New York, NY
52. 3M Pharmaceuticals, St. Paul, MN
53. Upshur-Smith, Minneapolis, MN
54. The Upjohn Company, Kalamazoo, MI
55. U.S. Pharmaceutical Corporation, Decatur, GA
56. Vitaline Formulas, Ashland, OR
57. Warner-Lambert Company, Morris Plains, NJ
58. Whitby Pharmaceuticals, Inc., Richmond, VA
59. Whitehall Laboratories, Inc., New York, NY
60. Winthrop Consumer, New York, NY
61. Wyeth-Ayerst Laboratories, Philadelphia, PA

INDEX

azathioprine, 58
corticosteroids, 59
cyclosporine, 58
monoclonal antibodies, 59
In-center hemodialysis, 27
Indirect nutrition functions, 233–234
determination of, 236–237
Infants. *See* Children with renal disease
Insulin-dependent diabetes mellitus (IDDM), 12. *See also*
Diabetes mellitus
renal insufficiency with, 69–70
Insulin-like growth factor-1, 9
Interdialytic weight gains, controlling excessive, 192–193
Interdisciplinary note, 219–220
Intermittent feeding method, 105
Intermittent peritoneal dialysis (IPD), 37, 38, 92
Intradialytic parenteral nutrition (IDPN)
determining appropriate formula for, 117–118
indices for identifying candidates and monitoring
patients receiving, 117
for patient with renal failure, 117–118
solution composition, 119
Intraperitoneal parenteral nutrition (IPPN)
concerns with, 119–120
for patient with renal failure, 118–120
Iron
effects of, on biochemical indices, 141
evaluation of serum levels of, 12
in hemodialysis, 28, 33
Iron overload, 33
Iron preparations
iron and vitamin content of, 146
and nutritional status, 134–135

J

Jejunostomy feeding tubes, 101
Joint Commission on Accreditation of Healthcare
Organizations (JCAHO), requirements for nutrition
care, 226

K

Kayexalate, 31, 91
Kidney, functions of, 1
Kidney failure. *See* Acute renal failure; Chronic renal
failure; Renal failure
Kidney stones. *See* Urolithiasis
Kilocalories in hemodialysis, 28, 29–30
Kinetic modeling in peritoneal dialysis, 39
Kt/V
in assessing adequacy of dialysis, 12–13
in assessing peritoneal dialysis, 38, 39

L

Laxatives, 11
Leaching, 30
Lipid metabolism
and continuous ambulatory peritoneal dialysis, 173
evaluation of serum levels of, 12
and hemodialysis, 172–173
predialysis, 172–173
with renal disease, 171
Lipids, effects of, on biochemical indices, 141
Low phosphorus diet for renal bone disease, 154, 156

M

Magnesium
evaluation of serum levels of, 11
in hemodialysis, 26, 32–33
Magnesium-containing phosphate binders, 160–161
Magnesium oxide, 145
Malnutrition
and dialysis in presence of hyperglycemia, 74
effect on patient outcome, 188
in renal failure, 187
Manufacturers, reference index for, 230–232
Mechanical complications in tube feedings, 106
Medicaid, coverage for dietary management, 17
Medical review criteria, dietitian's checklist for, 213–214,
216
Medicare, coverage for dietary management, 17
Medications
aluminum-containing, 159
anticonvulsant, 125
antihypertensive drugs, 125–128
cardiac, 130–131
for chronic renal failure, 123–139
effects of, on biochemical indices, 140–141
iron and vitamin content of iron preparations, 146
mineral content of, 144–145
percentage of iron, calcium, and aluminum, 146–147
sample patient information card, 148
reference index for, 243–244
Medium chain triglyceride (MCT), 86
Metabolic acidosis, 113
Metabolic complications, with tube feedings, 107
Metabolism
altered vitamin D, 152
carbohydrate, 95
lipid, 171–173
Metastatic calcification, 69
Microalbuminuria, 66
Midarm circumference (MAC) measurements, in patients
undergoing dialysis, 5
Minerals
in acute posttransplantation period, 61, 62
for children with end–stage renal disease
in hemodialysis, 83, 91–92
in peritoneal dialysis, 84, 94
posttransplantation, 85, 96
predialysis, 82, 89
in chronic renal failure, 21, 22
in peritoneal dialysis, 43, 48
Mixed lesions, 153
Modification of Diet in Renal Disease study, 17
Monoclonal antibodies, in acute posttransplantation period,
59
Mucormycosis, 33